A. LEE OSTERMAN, MD, CONSULTING EDITOR

ATLAS OF THE HAND CLINICS

Nerve Repair and Reconstruction: A Practical Guide

DAVID J. SLUTSKY, MD, FRCS(C), GUEST EDITOR

VOLUME 10 • NUMBER 1 • MARCH 2005

W.B. SAUNDERS COMPANY
A Division of Elsevier Inc.
PHILADELPHIA LONDON TORONTO MONTREAL SYDNEY TOKYO

W.B. SAUNDERS COMPANY
A Division of Elsevier Inc.

The Curtis Center • Independence Square West • Philadelphia, Pennsylvania 19106
http://www.TheClinics.com

ATLAS OF THE HAND CLINICS
March 2005
Editor: Debora Dellapena

Volume 10, Number 1
ISSN 1082-3131
ISBN 1-4160-2641-X
Chief Medical Illustrator:
Ron Boisvert, MS, CMI, Delaware, Ohio

Atlas of the Hand Clinics (ISSN 1082-3131) is published biannually by the Elsevier Inc. Corporate and editorial offices: 170 S Independence Mall W 300 E, Philadelphia, PA 19106-3399. Accounting and circulation offices: 6277 Sea Harbor Drive, Orlando, FL 32887-4800. For concurrent subscribers to the *Hand Clinics,* subscription prices for the *Atlas* are $121.00 per year (US subscribers), $152.00 per year (US nonsubscribers), $152.00 per year (other countries, subscribers), $185.00 per year (other countries, nonsubscribers), $93.00 (single issue price). Foreign air speed delivery is included in all Clinics' subscription prices. All prices are subject to change without notice. POSTMASTER: Send address changes to the *Atlas of the Hand Clinics,* W.B. Saunders Company, Periodicals Fulfillment, Orlando, FL 32887-4800. **Customer Service: 1-800-654-2452 (US). From outside of the US, call 1-407-345-4000.** E-mail: hhspcs@harcourt.com.

Printed in the United States of America.

CONSULTING EDITOR

A. LEE OSTERMAN, MD, Professor of Orthopaedic and Hand Surgery, Thomas Jefferson University Hospital; and President, The Philadelphia Hand Center and Fellowship Program, Philadelphia, Pennsylvania

GUEST EDITOR

DAVID J. SLUTSKY, MD, FRCS(C), Private Practice, South Bay Hand Surgery Center, Torrance California; and Professor of Clinical Electrophysiology, Rocky Mountain University of Health Professionals, Provo, Utah

CONTRIBUTORS

CHRISTOPHER H. ALLAN, MD, Assistant Professor, Department of Orthopaedics and Sports Medicine, Harborview Medical Center, University of Washington School of Medicine, Seattle, Washington

MARK ASHKAN, Undergraduate, Department of Bioengineering, University of California–Berkeley/ University of California–San Francisco, Ventura, California

DAVID T. W. CHIU, MD, FACS, Professor of Plastic Surgery and Director, New York Nerve Center, Institute of Reconstructive Plastic Surgery, New York University Medical Center, New York, New York

A. LEE DELLON, MD, Professor, Department of Plastic Surgery and Neurosurgery, Johns Hopkins University, Baltimore, Maryland; Clinical Professor, Department of Plastic Surgery and Neurosurgery, and Anatomy, University of Arizona, Tucson, Arizona; and Director, Dellon Institutes of Peripheral Nerve Surgery™, Baltimore, Maryland

EDWARD DIAO, MD, Professor, Department of Orthopaedic Surgery and Neurosurgery; Chief, Division of Hand, Upper Extremity and Microvascular Surgery; and Medical Director, University of California–San Francisco/Mount Zion Orthopaedic Faculty Practice, University of California, San Francisco, California

JOHN F. DIAZ, MD, Resident Instructor, Department of Plastic and Reconstructive Surgery, Albert Einstein College of Medicine and Montefiore Medical Center, Bronx, New York

PETER J. EVANS, MD, PhD, FRCSC, Director, Cleveland Combined Hand Fellowship and Peripheral Nerve Center, Hand, Elbow & Shoulder Surgery, Department of Orthopaedic Surgery, Cleveland Clinic Foundation, Cleveland, Ohio

CHARLES K. HERMAN, MD, Resident Instructor, Department of Plastic and Reconstructive Surgery, Albert Einstein College of Medicine and Montefiore Medical Center, Bronx, New York

VASILEIOS K. KOSTOPOULOS, MD, Orthopaedic Surgeon, Athens Naval Hospital, Greece; Microsurgery Fellow, Microsurgery Program, Eastern Virginia Medical School, Norfolk, Virginia

W.P. ANDREW LEE, MD, Professor and Chief of Plastic Surgery, University of Pittsburgh Medical School, Pittsburgh, Pennsylvania

JAMES M. SAVUNDRA, MBBS, FRACS, Hand Surgery Fellow, Institute of Reconstructive Plastic Surgery, New York University Medical Center, New York, New York

DAVID J. SLUTSKY, MD, FRCS(C), Private Practice, South Bay Hand Surgery Center, Torrance California; and Professor of Clinical Electrophysiology, Rocky Mountain University of Health Professionals, Provo, Utah

BERISH STRAUCH, MD, Professor and Chair, Department of Plastic and Reconstructive Surgery, Albert Einstein College of Medicine and Montefiore Medical Center, Bronx, New York

JULIA K. TERZIS, MD, PhD, FACS, FRCS(C), Professor of Surgery, Division of Plastic and Reconstructive Surgery, Director, Microsurgical Program, Microsurgical Research Center, Norfolk, Virginia

ERIC VANDERHOOFT, MD, Clinical Assistant Professor, Department of Orthopedic Surgery, Salt Lake Orthopedic Clinic, University of Utah Medical Center, Salt Lake City, Utah

BRADON J. WILHELMI, MD, Assistant Professor, Plastic Surgery Institute, Southern Illinois University School of Medicine, Springfield, Illinois

CONTENTS

FORTHCOMING ISSUES

September 2005

Rheumatoid Arthritis of the Wrist
Barry Katzman, MD, and Paul Feldon, MD
Guest Editors

March 2006

Sports Injuries
Kevin D. Plancher, MD, *Guest Editor*

RECENT ISSUES

September 2004

Disorders of the Wrist
Munir A. Shah, MD, *Guest Editor*

March 2004

Disorders of the Lunotriquetral Joint
David S. Ruch, MD, *Guest Editor*

September 2003

Scapholunate Ligament Injuries
Mark S. Cohen, MD, *Guest Editor*

ELSEVIER
SAUNDERS

Atlas Hand Clin 10 (2005) ix

Atlas of the
HAND
CLINICS

Dedication

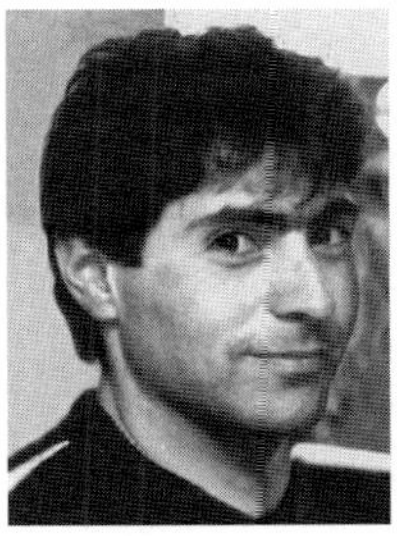

Morley Slutsky, MD, MPH

This issue is dedicated to Morley Slutsky, MD, MPH: A new father, a most loyal brother and a lifelong friend.

doi:10.1016/j.ahc.2004.09.003

ELSEVIER
SAUNDERS

Atlas Hand Clin 10 (2005) xi

Atlas of the
HAND
CLINICS

Foreword

Nerve Repair and Reconstruction: A Practical Guide

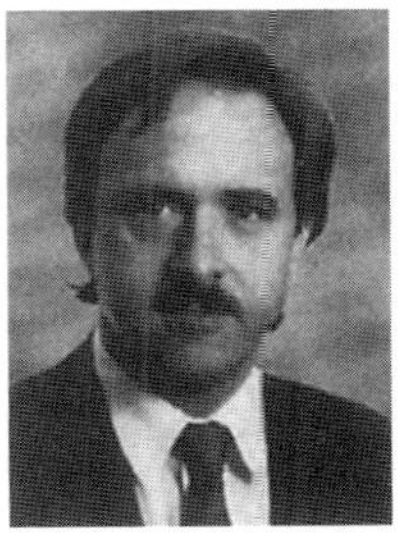

A. Lee Osterman, MD
Consulting Editor

As peripheral nerve surgeons, we are fortunate that peripheral nerve injuries can regenerate. Our goal is to maximize and augment that biologic healing response. The 1960s and 1970s saw advances in our care of nerve injury, including a better understanding of injury pathophysiology, microsurgical techniques, and nerve grafting.

Dr. David J. Slutsky has coerced the all-stars of peripheral nerve surgery to share their experiences and give us practical points regarding nerve repair and reconstruction. This issue of the *Atlas of the Hand Clinics* organizes and updates procedures such as vascularized nerve grafting and nerve conduits including synthetic, venous, and allograft techniques. The articles on neurosensory flaps detail the usefulness of these procedures.

In short, Dr. Slutsky and his coauthors have given us a reason to be enthusiastic about treating these difficult nerve injures.

A. Lee Osterman, MD
The Philadelphia Hand Center
834 Chestnut Street
Philadelphia, PA 19107, USA

E-mail address: loster51@bellatlantic.net

doi:10.1016/j.ahc.2004.10.004

ELSEVIER
SAUNDERS

Atlas Hand Clin 10 (2005) xiii–xiv

Atlas of the HAND CLINICS

Preface

Nerve Repair and Reconstruction: A Practical Guide

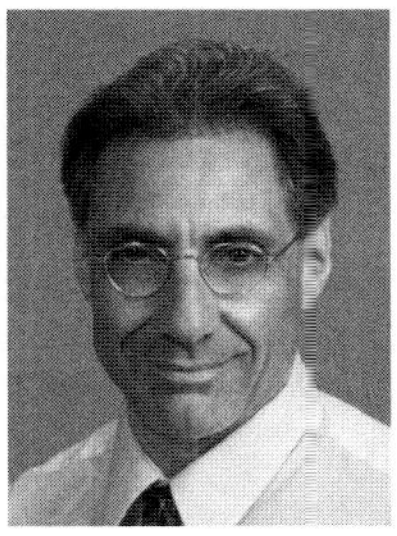

David J. Slutsky, MD FRCS(C)
Guest Editor

The management of nerve injuries is in the midst of a renaissance. The treatment focus is shifting from the operating theater toward the culture tube. Although repair by suture must appear inherently crude from the nerve's standpoint, the techniques have been refined to the point of eloquence.

This issue of *Atlas of the Hand Clinics* is a mixture of old time-honored methods and newer procedures that work in concert with the biochemical events that accompany nerve regeneration rather than in spite of them. The articles range from the succinct discussion by Drs. Mark Ashkan and Edward Diao on primary nerve repair to the elegant summation of the expected standards for nerve grafting by Drs. Christopher Allan and Eric Vanderhoot. Dr. Julia Terzis and coauthor reprise her seminal work on vascularized nerve grafting which helped usher in a whole new discipline in nerve reconstruction. Dr. Berish Strauch and Dr. David Chiu and their coauthors share their knowledge gleaned from more than two decades of experience with biologic and man-made nerve conduits in harnessing the regenerative capacities of injured nerve tissue.

Soft tissue reconstruction of the hand differs from other anatomic regions by the requirement for sensibility. Drs. Bradon Wilhelmi and W.P. Andrew Lee's imaginative use of innervated free flaps compliments a like-minded article on pedicled neurosensory flaps. Dr. Peter Evans illuminates us with the possible windfalls and potential perils that accompany the use of allograft nerve material.

Electrodiagnostic testing has become a gold standard in the assessment of nerve disorders, perhaps undeservedly so. Dr. A. Lee Dellon methodically points out the relative insensitivity of electrodiagnostic testing for quantitating peripheral nerve function. Through the use of his ingenious Pressure-Specified Sensory Device^{TM} he has boldly gone where no electromyographer has been before. Despite their shortcomings though, electrodiagnostic tests are still in wide use. Although these tests are invaluable extensions of the physical examination, the techniques for recording the electrophysiologic events in nerve and muscle carry with them a number of potential pitfalls. The methodology underlying the standard nerve conduction studies are reviewed with this in mind, as well as some of the newer techniques that have special application to hand surgeons.

It was a joy to collaborate with some of the true pioneers in the field of nerve repair as well as some of the up-and-coming stars. I hope the reader of this issue experiences the same. I owe a debt of gratitude to Dr. A. Lee Osterman for allowing me to head this effort as well as Deb

1082-3131/05/$ - see front matter
doi:10.1016/j.ahc.2004.09.001

Dellapena and Patrick Manley, the editors of this issue of *Atlas of the Hand Clinics*, for their gentle guidance and labors on my behalf.

David J. Slutsky, MD, FRCS(C)
South Bay Hand Surgery Center
3475 Torrance Boulevard, Suite F
Torrance, CA 90503, USA

E-mail address: d-slutsky@msn.com

ELSEVIER
SAUNDERS

Atlas Hand Clin 10 (2005) 1–31

Atlas of the
HAND
CLINICS

Measuring Peripheral Nerve Function: Electrodiagnostic Versus Neurosensory Testing

A. Lee Dellon, MD*

Department of Plastic Surgery and Neurosurgery, Johns Hopkins University, Suite 370, 3333 North Calvert Street, Baltimore, MD 21218, USA
Department of Plastic Surgery and Neurosurgery, and Anatomy, University of Arizona, Tucson, AZ 85721, USA
Dellon Institutes of Peripheral Nerve Surgery, Suite 370, 3333 North Calvert Street, Baltimore, MD 21218, USA

Electrodiagnostic testing (EDT) was introduced in the early 1950s to evaluate peripheral nerve function and has become an accepted standard among medical professionals. EDT includes nerve conduction studies (NCS) and electromyography (EMG). The testing usually is done by neurologists and physiatrists and may require an assistant. There are standard textbooks on EDT [1–3], journals related to electrodiagnostic testing, and articles in hand surgery journals explaining electrodiagnostic testing [4–7]. On the positive side, EDT is objective, specific, and can evaluate sensory and motor nerve function. EMG is able to detect myopathy and, by being able to sample select muscle groups based on known patterns of innervation, permits identification of nerve root problems and anomalous innervation [8–11].

From the vantage point of time, however, negative aspects of EDT are now evident. EDT has many false negatives: in a meta-analysis by neurologists, 33% of patients who clinically had signs and symptoms of carpal tunnel syndrome had normal EDT [12]. The false negative percentage is approximately 50% for cubital tunnel syndrome [13] and is much higher in many studies related to pronator syndrome (Table 1). EDT is expensive, often costing $700–$2500 per test, depending on how many different nerves and muscles are examined. Unfortunately the clinical experience of having an EDT study is often so painful that patients do not undergo a second test, thereby limiting electrodiagnostic testing from clinical use in following patient progress. Furthermore, the large myelinated fibers that are evaluated with electrodiagnostic testing must have an advanced degree of demyelination to demonstrate abnormalities in latency and conduction velocity: as long as there are some normally myelinated large fibers present in the peripheral nerve, the first pickup by the recording electrode detects a normal conduction velocity despite that many other nerve fibers within the peripheral nerve are demyelinated already from the pathologic process. There are many standard conventions that may not be properly included in routine clinical EDT, such as warming or cooling the extremity to the proper temperature, measuring distances between electrode placements, laboratory-adjusted reference values, and adjusting for anthropomorphic differences, like extremes of height [14–19]. These inherent aspects of NCS limit the ability to identify the earliest stages of nerve compression and neuropathy (Table 2). Finally there are simply some nerves that, because of their depth in tissues, anatomic variability, or short length, are difficult for electrodiagnostic evaluation, such as the median nerve in the forearm (pronator syndrome) [20], brachial plexus compression in the thoracic inlet (thoracic outlet syndrome) [21], calcaneal nerve entrapment (heel pain syndrome) [22], and deep peroneal nerve entrapment over the dorsum of the foot [23].

Conflict of interest statement: the author has a proprietary interest in the Pressure-Specified Sensory Device and the Neurotube.

* Correspondence: Dellon Institutes for Peripheral Nerve Surgery™, Suite 370, 3333 North Calvert Street, Baltimore, MD, 21218.

E-mail address: aldellon@erols.com

1082-3131/05/$ - see front matter
doi:10.1016/j.ahc.2004.09.002

Table 1
False-negative electrodiagnostic findings in pronator syndrome

	No of patients with pronator syndrome	No of positive EDT	Percent of false negative EDT
Buchtal et al, 1974 [103]	11	3	71%
Johnson et al, 1979 [104]	51	0	100%
Hartz et al, 1981 [105]	36	6	84%
Briedenbach et al, 1985 [106]	21	14	33%
Olehnik et al, 1994 [107]	37	12	67%
Borud et al, 2000 [108]	65	6	91%

Quantitative sensory testing

In the late 1970s neurologists led by the group at the Mayo Clinic began documenting the validity and reliability of tests that quantitated peripheral nerve function without electrodiagnostic testing [24]. These tests used a mechanical rather than an electrical stimulus. As a group these evaluations were described as quantitative sensory testing (QST). Primarily because EDT has false negatives, does not correlate well with patient symptomatology, and is painful and expensive, a group of neurologists met in 1982 at a conference in San Antonio, reviewed the available information, and gave QST a formal acceptance [25]. They concluded that this testing was valid, reliable, correlated with symptoms, and was suitable for clinical research and following clinical disease states. QST, instead of measuring the response of a peripheral nerve or muscle at one point to an electrical stimulus delivered to the skin at a different, remote point, relies on the patient's verbal response for the cortical interpretation of different sensory stimuli applied to the skin. Instrumentation is available for each form of QST. For example, a stimulus that is related to different temperatures (hot or cold) measures the thermal threshold, a small fiber response not possible with EDT, and this type of instrument has been well described [26]. A stimulus related to different oscillating intensities measures the cutaneous vibratory threshold for a given frequency, a large fiber, quickly adapting response. Generically these instruments are called vibrometers [27]. A stimulus related to different static intensities measures the cutaneous pressure threshold for one-point static touch, a large fiber, slowly adapting response. Classically this testing instrument was called a Von Fry Hair and has been replaced today by the Semmes-Weinstein nylon monofilaments (SWM) [28]. A disadvantage of the set of nylon filaments is that it permits only an estimate of a range for the one-point static-touch threshold, with the true threshold being somewhere between the marking of the filament that cannot be perceived and the filament that can be perceived. By contrast, an instrument is available that evaluates a continuous range for the cutaneous pressure threshold: a stimulus related to distinguishing one from two different static or moving intensities, measures the one- and two-point moving and one- and two-point static cutaneous pressure thresholds, which are large fiber, quickly and slowly adapting responses, respectively. This instrument is called a Pressure-Specified Sensory

Table 2
Neurophysiologic causes of failure of electrodiagnostic testing to correlate with clinical peripheral nerve function

Incomplete remyelination (slow conduction velocity and increased distal latency)
- After nerve repair
  - Better clinical function than expected from EDT results
- After nerve decompression
  - Suggests failure when a proximal lesion may be the cause of symptoms

Detection of fastest conducting fibers while total number of fibers is reduced
- After nerve repair
  - Clinical use if much worse than expected from EDT results
- With nerve compression
  - Clinical symptoms with normal EDT, the false negative report

Room temperature at time of recording (conduction decreases in the cold)
- With nerve compression
  - If limb is not warmed in winter, false positives are recorded
  - If limb is not cooled in summer, false negatives are recorded

Device (PSSD) [29]. A multiple device instrument is available that incorporates a thermal detection unit, a one-point static pressure device, and a vibrometer at 128 Hz is the Computer-Assisted Sensory Evaluation device (CASE IV) [30].

QST has been demonstrated to be valid, reliable, and painless, and therefore reasonable to use for clinical problems that require more than one evaluation and that do not require identification of specific muscle or motor nerve problems. QST has the negative inherent limitation that it requires the patient's cooperation, because a verbal response to the stimulus is necessary. QST, despite giving meaningful quantitative data in cutaneous thresholds, therefore is subjective in nature. Patients who cannot mentally understand the test or who are under the influence of narcotic, alcoholic, or neuropathic pain medications such that they are not sufficiently alert cannot give appropriate answers. One form of QST, like the PSSD, can identify the patient who is malingering, because there is a true physiologic response, a pattern of test results, for nerve compression or neural regeneration that can be detected when the subject gives less than their maximal effort during the evaluation [31].

Nylon monofilaments

Some forms of QST, like the SWM, are best suited for screening examinations, because they are quick and do not make an actual measurement, but rather give an estimate of a range. Interpreting the numeric value obtained with a nylon filament is often misleading. The marking on the filament is a log value to the base ten of the force applied by the filament in tenths of a milligram. To obtain the pressure applied by a given filament, its cross-sectional area must be divided into the value for the force [28,32]. The marking on the filament obtained as the threshold for a given series of patients therefore cannot be averaged or used for statistic purposes without converting the logarithm first. These values cannot be used to define a normal population by its mean or 99% confidence limit. Because, as noted earlier, the true one-point static threshold, obtained with the SWM approach, lies somewhere between the lower and the higher log value determined with the set of filaments, an individual patient actually may improve between the values of the two adjacent filaments in a set, and this improvement or worsening can go without notice. With increasing use of the SWM for screening of patients with diabetes for loss of protective sensibility in the feet [33–35], additional engineering studies have been done on the commercially available filaments. These have demonstrated that for a given filament like the 5.07, which is supposed to deliver 10 gm of force, the actual filaments range from 9–11 gm and that with repeated use, the force applied decreases as the mechanical properties of the filament degrade, so that the filament often does not apply the force it is calibrated to apply [36,37].

Vibrometry

The vibratory threshold measurement, although valid for evaluating populations of patients related to a specific disease process like a neuropathy, cannot identify a problem with a specific peripheral nerve; the vibratory stimulus is a wave form and, if applied to the thumb, stimulates the radial sensory and the median nerve. Testing the thumb would be valid for vibrometry if one were testing the C-6 nerve root, because this nerve root innervates the entire thumb. As another example, when the hand surgeon attempts to distinguish whether the numbness in the little finger originates from a problem with the ulnar nerve at the wrist or the elbow, the presence of abnormal sensibility over the ulnar dorsum of the hand localizes the lesion to somewhere proximal to the wrist. If the little finger pulp were tested with a vibratory stimulus, the test would be valid for the C-8 nerve root, which innervates the entire little finger, but vibrometry could not distinguish between an ulnar nerve problem at the wrist or at the elbow because it simultaneously stimulates the dorsal and the volar surface. Similar analysis can be applied to vibrometry testing of the big toe; the waveform stimulates the peroneal and the tibial nerves simultaneously. Use of the tuning fork, which is qualitative instead of quantitative, is still a valid screening test for identifying a digital nerve injury or a unilateral median versus an ulnar nerve entrapment, because the examiner can ask the patient to compare one test site to another, presumed normal, test site [38]. A diagnostic problem occurs with the patient with bilateral peripheral nerve problems, because there is no absolute threshold measurement for the normal population with tuning forks. This is similar to using the TEN test to evaluate peripheral nerve function [39].

Thermal testing

Thermal threshold testing can be used for a specific nerve, because it stimulates the single piece of skin to which the stimulus is applied. Thermal testing, however, because it evaluates small diameter nerve fibers, is not generally a useful modality for the surgeon interested in peripheral nerve function; with nerve compression problems, the small fiber function is the last to become involved, and with neural regeneration, small fiber function almost always recovers and therefore is not a useful predictor of outcome from nerve repair or grafting [40]. There is a form of small fiber neuropathy that, though rare, is important to identify, because it causes a painful neuropathy that is not known to be helped by surgical intervention [41]. Small fiber neuropathy can be identified with QST [42] and also by a skin biopsy, quantifying the intraepidermal population of small myelinated nerve fibers [43,44]. In a patient with a painful small fiber neuropathy an abnormal thermal threshold would be present, whereas large fiber function would be normal. An abnormal large fiber measurement such as cutaneous vibratory or pressure threshold measurement, or EDT, excludes the presence of a small fiber neuropathy. Small fiber testing therefore is not a necessary test for the surgeon interested in managing peripheral nerve function to identify nerve compression or neuropathy.

Pressure-specified sensory device

The Pressure-Specified Sensory Device (PSSD) can be used to evaluate a specific peripheral nerve, because it stimulates the single piece of skin to which the stimulus is applied. For example, to evaluate ulnar nerve function, the little finger pulp and the dorsal ulnar sensibility of the hand are tested; if the little finger pulp is abnormal but the dorsum is normal, the site of compression is at the wrist, but if both are abnormal, the site of compression is proximal to the wrist [29]. As another example, to evaluate median nerve function, the index finger pulp and the sensibility of the thenar eminence are tested; if the index pulp is abnormal but the thenar eminence is normal, the site of compression is at the wrist, but if both are abnormal, the site of compression is proximal to the wrist [20]. The PSSD has been demonstrated to be useful for monitoring peripheral nerve function: with nerve compression problems, the large fiber function is the first to become involved, and with neural regeneration, recovery of functional sensation is related to the innervation density of the large fiber populations [45,46]. Because the PSSD differs from the other forms of QST in its diagnostic ability (as described later), it is useful to distinguish the PSSD from other forms of QST instruments by describing it with the term neurosensory testing (NST).

Neurosensory testing (Pressure-Specified Sensory Device) versus electrodiagnostic testing

The theoretic advantages of using the PSSD instead of EDT are given in Table 3 and restate the points described earlier, namely (1) that a quantitative method of measuring large fiber function in a single skin site is painless and therefore can be used to follow clinical peripheral nerve problems, (2) that the large nerve fiber population is the critical one to measure during nerve regeneration, because it correlates with the recovery of functional sensation, (3) that the ability to select individual skin sites for testing permits localization of nerve compression sites, (4) that the ability to measure function of a peripheral nerve permits staging of the degree of nerve compression and neuropathy, (5) that the ability to stage peripheral nerve function permits clinical, therapeutic decision making, and (6) that there are certain peripheral nerve problems that simply cannot be evaluated adequately by EDT.

Table 3
Theoretic benefits of the PSSD over EDT

Measuring large fiber function in a single skin site is painless and therefore can be used to follow clinical peripheral nerve problems
Perception of sensory recovery occurs before electrical evidence of sensory nerve function and before evidence of muscle reinnervation
Ability to measure wide range of sensory function of a peripheral nerve permits staging of the degree of nerve compression and neuropathy
Ability to stage peripheral nerve function permits clinical, therapeutic, decision making
Ability to measure function of small, distal peripheral nerves, like the palmar cutaneous nerve, deep peroneal nerve, and calcaneal nerves
Ability to provoke the brachial plexus to identify compression at the thoracic inlet
Less expensive

Neural regeneration after nerve repair

EDT has been demonstrated not to correlate with clinical evidence of recovery of sensory and motor function in patients having median or ulnar nerve repairs. In a study of 29 nerve repairs, each of which was evaluated with clinical examination of the sensory and the motor function and with EDT every 3 months for 24 months, only 8 of the nerve repairs demonstrated a correlation between all three parameters, and in none of the 29 repairs was EDT the first to detect recovery [47]. This confirmed one of the earliest observations (1970) of the failure of EDT to predict clinical recovery after nerve repair, in which it was demonstrated that sensory nerve conduction velocity did not correlate with static two-point discrimination [48]. Similar findings were made a decade ago for the motor system; although EDT evidence of reinnervation of intrinsic muscles was identified after nerve repair, this finding did not correlate with the functional use of these muscles [49]. The theoretic basis for these failures of EDT to predict neural regeneration after nerve repair in a useful manner is given in Table 2 and was suggested by the work of Tackmann et al in 1983 [50]; the number and myelination of reinnervated fibers may be sufficient to give normal conduction velocities even though this number of fibers is insufficient to allow voluntary muscle contraction. Those investigators concluded that sensory electrophysiologic parameters are inadequate predictors of clinical sensory recovery. In contrast to this electrophysiologic limitation, evaluating the perception of sensation caused by mechanical stimuli to the skin during neural regeneration does correlate with hand function. It was demonstrated in 1972 that following nerve repair the sequence of recovery of large nerve fiber touch perceptions is perception of moving-touch first and then constant-touch [51]. In 1978, it was demonstrated that moving two-point discrimination recovers before static two-point discrimination [52]. Because the PSSD can measure one- and two-point static- and moving-touch thresholds, the PSSD is able to evaluate the full clinical course of sensory reinnervation following nerve repair. This has been documented for a patient after ulnar nerve repair at the wrist; the order of recovery of sensibility was one-point moving-touch, then one-point static-touch, then two-point moving-touch, and finally two-point static-touch [46]. An example of this recovery for a median nerve repair at the wrist is given in Fig. 1. This demonstrates that the PSSD is superior to EDT in evaluating clinical recovery from nerve repair.

The medical necessity of doing neurosensory testing with the PSSD after a nerve repair is that a decision must be made as to the adequacy of the nerve repair. If the repair is not going to be successful, as determined by a failure to demonstrate a neural regeneration pattern, the decision is made to resect the nerve repair site and do a nerve reconstruction, typically with interposition fascicular grafts, or now with a neural conduit such as the Neurotube [53]. If the patient is having pain at the nerve repair site and the neurosensory testing with the PSSD demonstrates that neural regeneration is proceeding as expected for the time interval after that nerve repair (Figs. 1–4), a neurolysis with an interposition muscle flap would be indicated [54,55]. Furthermore, the timing of sensory re-education for rehabilitation is guided by the pattern of neural regeneration [56] (Fig. 3). For identifying neural regeneration, the PSSD is better than the functional equivalent of EDT.

Index Finger Pulp

	Left Gm/mm2	Spacing mm	Right Gm/mm2	Spacing mm
1 Pt Static	.5		106.3	
2 Pt Static	.8	3.0	106.5	20.0*
1 Pt Moving	.8		106.3	
2 Pt Moving	.8	3.0	106.5	20.1*

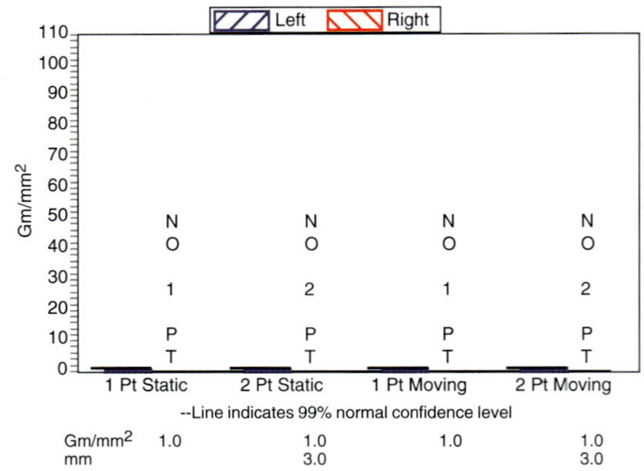

Thumb Pulp

	Left Gm/mm2	Spacing mm	Right Gm/mm2	Spacing mm
1 Pt Static	.7		109.7	
2 Pt Static	.9	3.0	105.8	20.0*
1 Pt Moving	.5		71.7	
2 Pt Moving	.7	3.0	105.0	20.1*

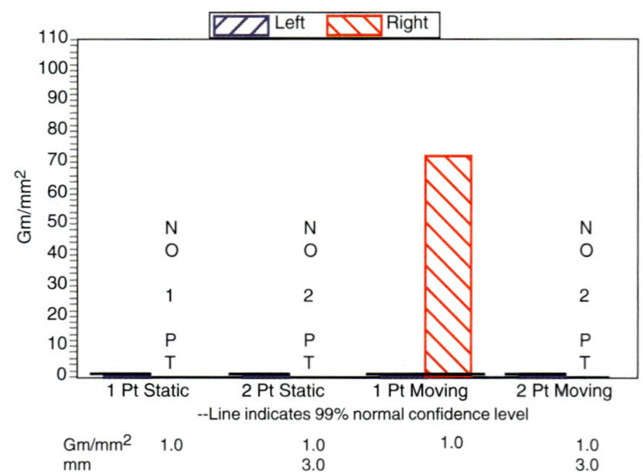

Fig. 1. Neural regeneration is illustrated for a patient 3 months after right median nerve repair at wrist. Note that blue denotes the left hand, normal values. Because the thumb is shorter, recovery should be reflected first in the right thumb, whereas the right index finger pulp lags behind. One-point moving touch is the first sensation to recover, and this is noted by the single red bar in the right thumb pulp. Note that the bar represents a high cutaneous pressure threshold typical of early regeneration. Normative data (99% confidence limit) is given numerically below each graph and by a black horizontal line for each measurement. Actual numeric values are given to the left of the graph. This is the earliest pattern of neural regeneration [46,101] and the clinical decision is made to continue to observe the patient and not to do a neurolysis or a nerve graft. Early phase sensory re-education is begun. From: Seiler D, Barrett SL, Dellon AL. Guide to interpretation of neurosensory testing with the pressure-specified sensory device. Baltimore: Sensory Management Services Pub.; 2004, and Cohen MD, Dellon AL. Computer-assisted sensorimotor testing documents neural regeneration after ulnar nerve repair at the wrist: case report. Plast Reconstr Surg 2001;107:501–5; with permission.

Carpal tunnel syndrome: diagnosis

Perhaps it can be said that never has so much been written by so many about just one nerve compression syndrome. If we restrict our discussion to the role of EDT versus NST with the PSSD, the following are the problems that remain in clinical practice relating to carpal tunnel syndrome: (1) how to document the presence of median nerve dysfunction in the patient with a history and physical examination consistent with carpal tunnel syndrome but in whom EDT is reported to be normal, (2) how to determine whether the patient who is not better after carpal tunnel decompression surgery has recurrent or persistent median nerve compression or another diagnosis, and (3) how to determine the presence of carpal tunnel syndrome in the patient with a coexisting neuropathy, like diabetic neuropathy.

We must begin with several statements with which most physicians interested in patients with peripheral nerve problems would agree. Taken together these statements clinically comprise the definition of carpal tunnel syndrome. The patient has complaints expressed as numbness or tingling in the thumb, index, and middle finger, which usually awakens the patient at night and

Index Finger Pulp

	Left Gm/mm²	Spacing mm	Right Gm/mm²	Spacing mm
1 Pt Static	.5		105.0	
2 Pt Static	.8	3.0	106.5	20.1*
1 Pt Moving	.6		67.5	
2 Pt Moving	.8	3.0	106.0	20.1*

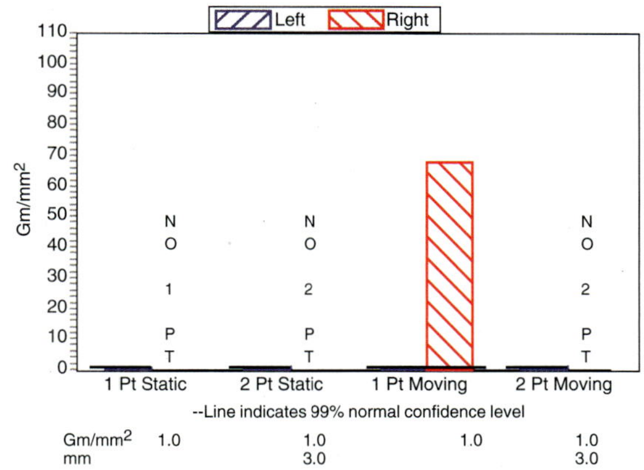

Thumb Pulp

	Left Gm/mm²	Spacing mm	Right Gm/mm²	Spacing mm
1 Pt Static	.5		71.9	
2 Pt Static	.7	3.0	104.9	20.1*
1 Pt Moving	.6		46.2	
2 Pt Moving	.6	3.1	105.2	20.0*

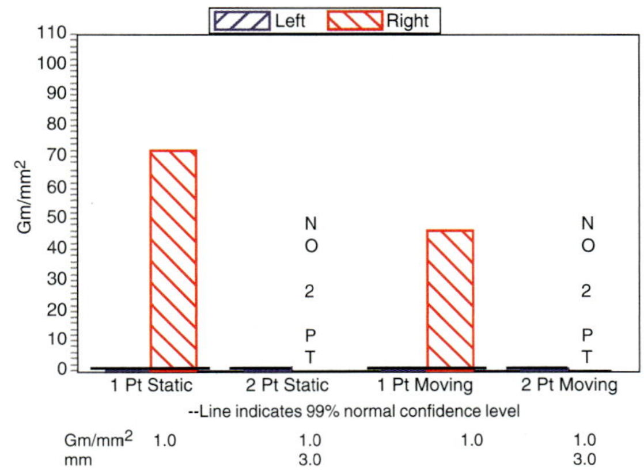

Fig. 2. Neural regeneration is illustrated for a patient 6 months after right median nerve repair at wrist. Note one-point moving-touch is now measurable at the index finger pulp, whereas for the thumb pulp, neural regeneration is proceeding with one-point static-touch threshold now being measured. Note that the threshold for one-point moving-touch is now lower, indicating further regeneration. This test result documents continued neural regeneration. The clinical decision is made not to do a neurolysis or a nerve graft, to continue to observe the patient, and because moving- and static-touch have begun to recover, it is appropriate to begin late phase sensory re-education.

is brought on or made worse with repetitive use of the hand during the day. There is usually no history of trauma, but trauma to the wrist can be a cause of this problem. The problem is often in the opposite hand. On physical examination there is most often a positive Tinel sign or a positive Phalen sign. Signs of thenar muscle wasting are usually not present unless the problem has been of considerable duration. Known predisposing problems are an underlying metabolic disease with a neuropathy, like diabetes, vasculitis, lupus, or rheumatoid arthritis, or a condition that retains fluid, like hypothyroidism. Laboratory studies are indicated if these clinical problems are suspected. Known associated peripheral nerve problems are a cervical radiculopathy with the C6 nerve root: if the patient has symptoms related to the neck, an EMG is indicated to determine if a radiculopathy is present. Certain occupations, such as assembly line work, meat packing, and computer data entry, or hobbies, such as sewing or knitting, have a known association with carpal tunnel syndrome. Nonoperative therapy, including splinting, changing activities of daily living, ergonomic changes, and cortisone injections, are known to relieve the symptoms in some patients for a variable amount of time.

In a patient who has this profile, many surgeons today would argue there is no need to do further diagnostic studies, because the diagnosis seems clear: the patient has carpal tunnel syndrome. Yet tradition has taught that EDT is indicated in the patient with peripheral nerve symptoms, and most patients have an EDT included in their evaluation, often before they are even referred to the hand surgeon. EDT is specific. Since the advent of the inching technique by

Index Finger Pulp

	Left Gm/mm2	Spacing mm	Right Gm/mm2	Spacing mm
1 Pt Static	.5		42.4	
2 Pt Static	.7	3.0	105.3	20.0*
1 Pt Moving	.7		3.2	
2 Pt Moving	.7	3.0	81.7	10.0*

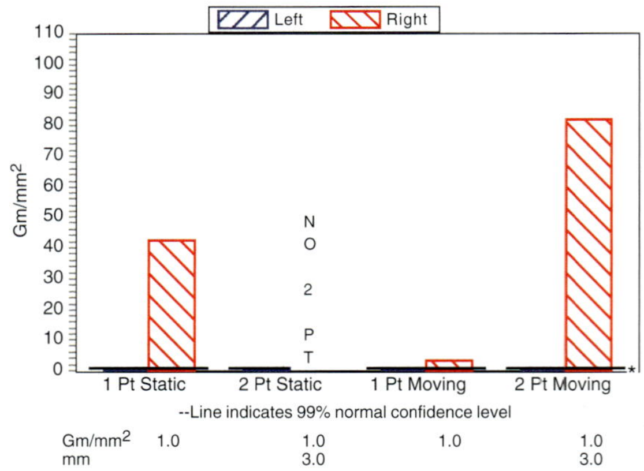

Thumb Pulp

	Left Gm/mm2	Spacing mm	Right Gm/mm2	Spacing mm
1 Pt Static	.5		4.3	
2 Pt Static	.8	3.0	70.9	6.0*
1 Pt Moving	.7		2.3	
2 Pt Moving	.7	3.0	36.1	4.1*

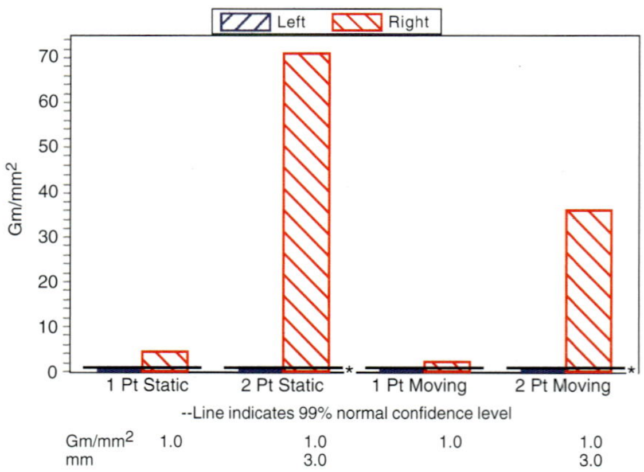

Fig. 3. Neural regeneration is illustrated for a patient 12 months after right median nerve repair at wrist. Note that with further regeneration there are increasing numbers of quickly adapting large fibers in the thumb pulp, represented by perception of two-point moving-touch in the thumb pulp. There is an asterisk next to this red bar, indicating that this measurement is not normal; reference to the absolute measured data indicates that this value is 4 mm, and a higher than normal pressure is required for the patient to distinguish one from two moving touch stimuli. Two-point static-touch also has begun to recover now, with an abnormal distance of 6 mm and a high threshold. Note also that neural regeneration is progressing in the more distant index pulp, in that one-point static-touch now can be perceived at 10 mm, and the threshold for one-point moving-touch has decreased. Two-point static-touch is not yet present in the index finger, even when a distance of 20 mm is given at a pressure greater than 100 gm/mm^2. No surgical intervention would be undertaken unless there were a painful neuroma-in-continuity, in which case, with this PSSD report, a neurolysis and muscle flap would be indicated and a graft would be contraindicated because of the excellent documented recovery of median nerve function.

Kimura in 1979 in which the distal latency is repeated every centimeter across the wrist looking for the location in which a change occurs (indicating the site of entrapment), the chance for EDT to be positive, identify a cause for the symptoms, increased [57]. When inching is combined with a comparison of the ulnar versus the median distal latency, the chance for a positive test further increases [7]. If the EDT is positive, the physician can be approximately 90% certain that the patient really has carpal tunnel syndrome, and so EDT has become the so-called gold standard for diagnosis. The problem remains, however, that for diagnosis of median nerve compression at the wrist, when EDT is the best it can be for peripheral nerve compression problems, EDT is still just 66% specific, meaning the false negative problem occurs 33% of the time [12]. This happens because even if only a small percentage of the large myelinated fibers remain myelinated normally, they continue to conduct at a normal velocity, and the recording electrode picks up that signal in the normal range [7]. What further work-up should the medical physician order now? What decision should the hand surgeon make: is it within the standard of care for the hand surgeon to decompress the carpal tunnel in the patient with a "normal" EDT?

Index Finger Pulp

	Left Gm/mm²	Spacing mm	Right Gm/mm²	Spacing mm
1 Pt Static	.6		.7	
2 Pt Static	.8	3.0	76.1	7.0*
1 Pt Moving	.5		.8	
2 Pt Moving	.7	3.0	6.0	3.0

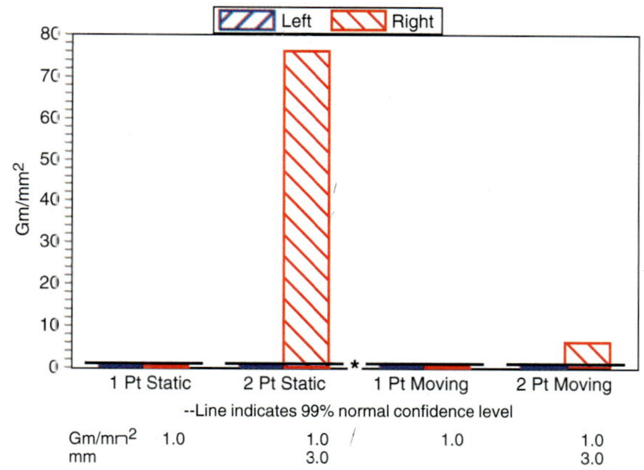

Thumb Pulp

	Left Gm/mm²	Spacing mm	Right Gm/mm²	Spacing mm
1 Pt Static	.6		.8	
2 Pt Static	.8	3.0	65.4	3.0
1 Pt Moving	.6		.7	
2 Pt Moving	.8	3.0	.9	3.0

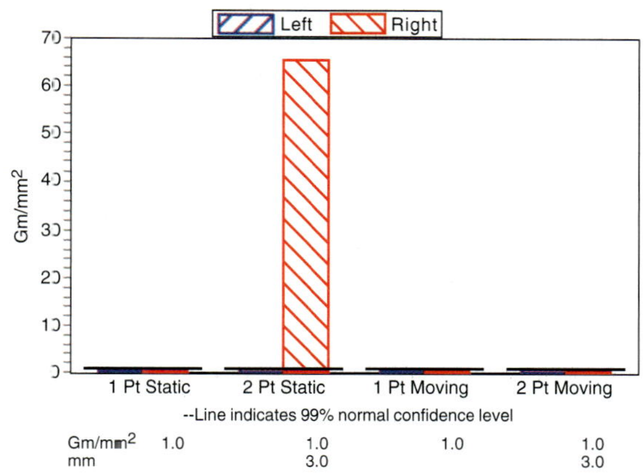

Fig. 4. Neural regeneration is illustrated for a patient 2 years after right median nerve repair at wrist. The neural regeneration pattern is completed for the thumb and almost completed for the index finger, as denoted by static two-point discrimination being recovered in the index and the thumb pulp. The thresholds may remain abnormal and the distance at which one from two points can be distinguished may never return to normal. Functional capacity determinations for the hand can be made from these measurements, because the PSSD has been validated for hand function [102]. From: Dellon ES, Keller KM, Moratz V, Dellon AL. Validation of cutaneous pressure threshold measurements for the evaluation of hand function. Ann Plast Surg 1997;38:485–92; with permission.

If the hand surgeon should have a complication doing the carpal tunnel decompression in such a "normal" person, what is the position of his legal defense counsel? Certainly the person with symptoms that are not relieved by the nonoperative therapies described will continue to seek help. It is in this setting that NST with the PSSD should be considered. In the future, it would be advisable to request the test that is the most sensitive, least painful and least expensive as the first test, not when the traditional testing detects no problem.

In 1997 the first description of the PSSD to evaluate patients with symptoms of median nerve compression at the wrist was published [29]. Normative data were reported that contained the 99% confidence level for the upper limit of confidence for populations younger and older than the age of 45 years, and compared these to a clinical series of patients with carpal tunnel syndrome. Regression analysis demonstrated that the first parameter that could be measured with the PSSD to change in chronic nerve compression was the pressure required to distinguish one from two static-touch paired stimuli. The two populations, normal versus diseased, had distribution curves for the index finger cutaneous pressure threshold for distinguishing one from two static points that did not overlap. This implied that repetitive, paired stimuli to the sensory end-organs in a given piece of skin with the PSSD would have a high degree of sensitivity and specificity for identifying chronic nerve compression. Furthermore, the PSSD test was painless, using a mechanical instead of an electrical stimulus. The change in the pressure required to

Table 4
Relationships between electrodiagnostic and neurosensory report parameters

	Nerve conduction study	Pressure-Specified Sensory Device
Parameter		
Stimulus	Single, electrical	Paired, mechanical
Application site	Peripheral nerve	Skin end-organ
Threshold	Distal latency (msec)	Cutaneous pressure threshold (gm/mm^2)
Number of nerve fibers	Amplitude (mv)	Innervation density (mm)
Graphic representation	Waveform	Bar graph

discriminate one from two static stimuli was the analog of the distal latency measurement of the EDT. It was found using the PSSD that, as the clinical degree of severity became worse, the ability to distinguish one from two, regardless of applied pressure, changed, indicating a decrease in innervation density, which was the analog of the amplitude measurement of the EDT. Instead of presenting the data as a waveform, as indicated for electrical stimuli, the data were presented as bar graphs, as indicated for mechanical pressure stimuli (Table 4).

Recognition of this ability of NST with the PSSD to document different degrees of peripheral nerve pathology provided a basis for a numeric grading scale that permitted the staging of the degree of compression of the median nerve at the wrist and the ulnar nerve at the elbow [58]. The pathophysiologic and historic progression of this numeric grading scale is given in Tables 5–9.

As patients who had EDT were evaluated with NST using the PSSD, it became clear that for many different nerve compression sites, the PSSD was able to identify impaired peripheral nerve function at a time when the traditional electrophysiologic approach indicated that the nerve was functioning normally. This was reported in 1996 for a series of patients who had their EDT done by different doctors within the community from which they were referred [59]. The results of this cross-sectional, retrospective study had limitations, but were the first to bring attention to the value of PSSD testing versus EDT (Table 10). A prospective study in which one neurologist did all the EDT was reported in 1999 to the American Society for Peripheral Nerve Surgery at their annual meeting in San Diego [60]. In that study, 15 patients who were suspected clinically to have nerve compression but who had normal nerve conduction studies then went on to have testing with the PSSD, done by that same neurologist. In all 15 patients, the PSSD measurements were abnormal. Furthermore, in 8 of the 15 patients EMGs were done, and in all of these 8 the EMGs were "normal," whereas the PSSD was abnormal. The investigator concluded that the PSSD was more sensitive than the EDT for patients with carpal, cubital, and tarsal tunnel syndrome. In 2000, a prospective, randomized, blinded study of EDT versus the PSSD was done at the Scott and White Clinic in Texas. A neurologist and a hand therapist each

Table 5
The British system [109]

Sensory recovery within the autonomous zone of the nerve	
S0	Absence of sensibility
S1	Recovery of deep cutaneous pain sensibility
S1+	Recovery of superficial pain sensibility
S2	Return of some degree of superficial pain and tactile sensibility
S2+	As in S2, but with an over-response
S3	Return of superficial pain and tactile sensibility; no over-response
S3+	As in S3 but good stimulus localization and some two-point discrimination
S4	Complete recovery
Motor recovery of muscles innervated by this nerve	
M0	No contraction of any muscle
M1	Perceptible contraction in proximal muscles
M2	Perceptible contraction in proximal and distal muscles
M3	M2 plus all muscles can act against resistance
M4	M3 plus synergistic and isolated movements are possible
M5	Complete recovery

From: Seddon HJ. Peripheral nerve injury. Medical Research Council Special Report Series 282. London: Her Majesty's Stationery Office; 1954; with permission.

Table 6
Pathophysiologic basis for Peripheral nerve grading scale

Degree of severity	Pathophysiology	Clinical
Mild	Blood–nerve barrier breakdown	Symptoms, no signs
Moderate	Demyelination	Symptoms, signs of abnormal threshold
Severe	Axonal loss	Symptoms, signs of decreased innervation density

From: Dellon AL. Management of peripheral nerve problems in the upper and lower extremities using quantitative sensory testing. Hand clin 1999;15:697–715; with permission.

Table 7
Prototype numeric grading scale for any peripheral nerve

Grade	Description
0	Normal
1	Intermittent sensory symptoms
2	Increased sensorimotor threshold
3	Increased sensorimotor threshold
4	Increased sensorimotor threshold
5	Persistent sensory symptoms
6	Sensorimotor degeneration
7	Sensorimotor degeneration
8	Sensorimotor degeneration
9	Anesthesia
10	Muscle atrophy, severe

From: Dellon AL. Management of peripheral nerve problems in the upper and lower extremities using quantitative sensory testing. Hand clin 1999;15:697–715; with permission.

tested the same group of subjects, 25 of whom were asymptomatic and 25 of whom met the clinical criteria for having carpal tunnel syndrome [61]. The EDT was found to be 81% sensitive and 72% specific. The PSSD was found to be 91% sensitive and 82% specific. These differences were not statistically significant. The PSSD, however, was found to be significantly less painful using a visual analog scale ($P < 0.001$). This study, using the highest degree of evidence-based medicine, demonstrated that the same degree of sensitivity and specificity could be obtained with the PSSD as with the EDT but for less cost and with significantly less pain. The most recent

Table 8
Numeric grading scale for the median nerve at the wrist level

Numeric score Sensory	Motor	Description of impairment
0	0	None
1		Paresthesia, intermittent
2		Abnormal pressure threshold, (Pressure-Specified Sensory Device) <45 years old; ≤ 3 mm, at 1.0–20.0 gm/mm^2 ≥ 45 years old; ≤ 4 mm, at 2.2–20.0 gm/mm^2
	3	Weakness, thenar muscles
4		Abnormal pressure threshold, (Pressure-Specified Sensory Device) <45 years old; ≤ 3 mm, at >20.0 gm/mm^2 ≥ 45 years old; ≤ 4 mm, at >20.0 gm/mm^2
5		Paresthesias, persistent
6		Abnormal innervation density (Pressure-Specified Sensory Device) <45 years old; ≥ 4 mm <8 mm, at any gm/mm^2 ≥ 45 years old; ≥ 5mm <9 mm, at any gm/mm^2
	7	Muscle wasting (1–2/4)
8		Abnormal innervation density (Pressure-Specified Sensory Device) <45 years old; ≥ 8 mm, at any gm/mm^2 ≥ 45 years old; ≥ 9 mm, at any gm/mm^2
9		Anesthesia
	10	Muscle wasting (3–4/4)

From: Dellon AL. Management of peripheral nerve problems in the upper and lower extremities using quantitative sensory testing. Hand clin 1999;15:697–715; with permission.

Table 9
Numeric grading scale for the ulnar nerve at the elbow level

Numeric score Sensory	Motor	Description of impairment
0	0	None
1		Paresthesia, intermittent
	2	Weakness Pinch/grip (lbs) Female 10–14/26–39 Male 13–19/31–59
3		Abnormal pressure threshold (Pressure-Specified Sensory Device) <45 years old; <3 mm, at 10–20.0 gm/mm^2 ≥45 years old; ≤4 mm, at 19–20.0 gm/mm^2
	4	Weakness Pinch/grip (lbs) Female 6–9/15–25 Male 6–12/15–30
5		Paresthesia, persistent
6		Abnormal innervation density (Pressure-Specified Sensory Device) <45 years old; ≥4 mm <8 mm, at any gm/mm^2 ≥45 years old; ≥5 mm <9 mm, at any gm/mm^2
	7	Muscle wasting (1–2/4)
8		Abnormal innervation density (Pressure-Specified Sensory Device) <45 years old; ≥8 mm, at any gm/mm^2 ≥45 years old; ≥9 mm, at any gm/mm^2
9		Anesthesia
	10	Muscle wasting (3–4/4)

From: Dellon AL. Management of peripheral nerve problems in the upper and lower extremities using quantitative sensory testing. Hand Clin 1999;15:697–715; with permission.

study, published in 2004, demonstrated that the PSSD could document the presence of carpal tunnel syndrome in the presence of normal EDT in patients with underlying medical problems, like diabetes, who were involved in motor vehicle and worker's compensation litigation [62]. Finally, the recent conclusion of a university electrophysiologist who does EDT is instructive: "supporters of routine preoperative nerve conduction studies ignore their shortcomings, which include lack of standardization, absence of population-based reference intervals, and lack of sensitivity and specificity" [63].

The medical necessity for PSSD testing in carpal tunnel syndrome follows from these considerations. In the patient with symptoms of carpal tunnel syndrome, the initial diagnostic testing with the PSSD demonstrates a cutaneous pressure threshold for the index finger that is greater than the 99% confidence limit, age adjusted. If the two-point static discrimination is still within normal limits for distance (millimeters between the prongs), then axonal loss has not occurred yet, and a nonoperative approach is justified. If the symptoms persist despite nonoperative therapy for 3 months, the PSSD test is repeated. If progression of the median nerve compression is demonstrated (if the distance between the prongs has now increased beyond the 99% confidence limit), then axonal loss has begun and surgical decompression is justified. Figs. 5 and 6 illustrate the typical PSSD report for carpal tunnel syndrome of differing degrees of severity. For carpal tunnel syndrome, the PSSD is the functional equivalent of EDT.

Table 10
Sensitivity of EDT versus PSSD for different peripheral nerves

	Sensitivity for diagnosis	
	Electrodiagnosis NCV/EMG	Neurosensory testing Pressure-Specified Sensory Device
Median nerve (n = 23)	87%	100%
Ulnar nerve (n = 23)	39%	100%
Tibial nerve (n = 16)	81%	100%
Peroneal nerve (n = 10)	70%	90%

A

Index Finger Pulp

	Left Gm/mm²	Spacing mm	Right Gm/mm²	Spacing mm
1 Pt Static	.7		.8	
2 Pt Static	1.0	3.0	36.4	3.0
1 Pt Moving				
2 Pt Moving				

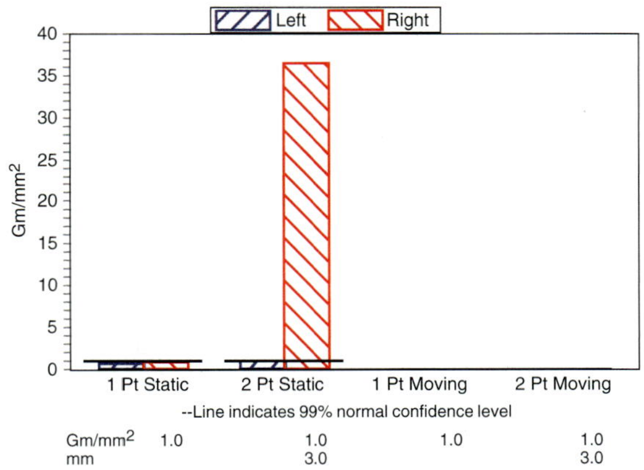

Little Finger Pulp

	Left Gm/mm²	Spacing mm	Right Gm/mm²	Spacing mm
1 Pt Static	.5		.7	
2 Pt Static	.9	3.0	.8	3.0
1 Pt Moving				
2 Pt Moving				

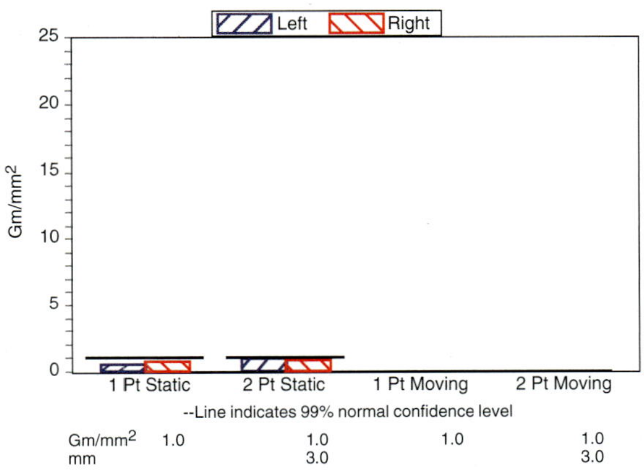

Fig. 5. (*A*, *B*) Documentation of carpal tunnel syndrome with the Pressure-Specified Sensory Device. Early degree of right median nerve compression. Note that the blue bars for the left side are normal for the index finger and little finger pulp, for the thenar eminence, and for the dorsal radial skin territory. Note that the red bar is normal for all these territories except the right index pulp, representing the median nerve territory at the wrist level. This is the red bar for the right cutaneous pressure threshold for two-point static-touch. Note there is no asterisk next to this elevated red bar, so the distance at which one from two static points is distinguished is still normal in distance, although the threshold is abnormal for pressure. This is the earliest abnormal finding in a patient with a right carpal tunnel syndrome tested with the PSSD. Nonoperative therapy is indicated at this stage.

Recurrent carpal tunnel syndrome or different diagnosis?

EDT is not able to determine with certainty the cause of the problems related to persistent or recurrent numbness in the thumb and index finger after carpal tunnel decompression surgery. The reason for this is that once a compressed nerve is decompressed, it does not usually remyelinate to its normal thickness. Even the patient who has a successful decompression of the carpal tunnel therefore still may have an abnormal postoperative EDT. EDT can show, however, a worsening of the condition when compared with the preoperative condition. In general, however, postoperative abnormalities must be interpreted with caution in the patient who has had a nerve decompression. If a cervical root compression is suspected by history or if there is a positive Spurling sign on physical examination (pain radiating into the shoulder or upper extremity with pressure applied to the top of the head), then an EMG, as noted, is indicated to identify a specific pattern of muscle involvement.

All too often the patient who still has symptoms of numbness in the thumb and index finger after carpal tunnel decompression does not have recurrent or persistent median nerve

B

Radial Hand Dorsum

	Left Gm/mm²	Spacing mm	Right Gm/mm²	Spacing mm
1 Pt Static	.6		.7	
2 Pt Static	.8	3.0	.9	3.0
1 Pt Moving				
2 Pt Moving				

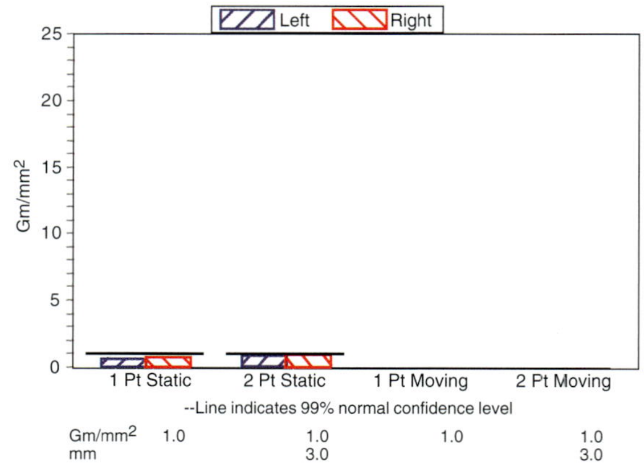

Thenar Eminence

	Left Gm/mm²	Spacing mm	Right Gm/mm²	Spacing mm
1 Pt Static	.7		.6	
2 Pt Static	1.7	6.0	1.4	6.0
1 Pt Moving				
2 Pt Moving				

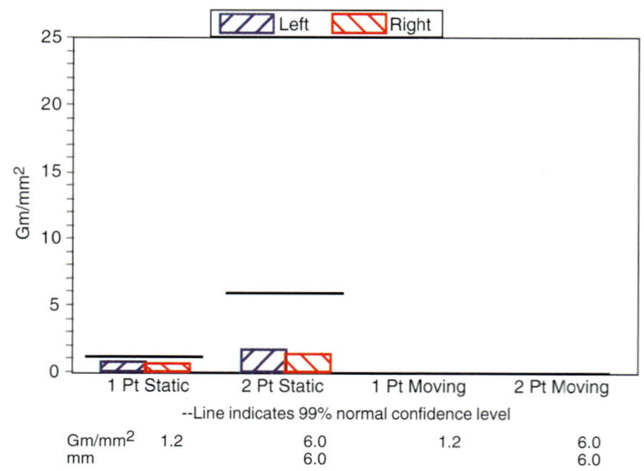

Fig. 5 (*continued*)

compression at the wrist, but has a second, different, nerve compression present. The differential diagnosis must include a proximal median nerve compression, the pronator syndrome, or a radial sensory nerve compression. These two nerve compressions are difficult to demonstrate with traditional EDT. Table 1 illustrates the high false negative rate of EDT for documenting compression of the median nerve in the forearm. The problem with documenting radial sensory nerve compression in the forearm is that its skin territory is not unique, being overlapped by the lateral antebrachial cutaneous nerve in 75% of patients [64]. It may be possible to create an abnormal EDT using provocative tests, an attempt to produce decreased blood flow to the proximal median or radial nerve by increasing muscle pressure on these nerves [65,66], which further demonstrates how difficult it is to identify these problems with EDT.

In contrast to EDT, NST with the PSSD can identify the presence of persistent carpal tunnel syndrome by persistent abnormality in the cutaneous pressure threshold for the index finger pulp or worsening of this condition.

In contrast to EDT, NST with the PSSD can identify proximal median nerve compression by using the knowledge that the palmar cutaneous nerve arises 5–7 cm proximal to the wrist crease [67]. The thenar eminence, which is innervated by the palmar cutaneous branch of the median nerve, therefore has normal sensibility in the patient with carpal tunnel syndrome or recurrent carpal tunnel syndrome, but abnormal sensibility in the patient with a pronator syndrome (Fig. 7). If there has been a history of blunt trauma to the wrist or previous wrist surgery, the palmar cutaneous branch can be entrapped in its course alongside the flexor carpi radialis tunnel and into the thenar eminence [68]. This rare condition can be determined from the more

A

Index Finger Pulp

	Left Gm/mm2	Spacing mm	Right Gm/mm2	Spacing mm
1 Pt Static	.7		.6	
2 Pt Static	.8	3.0	55.9	6.1*
1 Pt Moving				
2 Pt Moving				

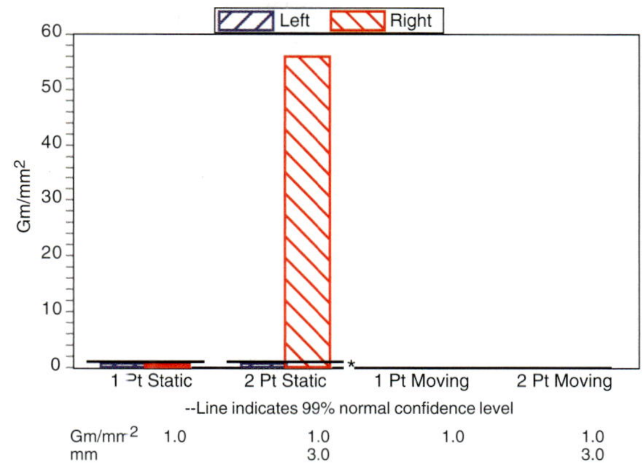

Little Finger Pulp

	Left Gm/mm2	Spacing mm	Right Gm/mm2	Spacing mm
1 Pt Static	.6		.7	
2 Pt Static	.8	3.0	.8	3.0
1 Pt Moving				
2 Pt Moving				

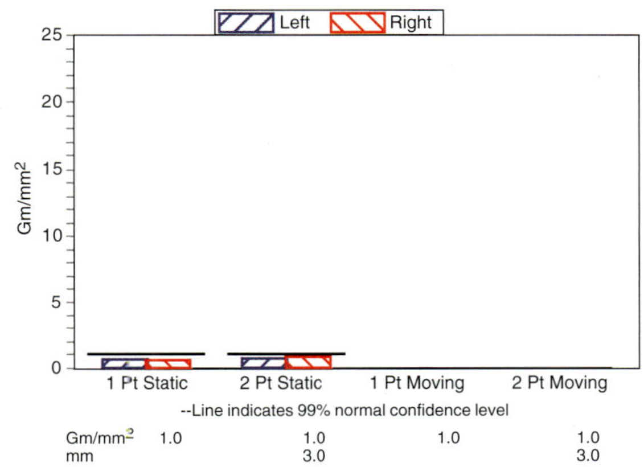

Fig. 6. (*A*, *B*) Documentation of carpal tunnel syndrome with the Pressure-Specified Sensory Device. Severe degree of right median nerve compression. Note that the blue bars for the left side are normal for the index finger and little finger pulp, for the thenar eminence, and for the dorsal radial skin territory. Note that the red bar is normal for all these territories except the right index pulp, representing the median nerve territory at the wrist level. This is the red bar for the right cutaneous pressure threshold for two-point static-touch. Note there is an asterisk next to this elevated red bar, so the distance at which one from two static points is distinguished is not normal in distance; it is 6 mm, consistent with axonal loss. At this stage surgical decompression is indicated.

proximal median nerve location by the classic physical examination maneuvers that identify the site of the median nerve entrapment between the medial humeral epicondyle and a fibrous arcade of the superficialis muscle [69–71]. The PSSD therefore can identify the presence of a proximal median nerve compression with or without a coexisting or recurrent distal median nerve compression (Fig. 7 compared with Fig. 8).

In contrast to EDT, NST with the PSSD can identify the presence of radial sensory nerve compression by testing the skin over the dorsal radial aspect of the hand. Even though this skin may be innervated also by the lateral antebrachial cutaneous nerve, there is not a common entrapment of this nerve, and so abnormal cutaneous pressure threshold for this skin indicates a problem with the sensory branch of the radial nerve (Fig. 9). The physical examination demonstrates a positive Tinel sign where the radial sensory nerve exits the fascia between the brachioradialis tendon and the extensor carpi radialis longus [72].

The medical necessity for NST with the PSSD is the differential diagnosis for the patient with paresthesias in the distribution of the median nerve following carpal tunnel decompression. The differential diagnosis includes pronator syndrome, radial sensory nerve compression, and

B

Radial Hand Dorsum

	Left Gm/mm²	Spacing mm	Right Gm/mm²	Spacing mm
1 Pt Static	.5		.6	
2 Pt Static	.9	3.0	.8	3.0
1 Pt Moving				
2 Pt Moving				

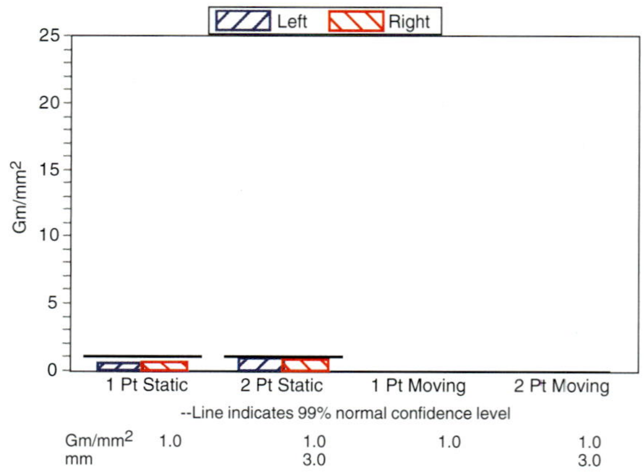

Thenar Eminence

	Left Gm/mm²	Spacing mm	Right Gm/mm²	Spacing mm
1 Pt Static	.8		.7	
2 Pt Static	2.8	6.0	2.6	6.0
1 Pt Moving				
2 Pt Moving				

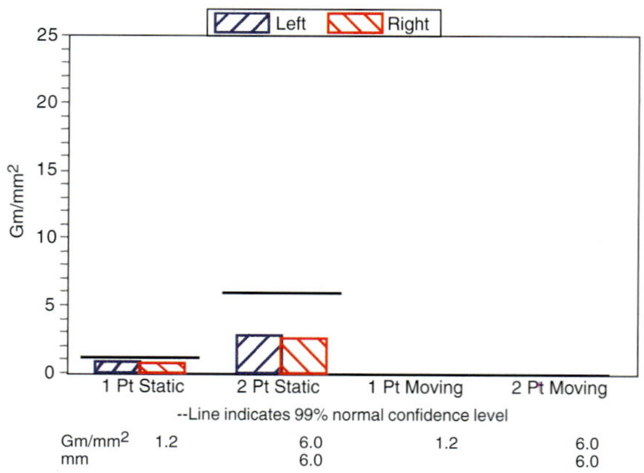

Fig. 6 (*continued*)

recurrent distal median nerve compression in the carpal tunnel. In this clinical situation, the PSSD is better than the functional equivalent of EDT.

Carpal tunnel syndrome in the patient with neuropathy

In the patient with an underlying neuropathy, how can the presence of a nerve compression be identified and documented? Traditionally EDT is obtained. Recently a team consisting of a neurologist, an endocrinologist, and a statistician attempted to answer this question for the population of patients with diabetes [73]. Their clinical diagnosis of carpal tunnel syndrome was made using the criteria listed earlier. Their reference population had an incidence of carpal tunnel syndrome of 2%. Their diabetic population, who did not have neuropathy, had an incidence of carpal tunnel syndrome of 14%. Their population with diabetic neuropathy had an incidence of carpal tunnel syndrome of 30%. They used the most sophisticated analysis of their EDT data to identify carpal tunnel syndrome. When they did their regression analysis to attempt to determine if EDT could identify the patient with carpal tunnel syndrome in the presence of neuropathy, they concluded "electrodiagnostic parameters are not significant predictors of clinical carpal tunnel syndrome in diabetics." They further concluded that "therapeutic decisions for carpal tunnel syndrome can be made independently of electrodiagnostic findings." They used a Tinel sign to localize the site of nerve compression clinically. In the anatomic region in which EDT is most reliable, the wrist, it was concluded therefore that EDT cannot be used to identify a superimposed nerve compression in the patient with an underlying neuropathy.

A

Index Finger Pulp

	Left Gm/mm2	Spacing mm	Right Gm/mm2	Spacing mm
1 Pt Static	.7		.9	
2 Pt Static	.9	3.0	42.7	3.0
1 Pt Moving				
2 Pt Moving				

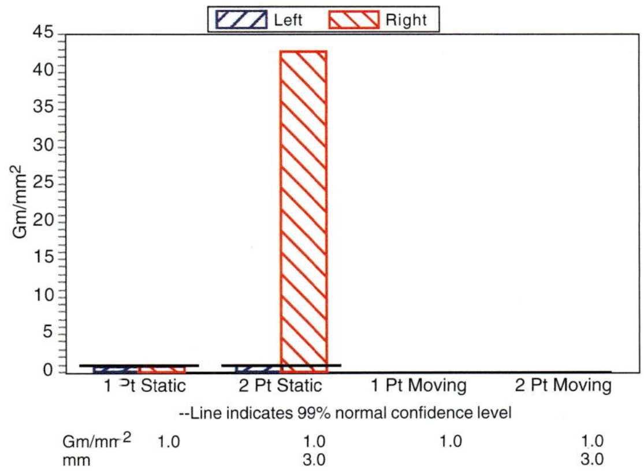

Little Finger Pulp

	Left Gm/mm2	Spacing mm	Right Gm/mm2	Spacing mm
1 Pt Static	.6		.6	
2 Pt Static	.8	3.0	.8	3.0
1 Pt Moving				
2 Pt Moving				

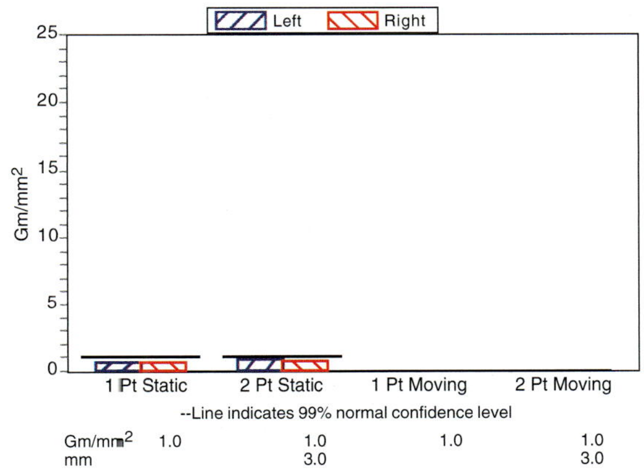

Fig. 7. (*A*, *B*) Documentation of a right pronator syndrome with the Pressure-Specified Sensory Device. Note that for the left side all blue bars are within normal limits. On the right side the red bars for the little finger pulp and the radial sensory skin are also normal. The presence of a mildly elevated index finger pulp plus an elevated bar for the right, red, thenar eminence demonstrates a proximal compression of the median nerve.

In contrast, NST with the PSSD in combination with the physical examination can identify a superimposed nerve compression in the patient with neuropathy and can document the degree of the neuropathy. For the neuropathy patient who has been involved with trauma and has symptoms in one extremity that are different from the other, the PSSD has been demonstrated to document an asymmetric pattern of sensory loss that is consistent with trauma [61]. Neuropathy is documented with the PSSD by a pattern of sensory abnormalities that involves multiple upper or lower extremity nerves that are bilaterally symmetrically abnormal (Fig. 10). If there is a positive Tinel sign over a known site of nerve compression, such as over the median nerve at the wrist for the carpal tunnel or the over the tibial nerve at the ankle for the tarsal tunnel, there is nerve compression at that site.

In the patient with symptoms of bilateral upper or lower extremity numbness or paresthesias with or without burning pain, the diagnosis is going to be neuropathy. It is determined by the medical evaluation as to whether this neuropathy is caused by diabetes, thyroidism, collagen vascular disease, or if the etiology is unknown. EDT cannot establish the etiology of the neuropathy, nor can NST with the PSSD. For neuropathy, the PSSD is the functional equivalent of EDT. The medical necessity for the PSSD measurement is that in addition to documenting the presence of a neuropathy, it can indicate if there is sufficient axonal degeneration to consider nerve decompression in the patient with neuropathy, just as it can for the patient with a nerve compression without a neuropathy.

B

Radial Hand Dorsum

	Left Gm/mm2	Spacing mm	Right Gm/mm2	Spacing mm
1 Pt Static	.6		.6	
2 Pt Static	.8	3.0	.9	3.0
1 Pt Moving				
2 Pt Moving				

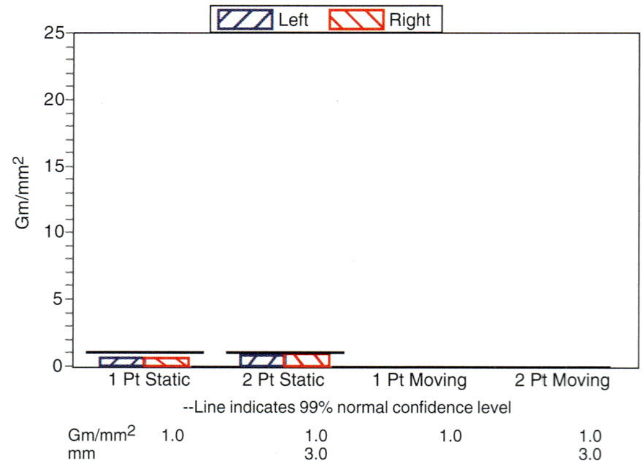

Thenar Eminence

	Left Gm/mm2	Spacing mm	Right Gm/mm2	Spacing mm
1 Pt Static	.8		.9	
2 Pt Static	1.6	6.0	<u>70.1</u>	9.0*
1 Pt Moving				
2 Pt Moving				

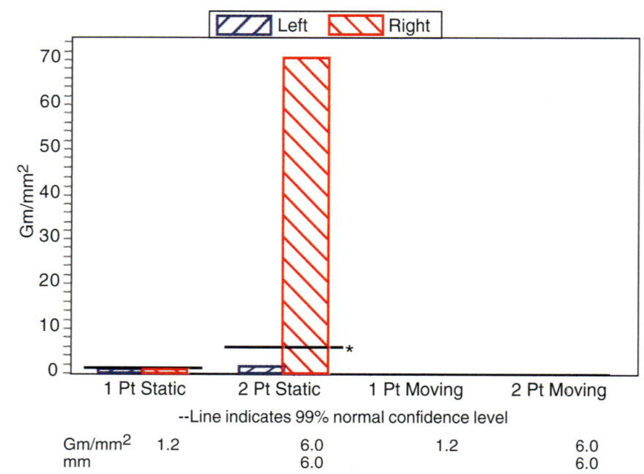

Fig. 7 (*continued*)

Brachial plexus compression

A critical area relating EDT to the PSSD concerns the diagnosis of brachial plexus problems. When brachial plexus problems are of sudden onset and without a history of trauma, a brachial plexitis, such as the Parsonage-Turner syndrome, is probably the cause. This is not a surgical condition, because the inflammation usually resolves. The diagnosis is best made by an EMG demonstrating an incomplete pattern of muscle involvement, often simulating an anterior interosseous nerve syndrome or an upper trunk plexopathy [74]. The second diagnosis in which the EDT can identify the cause of a brachial plexus problem is when the lower trunk is involved. In this situation the EMG can demonstrate denervation in median and ulnar innervated intrinsic muscles, whereas the sensory conduction studies demonstrate a decrease in amplitude of C8 (little finger) but normal amplitude in C6 (index finger) digital nerves. This has been called the true neurogenic form of thoracic outlet syndrome [75]. The EMG also is helpful if an isolated brachial plexus motor branch is involved, such as entrapment of the suprascapular nerve in the suprascapular notch or the axillary nerve in the quadrangular space [76]. Each of these four clinical entities is almost rare, however (Table 11).

The most common clinical problem with the brachial plexus is compression in the thoracic inlet, usually called by its misnomer, thoracic outlet syndrome [77–79]. EDT cannot identify this site of nerve compression, because the large number of anatomic anomalies related to this condition (Table 10), the variable thickness of the chest wall, and the inability to measure the distance required for calculations combine to make EDT unreliable for diagnosis for this clinical problem [80–82]. Indeed, it is the very problem with diagnosis of brachial plexus compression

Table 11
Anatomic anomalies in the thoracic inlet that contribute to brachial plexus compression

Cervical rib
Fibrous bands from C7 transverse process
Extra origins for scalene muscles
Pre- or post-fixed brachial plexus
Intra-plexus anomalous connections
Elevated position of subclavian artery
Muscle of albinus (scalenus minimus)
Fibrous edges of scalene muscles
Anomalous vessels crossing plexus
Sibson fascia crossing T1 nerve root
Proximal junction of T1 to C8

From: Tassler PL, Dellon AL. Correlation of measurements of pressure perception using the pressure-specified sensory device with electrodiagnostic testing. J Occup Environ Med 1995;37:862–6; with permission.

that makes its existence doubted even today. Yet the appropriate diagnosis opens the clinical pathway for effective nonoperative treatment [82–86], and, for those failing to improve from therapy, the possibility exists for surgical decompression of the brachial plexus [87–90].

The diagnostic evaluation of the patient with symptoms of headache, neck and shoulder aching and pain, and numbness or heaviness throughout the upper extremity with or without

A

Index Finger Pulp

	Left Gm/mm2	Spacing mm	Right Gm/mm2	Spacing mm
1 Pt Static	.6		.7	
2 Pt Static	.9	3.0	68.8	8.0*
1 Pt Moving				
2 Pt Moving				

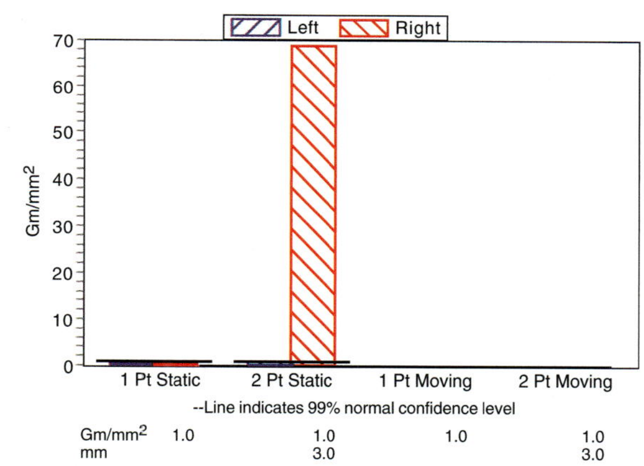

Little Finger Pulp

	Left Gm/mm2	Spacing mm	Right Gm/mm2	Spacing mm
1 Pt Static	.5		.6	
2 Pt Static	.8	3.0	.8	3.0
1 Pt Moving				
2 Pt Moving				

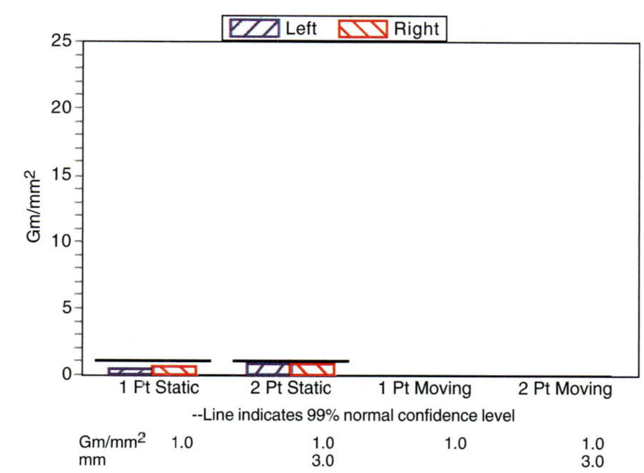

Fig. 8. (*A, B*) Documentation of a right pronator syndrome plus carpal tunnel syndrome with the Pressure-Specified Sensory Device. Note that for the left side all blue bars are within normal limits. On the right side the red bars for the little finger pulp and the radial sensory skin are also normal. The presence of a severely abnormal elevated index finger pulp bar (note the asterisk indicating axonal loss at 8 mm) plus an elevated bar for the right, red, thenar eminence demonstrates a proximal compression of the median nerve.

B

Radial Hand Dorsum

	Left Gm/mm^2	Spacing mm	Right Gm/mm^2	Spacing mm
1 Pt Static	.7		.5	
2 Pt Static	.8	3.0	.7	3.1
1 Pt Moving				
2 Pt Moving				

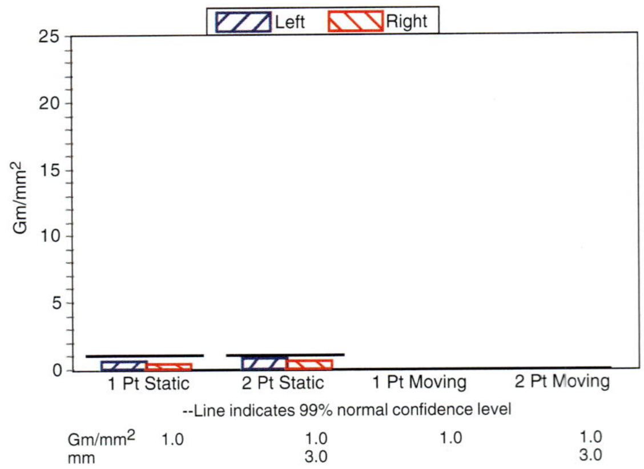

Thenar Eminence

	Left Gm/mm^2	Spacing mm	Right Gm/mm^2	Spacing mm
1 Pt Static	.6		.6	
2 Pt Static	2.0	6.0	60.6	9.0*
1 Pt Moving				
2 Pt Moving				

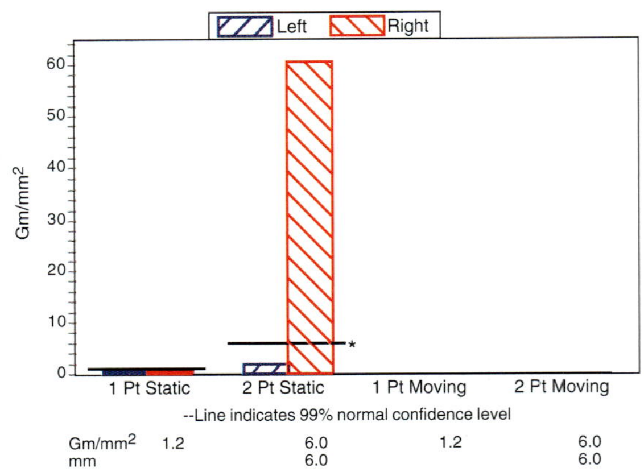

Fig. 8 *(continued)*

swelling or coldness in the arm must take into consideration compression of the brachial plexus in the thoracic inlet. The diagnostic workup should include an EMG and MRI of the cervical spine if cervical disc problems are considered, an MRI of the shoulder and musculoskeletal examination of the shoulder, and a routine chest radiograph [91,92]. The introduction to NST with the PSSD for diagnosis of brachial plexus compression in the thoracic inlet began with the appreciation that patients' symptoms are exacerbated when the arm is held over the head, placing the brachial plexus under stretch or tension. The pressure-provocative test of the supraclavicular plexus elicits symptoms [91] in the same manner as does the Roos test (holding the hands over the head while opening and closing the fingers [89]. Two independent studies have now demonstrated that the PSSD can identify patients who have compression of the brachial plexus in the thoracic inlet [21,93].

In 2000, noninvasive and nonpainful NST with the PSSD was combined with a provocative test (elevation of the hand above the shoulder for 3 minutes) to document compression of the brachial plexus [93]. Data from an asymptomatic group of 61 normal adults were compared with a group of 11 patients with symptoms of brachial plexus compression by testing the cutaneous pressure threshold of the index finger (reflecting the upper trunk of the plexus) and the little finger (reflecting the lower trunk of the plexus) before and after elevation of the hands. In the control subjects there was no change in the cutaneous pressure thresholds as measured with the PSSD. In contrast, the patients who clinically had a history and physical examination consistent with brachial plexus compression in the thoracic inlet had a significant increase in their baseline thresholds after their hands were elevated for one-point static touch of the index finger and of the little finger was significant at the $P < 0.001$ level for each finger. In 2003, this

A

Index Finger Pulp

	Left Gm/mm2	Spacing mm	Right Gm/mm2	Spacing mm
1 Pt Static	.8		.7	
2 Pt Static	.9	3.0	.9	3.0
1 Pt Moving				
2 Pt Moving				

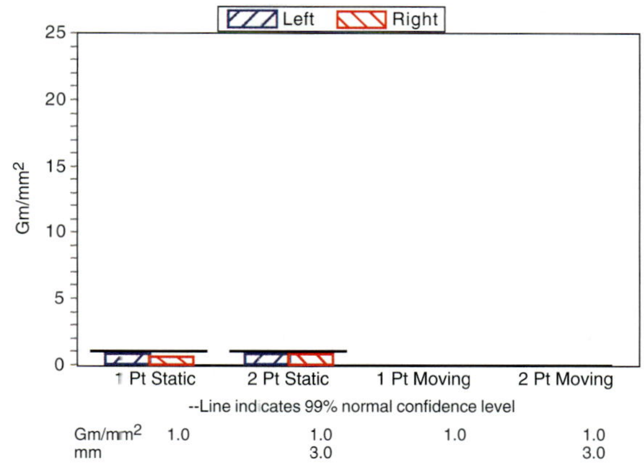

Little Finger Pulp

	Left Gm/mm2	Spacing mm	Right Gm/mm2	Spacing mm
1 Pt Static	.6		.5	
2 Pt Static	.8	3.0	.8	3.0
1 Pt Moving				
2 Pt Moving				

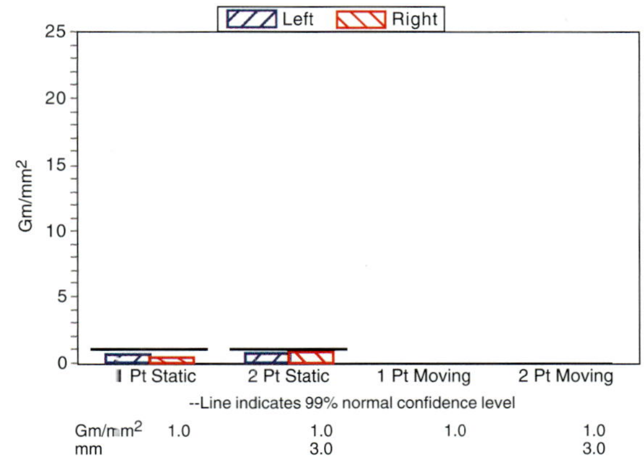

Fig. 9. (*A, B*) Documentation of right radial sensory nerve compression with the Pressure-Specified Sensory Device. Note that for the left, blue bar, side, all bars are within normal limits. Note that for the right, symptomatic side, only the red bar for the radial sensory nerve is elevated. This is the pattern for right radial sensory nerve compression. Note the asterisk next to the elevated red bar, indicating abnormal static two-point discrimination, meaning there is axonal loss. Surgical decompression is indicated.

approach was extended to include measurement of the change in not just one-point moving and static-touch, but also in two-point moving and static-touch thresholds and in pinch and grip strengths (eight separate parameters) for 16 normal control subjects and 42 patients with symptoms of brachial plexus compression [21]. The 99% upper limit for change in the normal population was used as a comparison to those patients with symptoms of brachial plexus compression. Those patients were dichotomized into those whose symptoms and findings were either mild or severe. Results demonstrated that when five or more of the eight possible parameters were greater than the 99% confidence limit for normal, this testing had a sensitivity of 82% and a specificity of 100% and a positive predictive value of 100% for the diagnosis of clinically severe brachial plexus compression. NST therefore is better than the functional equivalent of EDT for the diagnosis of brachial plexus compression in the thoracic inlet (Table 12).

The medical necessity of PSSD measurement of the patient with symptoms of brachial plexus compression is related to the inability of EDT to diagnosis this problem, and the ability of PSSD to identify patients with a mild degree of compression who would benefit from the nonoperative approach to management and identify either progression of compression in those who fail therapy or identify those at the outset whose compression is sufficiently severe so as to justify one of the surgical approaches to decompress the brachial plexus.

B

Radial Hand Dorsum

	Left Gm/mm^2	Spacing mm	Right Gm/mm^2	Spacing mm
1 Pt Static	.6		.7	
2 Pt Static	.8	3.0	67.0	8.0*
1 Pt Moving				
2 Pt Moving				

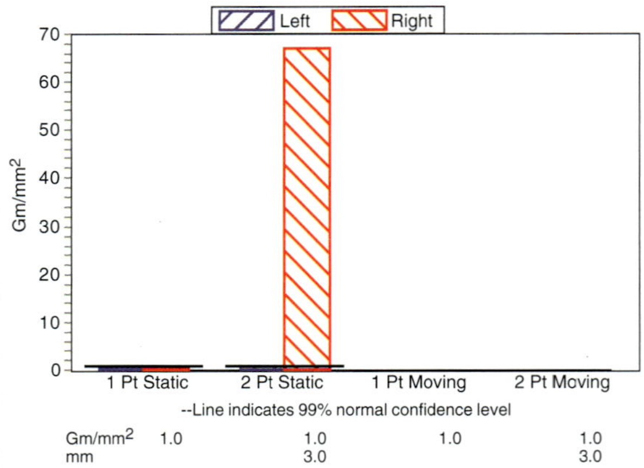

Thenar Eminence

	Left Gm/mm^2	Spacing mm	Right Gm/mm^2	Spacing mm
1 Pt Static	.6		.7	
2 Pt Static	1.9	6.0	1.7	6.0
1 Pt Moving				
2 Pt Moving				

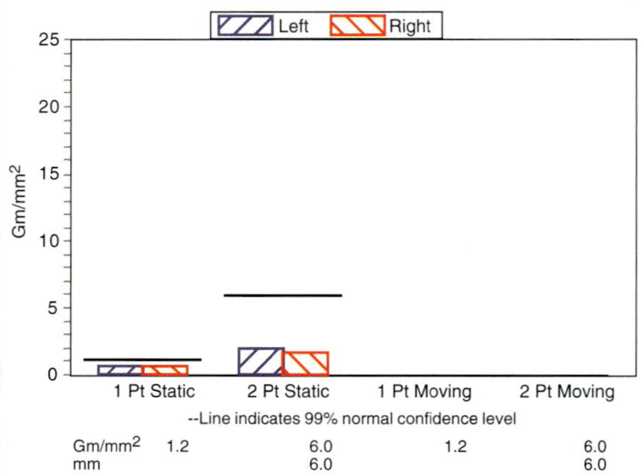

Fig. 9 (*continued*)

Lower extremity nerves

Hand surgeons, whether of an orthopedic or plastic surgery background, have experienced patients with lower extremity peripheral nerve problems. It may be related to care of the trauma patient. It may be the concern over numbness in the thigh following harvesting an iliac crest bone graft. It may be a neuroma of the sural nerve after harvesting a nerve graft. It may be a painful incision or persistent pain after an ankle or knee arthroscopy, ligament reconstruction,

Table 12
PSSD testing for brachial plexus compression

Sensitivity/specificity 99% confidence limit for normative data			
		Roos sign & scalene Tinel signs	
		Severe (≥3+)	Not severe (<3+)
Neurosensory & motor testing confidence limit			
≥5 tests >99%		14	0
≤4 tests >99%		3	3
		17	3 Total = 20 patients
Sensitivity = 82%	(18% false negatives)		
Specificity = 100%	(0% false positives)		
		Positive predictive value = 100	

Adapted from: Howard M, Lee C, Dellon AL. Documentation of brachial plexus compression in the thoracic inlet utilizing provocation with neurosensory and motor testing. J Reconstr Microsurg 2003;19:303–12.

Dorsal Web Space 1/2

	Left Gm/mm²	Spacing mm	Right Gm/mm²	Spacing mm
1 Pt Static	4.2		6.5	
2 Pt Static	40.4	12.1*	47.0	12.0*
1 Pt Moving				
2 Pt Moving				

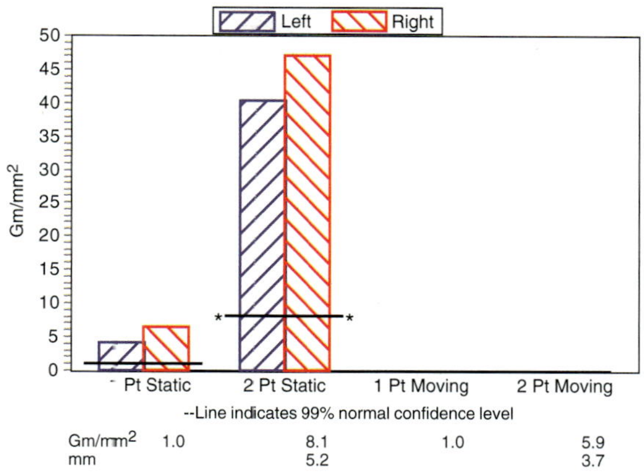

Great Toe Pulp

	Left Gm/mm²	Spacing mm	Right Gm/mm²	Spacing mm
1 Pt Static	7.5		8.7	
2 Pt Static	50.6	11.0*	55.6	12.0*
1 Pt Moving				
2 Pt Moving				

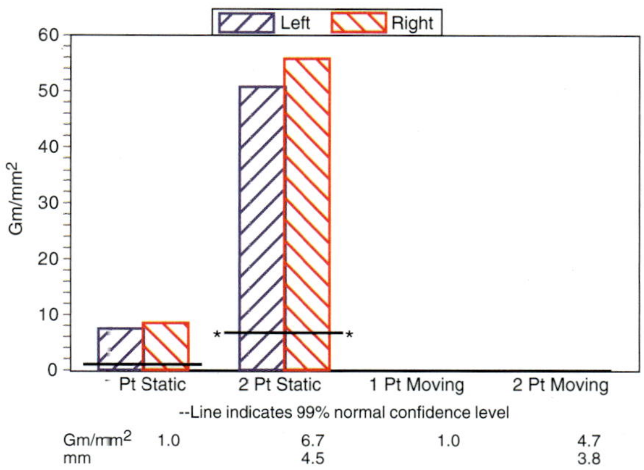

Fig. 10. Documentation of neuropathy with the Pressure-Specified Sensory Device. By definition neuropathy is present if there is a bilateral, symmetric, abnormal cutaneous pressure threshold for more than one nerve in the extremities. Because the commonest presentation of neuropathy is in the lower extremity, this is illustrated for the medial calcaneal (heel) and medial plantar (big toe pulp) branches of the tibial nerve and the deep peroneal and superficial peroneal branches of the common peroneal nerve. Note that the red (right side) and blue (left side) bars for static two-point discrimination are elevated above normal for each nerve. Because there is an asterisk present, this PSSD documentation is best evaluated as a sensory neuropathy with axonal loss. Note that at this stage of the neuropathy, one-point static-touch is still normal. Although the nylon monofilament would suggest this patient still has sufficient sensibility for protection, the beginning loss of two-point discrimination suggests otherwise. If a positive Tinel sign were present over known sites of nerve entrapment, decompression of the peroneal and tibial nerves therefore would be indicated.

or arthroplasty. It may be a peroneal nerve palsy. It may be that a patient with diabetes who has benefited from carpal tunnel decompression wishes to have sensibility restored to their feet [94]. There exists today a true deficit of surgeons appropriately trained to diagnosis and treat lower extremity peripheral nerve problems; it may be that the future will see hand surgeons filling this patient-care treatment gap. In this context it is important to appreciate that the problems experienced with EDT in the upper extremity are magnified in the lower extremity.

The only published material that compares EDT and the PSSD is the retrospective study whose results appear in Table 10 [59]. In this study the PSSD was more sensitive than EDT for identifying compression of the common peroneal nerve at the knee and the tibial nerve in the tarsal tunnel.

One anatomic area receiving increased attention related to entrapment in the region of the anterior hip is meralgia paresthetica. Although identified more often in the days when girdles were more commonly worn, today problems with the lateral femoral cutaneous nerve (LFCN) are seen after bone graft harvesting, car seatbelt injuries, lower abdominal wall procedures, and radiology interventional access to the groin vessels. Because of the wide anatomic variability of the location of the LFCN [95], EDT often cannot identify this entrapment site. It is

Dorsal Web Space 1/2

	Left Gm/mm2	Spacing mm	Right Gm/mm2	Spacing mm
1 Pt Static	.7		1.0	
2 Pt Static	2.6	5.2	2.8	5.2
1 Pt Moving				
2 Pt Moving				

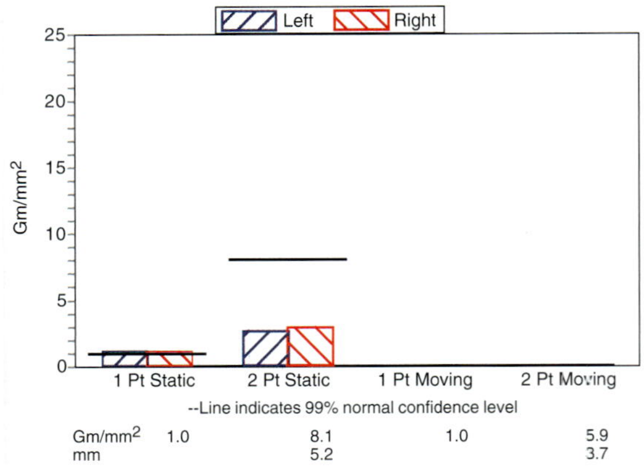

Great Toe Pulp

	Left Gm/mm2	Spacing mm	Right Gm/mm2	Spacing mm
1 Pt Static	.6		.8	
2 Pt Static	2.8	4.5	2.2	4.5
1 Pt Moving				
2 Pt Moving				

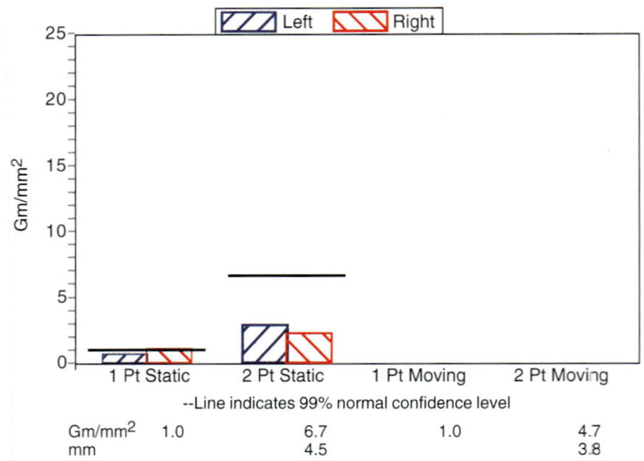

Heel (Medial)

	Left Gm/mm2	Spacing mm	Right Gm/mm2	Spacing mm
1 Pt Static	1.0		.8	
2 Pt Static	2.7	5.3	68.9	8.0*
1 Pt Moving				
2 Pt Moving				

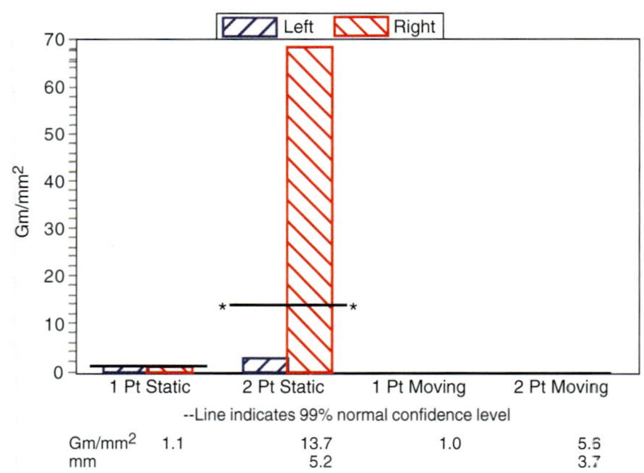

Fig. 11. Documentation of a right medial calcaneal nerve compression in heel pain syndrome and tarsal tunnel syndrome with the Pressure-Specified Sensory Device. Note that for the left, normal side, the blue bars for the medial calcaneal (heel), medial plantar (big toe pulp), and deep peroneal (dorsal web 0.5 interspace) nerve are in the normal range, below the black horizontal bar representing the 99% confidence upper limit of normal. On the symptomatic side, the right side, represented by the red bars, all the bars are in the normal range except the medial calcaneal nerve. This bar has an asterisk indicating axonal loss.

misdiagnosed frequently as being related to an L3 lumbar disc. Recently NST with the PSSD has established the ability to document entrapment of the LFCN [96], providing documentation needed to establish the diagnosis. There is a positive Tinel sign at the anterior superior iliac crest.

EDT has not been reported to be successful at identifying medial calcaneal nerve entrapment, and yet heel pain after diabetic foot problems is probably the second most common problem a

Great Toe Pulp

	Left Gm/mm2	Spacing mm	Right Gm/mm2	Spacing mm
1 Pt Static	.9		.8	
2 Pt Static	3.9	4.5	70.1	9.0*
1 Pt Moving				
2 Pt Moving				

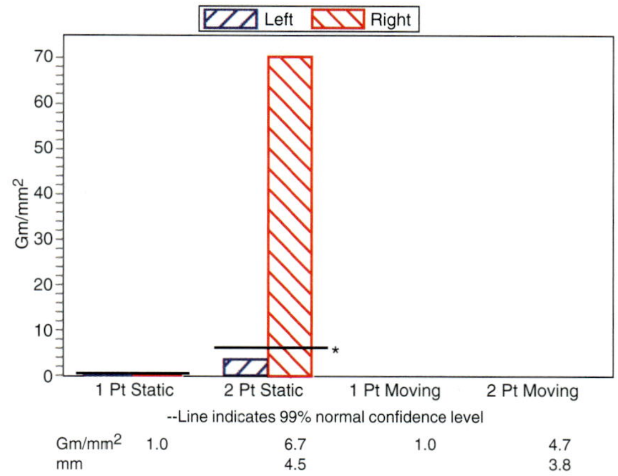

Heel (Medial)

	Left Gm/mm2	Spacing mm	Right Gm/mm2	Spacing mm
1 Pt Static	1.0		1.0	
2 Pt Static	7.2	5.3	66.4	8.0*
1 Pt Moving				
2 Pt Moving				

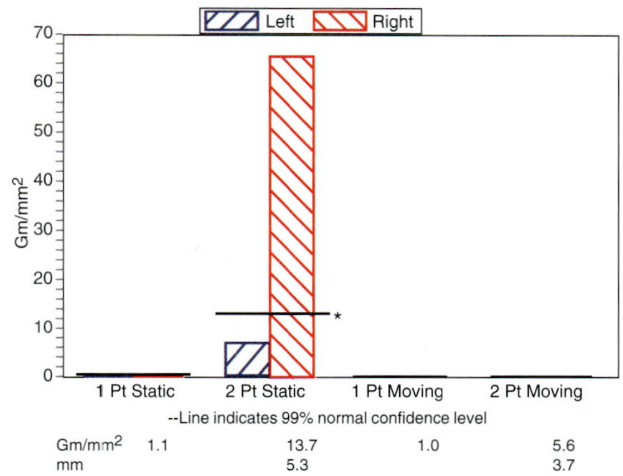

Dorsal Web Space 1/2

	Left Gm/mm2	Spacing mm	Right Gm/mm2	Spacing mm
1 Pt Static	.9		.7	
2 Pt Static	1.6	5.2	1.7	5.2
1 Pt Moving				
2 Pt Moving				

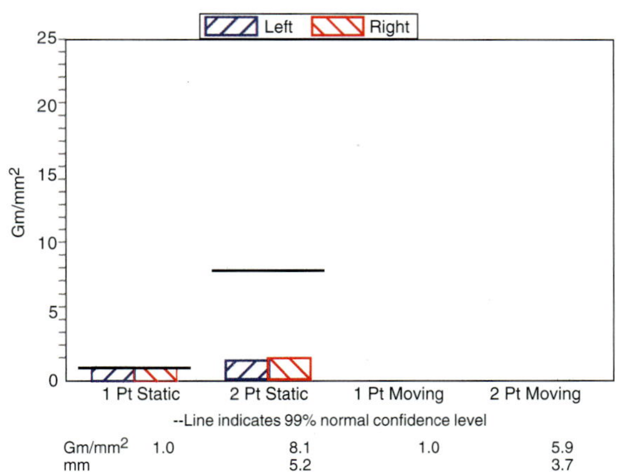

Fig. 12. Documentation of a right medial calcaneal nerve compression in heel pain syndrome and tarsal tunnel syndrome with the Pressure-Specified Sensory Device. Note that for the left, normal side, the blue bars for the medial calcaneal (heel), medial plantar (big toe pulp), and deep peroneal (dorsal web 0.5 interspace) nerve are in the normal range, below the black horizontal bar representing the 99% confidence upper limit of normal. On the symptomatic side, the right side, represented by the red bars, the deep peroneal nerve is normal but both the medial calcaneal and the big toe are abnormal. This is the pattern seen with tibial nerve compression in the tarsal tunnel, tarsal tunnel syndrome.

podiatric physician sees. By measuring the cutaneous pressure threshold of the medial calcaneal skin, the PSSD can identify calcaneal nerve compression as the source of heel pain [22] or calcaneal nerve dysfunction as part of tarsal tunnel syndrome [97,98]. Examples of PSSD reports related to these two peripheral nerve problems are given in Figs. 11 and 12. Recently the

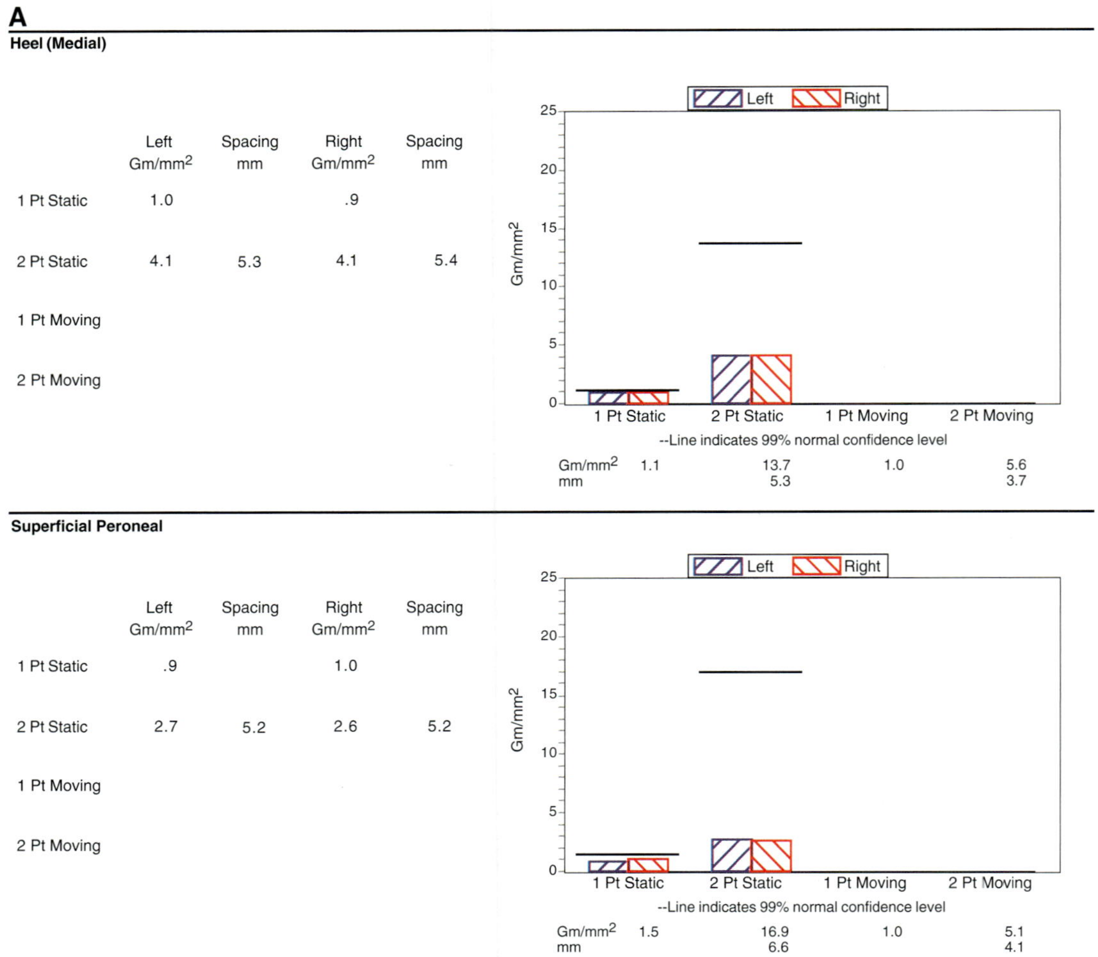

Fig. 13. (*A*, *B*) Documentation of a right deep peroneal nerve entrapment with the Pressure-Specified Sensory Device. Note that for the left, normal side, the blue bars for the medial calcaneal (heel), medial plantar (big toe pulp), and superficial and deep peroneal nerve are in the normal range, below the black horizontal bar representing the 99% confidence upper limit of normal. On the symptomatic side, the right side, represented by the red bars, all the bars are in the normal range except the deep peroneal nerve. This bar has an asterisk, indicating axonal loss. This severe degree of nerve injury is appropriate for neurolysis of the deep peroneal nerve over the dorsum of the foot. If the right superficial peroneal nerve bar were also abnormal, the site of compression most likely would be the common peroneal nerve at the fibular neck.

prevalence of medial calcaneal nerve abnormalities was evaluated in the population of a podiatric foot and ankle surgeon's routine practice: 23% of the patients at the time they presented were found to have abnormal heel sensibility alone, and another 49% were found to have abnormal heel and abnormal big toe pulp sensibility, demonstrating the value of the PSSD in identifying nerve problems as a contributing source of foot pain in this patient population [99]. EDT also has not been able to demonstrate entrapment of the distal deep peroneal nerve over the dorsum of the foot (Fig. 13), although it can identify the more proximal entrapment of this nerve by EMG identification of abnormalities in the extensor digiti minimi. Yet the distal site is a frequent source of pain related to straps from foot wear, fracture/dislocation of the second metatarsal (Lisfranc fracture), crush injury, and removal of ganglia and exostosis in this location [23]. By combining NST with the PSSD of the dorsomedial foot skin of the first/second webspace with that of the dorsolateral foot skin, the superficial peroneal nerve territory, identification of problems with the common peroneal nerve can be identified. This nerve often is involved in pain syndromes related to inversion sprains and knee injuries. Because of the inability of EDT to identify problems related to compression of the smaller nerves of the feet combined with its lack of sensitivity for identifying entrapment of the larger nerves of the lower extremity, the PSSD is more than the functional equivalent of EDT in the lower extremity.

B

Dorsal Web Space 1/2

	Left Gm/mm^2	Spacing mm	Right Gm/mm^2	Spacing mm
1 Pt Static	.7		1.7	
2 Pt Static	2.1	5.2	65.5	12.0*
1 Pt Moving				
2 Pt Moving				

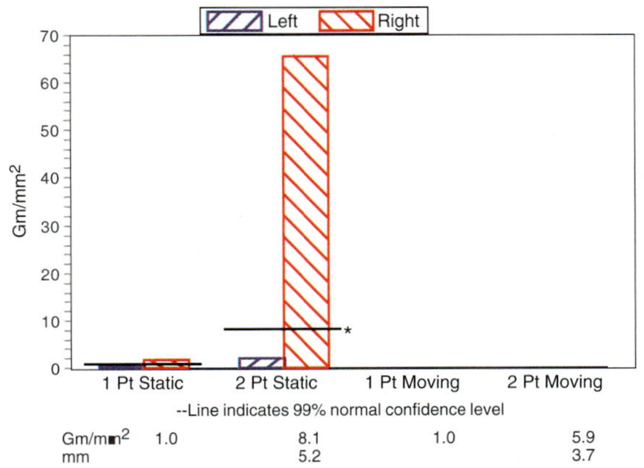

Great Toe Pulp

	Left Gm/mm^2	Spacing mm	Right Gm/mm^2	Spacing mm
1 Pt Static	.9		.8	
2 Pt Static	2.5	4.5	2.4	4.5
1 Pt Moving				
2 Pt Moving				

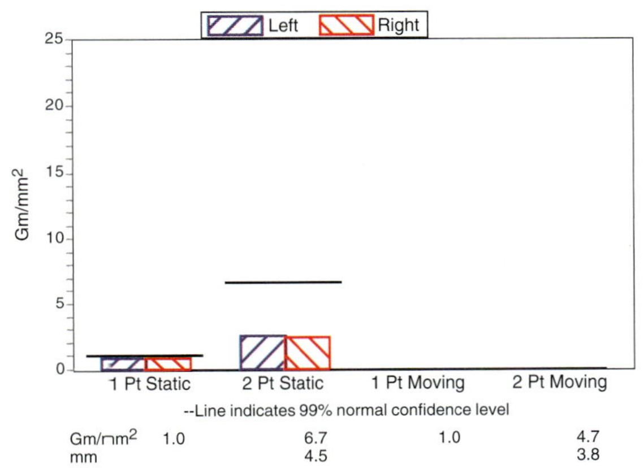

Fig. 13 (*continued*)

The medical necessity for using the PSSD in the lower extremity is the evaluation of complaints of pain or numbness that are not related to lumbosacral spine problems and when these complaints persist after traditional musculoskeletal approaches to relieve them have been exhausted.

Closed nerve injuries

Peripheral nerve problems after closed injuries are common. The classic problems are the radial nerve palsy after humeral fracture or median or ulnar nerve problems after elbow injuries. In the lower extremity, peroneal palsy after total hip or knee arthroplasty is especially difficult to manage clinically. The EDT problem is twofold: electrical evidence of muscle denervation does not occur until at least 3 weeks after nerve injury, delaying the time at which the earliest diagnosis can be made, and sensory recovery occurs before motor recovery, again delaying the time until clinical decision making can occur. In contrast, the neural regeneration pattern described is the ideal method using the PSSD to document soon after injury whether it is axonal loss or evidence of nerve regeneration. Because the PSSD is a painless test, the patient is compliant with more frequent monitoring. If a neural regeneration is present on the first test, which can be done as soon after injury as possible, a clinical period of waiting is likely to prove justified, because motor recovery is highly likely. If a neural regeneration pattern is not present at the 3-month follow-up evaluation with the PSSD, surgical intervention with neurolysis or possibly nerve reconstruction (depending on the intraoperative findings) is indicated, because functional recovery is not clinically likely to occur (presented to the American Society for

Peripheral Nerve meeting, 1999). For the management of closed nerve injuries, PSSD is the functional equivalent of EDT.

Limb lengthening

Limb lengthening in the upper and lower extremities is now a proven clinical modality. Nerve stretch traction injuries have been reported in up to 30% of patients undergoing this treatment, usually because the peripheral nerve is adherent along its course from the initial trauma or treatment that preceded the limb lengthening. Nerve decompression must be done during the course of the limb lengthening. Recently an approach using the PSSD to monitor peripheral nerve function during limb lengthening was reported [100]. This prospective study occurred over a span of 10 years and involved more than 900 limbs. The study concluded that the PSSD could identify nerve stretch/traction injuries earlier than EDT, and that by using the PSSD to monitor the patient during limb lengthening, stretch/traction injuries and the need for secondary peripheral nerve surgery can be decreased to the 1% level. That study establishes the PSSD as the standard of care in limb lengthening.

Summary

The surgeon involved with the evaluation and treatment of peripheral nerve problems must be aware of the critical indications for the use of electrodiagnostic testing and its true and unfortunately common limitations in providing guidance for clinical care of these patients. The Pressure-Specified Sensory Device has been proven and documented by an increasing body of clinical evidence to be the functional equivalent of EDT for all clinical peripheral nerve problems with the exception of identifying radiculopathy and is superior to EDT for many peripheral nerve problems for which EDT is simply unable to provide the critical information necessary for patient care.

References

[1] Kimura J. Electrodiagnosis in diseases of nerve and muscle. Philadelphia: FA Davis; 1983.
[2] Campbell WW. Diagnosis and management of common compression and entrapment neuropathies. Neurol Clin 1997;15:549–67.
[3] Dumitru D. Electrodiagnostic medicine. Philadelphia: Hanlery and Belfus, Inc.; 1995.
[4] Van Beek A, Hubble B, Kinkead L, Torros S, Suchy H. Clinical use of nerve stimulation and recording techniques. Plast Reconstr Surg 1983;71:225–40.
[5] Campion D. Electrodiagnostic testing in hand surgery. J Hand Surg 1962;21A:947–56.
[6] Brumback RA, Bobele GB, Rayan GM. Electrodiagnosis of compressive nerve lesions. Hand Clin 1992;8:241–54.
[7] Slutsky DJ. Nerve conduction studies in hand surgery. J Amer Soc Surg Hand 2003;3:152–69.
[8] Kaplan EB, Spinner M. Normal and anomalous innervation patterns in the upper extremity. In: Omer G, Spinner M, editors. Management of peripheral nerve problems. Philadelphia: WB Saunders; 1980. Chapter 6, pp. 75–99.
[9] Dorfman L. Quantitative clinical electrophysiology in the evaluation of nerve injury and regeneration. Muscle Nerve 1990;13:822–8.
[10] Kline D, Hudson A. Nerve action potential recordings. In: Kline D, Hudson A, editors. Nerve injuries. Philadelphia: WB Saunders Co.; 1995. pp. 102–15.
[11] Uchida YL, Sugioka YM. Electrodiagnosis of Martin-Gruber connection and its clinical importance in peripheral nerve surgery. J Hand Surg 1992;17A:54–9.
[12] AAEM Quality Assurance Committee. Literature review of the usefulness of nerve conduction studies and electromyography for the evaluation of patients with carpal tunnel syndrome. Muscle Nerve 1993;16:1392–414.
[13] Tomaino MM, Brach PJ, Vansickle DP. The rationale for and efficacy of surgical intervention for electrodiagnostic-negative cubital tunnel syndrome. J Hand Surg 2001;26A:1077–81.
[14] Braillar F. Electromyography: its use and misuse in peripheral nerve injuries. Orthop Clin N Am 1981;12:229–38.
[15] Halar EM, DeLisa JA, Soine TL. Nerve conduction studies in upper extremities: skin temperature corrections. Arch Phys Med Rehabil 1983;64:412–6.
[16] Dellon AL, Schlegel RW, Mackinnon SE. Validity of nerve conduction velocity studies after anterior transposition of the ulnar nerve. J Hand Surg 1987;12A:700–3.
[17] Corwin HK, Kasdan ML. Electrodiagnostic reports of median neuropathy at the wrist. J Hand Surg 1988;23A:55–7.

[18] Dellon AL. Pitfalls in interpretation of electrophysiological testing. In: Gelberman RH, editor. Operative nerve repair and reconstruction. Philadelphia: Lippincott; 1991. p. 185–96.
[19] Brown WF, Dellon AL, Campbell WW. Electrodiagnosis in the management of focal neuropathies: the WOG syndrome. Muscle Nerve 1994;17:1336–42.
[20] Rosenberg D, Conolley J, Dellon AL. Thenar eminence quantitative sensory testing in diagnosis of proximal median nerve compression. J Hand Ther 2001;14:258–65.
[21] Howard M, Lee C, Dellon AL. Documentation of brachial plexus compression (in the thoracic inlet) utilizing provocative neurosensory and muscular testing. J Reconstr Microsurg 2003;19:303–12.
[22] Dellon AL. Deciding when heel pain is of neural origin. J Foot Ankle Surg 2001;40:341–5.
[23] Dellon AL. Entrapment of the deep peroneal nerve on the dorsum of the foot. Foot Ankle 1990;11:73–80.
[24] Dyck PJ, Zimmerman IR, O'Brien PC, Ness A, Caskey PE, Karners J, Bushek W. Introduction of automated systems to evaluate touch-pressure, vibration, and thermal cutaneous sensation in man. Ann Neurol 1978;4:502–10.
[25] Arezzo JC, Boulton CF, Boulton A. Quantitative sensory testing: a consensus report from the Peripheral Neuropathy Association. Neurol 1993;43:1050–2.
[26] Jamal GA, Hansen S, Weir AL, Ballantyne JP. An improved automated method for the measurement of thermal thresholds. J Neurol Neurosurg Psychiatr 1985;48:354–60.
[27] Dellon AL. The vibrometer. Plast Reconstr Surg 1983;71:427–31.
[28] Levin S, Pearsall G, Ruderman RJ. von Frey's method of measuring pressure sensibility in the hand: an engineering analysis of the Weinstein-Semmes pressure aesthesiometer. J Hand Surg 1978;3:211–6.
[29] Dellon AL, Keller KM. Computer-assisted quantitative sensorimotor testing in patients with carpal and cubital tunnel syndromes. Ann Plast Surg 1997;38:492–502.
[30] Dyck PJ, Zimmerman IR, Johnson DM, Gillen D, Hokanson JHL, Karnes JL, Gruener G, O'Brien PC. A standard test of heat-pain responses CASE IV. J Neurol Sci 1996;136:54–63.
[31] Mitterhauser M, Muse VL, Dellon AL, Jetzer T. Detection of submaximal effort with computer-assisted grip strength measurement. J Occup Environ Med 1997;39:1221–7.
[32] Dellon AL, Mackinnon SE, Brandt KE. The Semmes-Weinstein nylon filaments' markings. J Hand Surg 1993; 18A:756–7.
[33] Kumar S, Fernando DJ, Veves A, et al. Semmes-Weinstein monofilaments: a simple, effective and inexpensive screening device for identifying diabetic patients at risk of foot ulceration. Diabetes Res Clin Pract 1991;13:63–6.
[34] Rith-Najarian SJ, Stolusky T, Gohdes DM. Identifying diabetic patients at high risk for lower-extremity amputation in a primary health care setting. A prospective evaluation of simple screening criteria. Diabetes Care 1992;15:1386–8.
[35] Armstrong DG, Lavery LA, Vela SA, Harkless L. Choosing a practical screening instrument to identify patients at risk for diabetic foot ulceration. Arch Intern Med 1998;158:289–92.
[36] McGill M, Molyneaux L, Spencer R, et al. Possible sources of discrepancies in the use of the Semmes-Weinstein monofilament; impact on prevalence of insensate foot and workload requirements. Diabetes Care 1999;22:598–600.
[37] Booth J, Young MJ. Differences in the performance of commercially available 10 gm monofilaments. Diabetes Care 2000;23:984–7.
[38] Dellon AL. Clinical use of vibratory stimuli to evaluate peripheral nerve injury and compression neuropathy. Plast Reconstr Surg 1980;65:466–76.
[39] Strauch B, Lang A, Ferder M, Keyes-Ford M, Freeman K, Newsein D. The ten test. Plast Reconstru Surg 1997;99: 1074–8.
[40] Dellon AL. Evaluation of sensibility and re-education of sensation in the hand. Baltimore: Williams and Wilkins; 1982.
[41] Mendell JR, Sahenk Z. Painful sensory neuropathy. N Engl J Med 2003;348:1243–55.
[42] Magda P, Norman L, Renard MV, Sander HW. Quantitative sensory testing: high sensitivity in small fiber neuropathy with normal NCS/EMG. J Periph Nerve Sys 2002;7:225–8.
[43] Hermann DN, Griffin JW, Hauer P, Cornblath DR, McArthur JC. Intraepidermal nerve fiber density and sural nerve morphometry in peripheral neuropathies. Neurol 1999;53:1634–0.
[44] Periquet MW, Novak V, Collins MP, Nagaraja HN, Ercem S, Nash SM, Freimer ML, Sahenk Z, Kissel JT, Mendell JR. Painful sensory neuropathy: prospective evaluation using skin biopsy. Neurol 1999;53:1641–7.
[45] Dellon AL. Clinical grading of peripheral nerve problems. Neurosurg Clin N Am 2001;12:229–40.
[46] Cohen MD, Dellon AL. Computer-assisted sensorimotor testing documents neural regeneration after ulnar nerve repair at the wrist: case report. Plast Reconstr Surg 2001;107:501–5.
[47] Van De Kar HJ, Jaquet JB, Meulstee J, Molenaar CBH, Schimsheimer RJ, Hovius SER. Clinical value of electrodiagnostic testing following repair of peripheral nerve lesions: a prospective study. J Hand Surgery 2002; 27B:345–9.
[48] Almquist E, Eeg-Olofsson O. Sensory nerve conduction velocity and two-point discrimination in sutured nerves. J Bone Joint Surg 1970;52A:791–6.
[49] Lester R, Smith P, Mott G, McAllister R. Intrinsic reinnervation—myth or reality? J Hand Surg 1993;18B:454–60.
[50] Tackmann W, Brennwald J, Nigst H. Sensory electroneuropathic parameters and clinical recovery of sensibility in sutured human nerves. J Neurol 1983;229:195–206.
[51] Dellon AL, Curtis RM, Edgerton MT. Evaluating recovery of sensation in the hand following nerve injury. Johns Hopkins Med J 1972;130:235–43.
[52] Dellon AL. The moving two-point discrimination test: clinical evaluation of the quickly-adapting fiber receptor system. J Hand Surg 1978;3:474–81.

[53] Weber RA, Breidenbach WC, Brown RE, Jabaley ME, Mass DP. A randomized prospective study of polyglycolic acid conduits for digital nerve reconstruction in human. Plast Reconstr Surg 2000;106(5):1036–45.
[54] Reisman NR, Dellon AL. The abductor digit minimi muscle flap: a salvage technique for palmar wrist pain. Plast Reconstr Surg 1983;72:859–63.
[55] Dellon AL, Mackinnon SE. The pronator quadratus muscle flap. J Hand Surg 1984;9A:423–7.
[56] Dellon AL. Somatosensory testing and rehabilitation. Bethesda MD: Am Occup Ther Assoc.; 1997.
[57] Kimura J. The carpal tunnel syndrome: localization of conduction abnormalities within the distal segment of the media nerve. Brain 1979;102:619–35.
[58] Dellon AL. Management of peripheral nerve problems in the upper and lower extremities using quantitative sensory testing. Hand Clin 1999;15:697–715.
[59] Tassler PL, Dellon AL. Correlation of measurements of pressure perception using the pressure-specified sensory device with electrodiagnostic testing. J Occup Environ Med 1995;37:862–6.
[60] Lobar B. A neurologist's perspective: improved documentation of clinically suspect nerve compression by adding quantitative sensory testing when traditional NCS/EMG tests are normal. J Reconstr Micro 1999;15:616.
[61] Weber R, Weber RA, Schuchmann JA, Ortiz J. A prospective blinded evaluation of nerve conduction velocity versus pressure-specified sensory device testing in carpal tunnel syndrome. Ann Plast Surg 2000;45:252–7.
[62] Coert JH, Meek MF, Gibeault D, Dellon AL. Documentation of posttraumatic nerve compression in patients with normal electrodiagnostic studies. J Trauma 2004;56:339–44.
[63] Smith NJ. Nerve conduction studies for carpal tunnel syndrome: essential prelude to surgery or unnecessary luxury? J Hand Surg 2002;27B:83–5.
[64] Mackinnon SE, Dellon AL. Overlap of lateral antebrachial cutaneous nerve and superficial sensory branch of the radial nerve. J Hand Surg 1985;10A:522–6.
[65] Mysiew WJ, Colachis SC III. The pronator syndrome. An evaluation of dynamic maneuvers for improving electrodiagnostic sensitivity. Am J Phys Med Rehab 1991;70:274–7.
[66] Kupfer DM, Bronson J, Lee GW, Beck J, Gillet J. Differential latency testing: a more sensitive test for radial tunnel syndrome. J Hand Surg 1998;23A:859–64.
[67] Naff N, Dellon AL, Mackinnon SE. The anatomic course of the palmar cutaneous branch of the median nerve, including a description of its own unique tunnel. J Hand Surg 1993;18B:316–7.
[68] Duncan GJ, Yospur G, Gomez-Garcia A, Lesavoy MA. Entrapment of the palmar cutaneous branch of the median nerve by a normal palmaris longus tendon. Ann Plast Surg 1995;35:534–6.
[69] Spinner M. Injuries to the major branches of the peripheral nerves of the forearm. 2nd edition. Philadelphia: WB Saunders; 1978.
[70] Dellon AL. Musculotendinous variations about the medial humeral epicondyle. J Hand Surg 1986;11B:175–81.
[71] Dellon AL, Mackinnon SE. Musculoaponeurotic variations along the course of the median nerve in the proximal forearm. J Hand Surg 1987;12B:359–63.
[72] Dellon AL, Mackinnon SE. Radial sensory nerve entrapment in the forearm. J Hand Surg 1986;11A:199–205.
[73] Perkins BA, Olaaleye D, Bril V. Carpal tunnel syndrome in patients with diabetic polyneuropathy. Diabetes Care 2002;25:565–9.
[74] Wong L, Dellon AL. Brachial neuritis presenting as anterior interosseous nerve compression—implications for diagnosis and treatment: a case report. J Hand Surg 1997;22A:536–9.
[75] Gilliatt RW, LeQuesne PM, Logue V, Sumner AJ. Wasting of the hand associated with a cervical rib or band. J Neurol Neurosurg Psychiatr 1970;33:615–9.
[76] Francel T, Dellon AL, Campbell JN. Quadrilateral space syndrome. Plast Reconstr Surg 1991;87:911–6.
[77] Leffert RD. Thoracic outlet syndromes. Hand Clin 1992;8:285–91.
[78] Mackinnon SE, Dellon AL. Surgery of the peripheral nerve. New York: Thieme; 1988 p. 175–91.
[79] Campbell JN, Naff N, Dellon AL. Thoracic outlet syndrome: a neurosurgical perspective. Neurosurg Clin N Am 1991;2:227–34.
[80] Wilbourn A, Urschel HC. Evidence for conduction delay in thoracic outlet syndrome is challenged. N Engl J Med 1984;310:1052–3.
[81] Roos D, Wilbourn AJ. Thoracic outlet syndrome is underrated/over-diagnosed. Arch Neurol 1990;47:228–30.
[82] Cherington M, Cherington C. Thoracic outlet syndrome reimbursement patterns and patient profiles. Neurol 1992; 42:492–5.
[83] Peet RM, Hendrickson JD, Anderson RP, Martin GM. Thoracic outlet syndrome: evaluation of a therapeutic exercise program. Mayo Clin Proc 1956;31:281–7.
[84] Kenny RA, Traynor GB, Withington D, Keegan DJ. Thoracic outlet syndrome: a useful exercise treatment option. Am J Surg 1993;165:282–4.
[85] Walsh MT. Therapist management of thoracic outlet syndrome. J Hand Ther 1994;7:131–44.
[86] Novak CB, Collins ED, Mackinnon SE. Outcome following conservative management of thoracic outlet syndrome. J Hand Surg 1995;20A:542–8.
[87] Urschel HC Jr, Razzuk MA. Management of the thoracic outlet syndromes. N Engl J Med 1972;286:1140–3.
[88] Sanders RJ. Thoracic outlet syndrome: a common sequelae of neck injuries. Philadelphia: JB Lippincott Co.; 1991.
[89] Roos DB, Owens JC. Thoracic outlet syndrome. Arch Surg 1996;93:71–4.
[90] Dellon AL. The results of supraclavicular brachial plexus neurolysis (without first rib resection) in management of post-traumatic "thoracic outlet syndrome." J Reconstr Microsurg 1993;9:11–7.
[91] Novak CB, Mackinnon SE, Patterson GA. Evaluation of patients with thoracic outlet syndrome. J Hand Surg 1993;18A:292–9.

[92] Levin LS, Dellon AL. Pathology of the shoulder as it relates to the differential diagnosis of thoracic outlet compression. J Reconstr Microsurg 1992;8:313–7.
[93] Lee GW, Massry DR, Kupfer DM, Abrams R. Documentation of brachial plexus compression in the thoracic inlet with quantitative sensory testing. J Reconstr Microsurg 2000;16:15–20.
[94] Dellon AL. Prevention of foot ulceration and amputation by decompression of peripheral nerves in patients with diabetic neuropathy. Ostomy Wound Management 2002;48:36–45.
[95] Aszmann OC, Dellon ES, Dellon AL. The anatomic course of the lateral femoral cutaneous nerve and its susceptibility to compression and injury. Plast Reconstr Surg 1997;100:600–4.
[96] Coert JH, Connolly J, Dellon AL. Documenting compressive neuropathy of the lateral femoral cutaneous nerve. Ann Plast Surg 2003;50:373–7.
[97] Dellon AL. Computer-assisted sensibility evaluation and surgical treatment of tarsal tunnel syndrome. Advanc Podiatr 1996;2:17–40.
[98] Tassler PL, Dellon AL. Pressure perception in the normal lower extremity and in tarsal tunnel syndrome. Muscle Nerve 1996;19:285–9.
[99] Rose JD, Malay DS, Sorrento DL. Neurosensory testing of the medial calcaneal and medial plantar nerves in patients with plantar heel pain. J Foot Ankle Surg 2002;42:173–7.
[100] Nogueira MB, Paley D, Bhave A, Herbert A, Nozenta C, Herzenberg J. Nerve lesions associated with limb lengthening. J Bone Joint Surg 2003;85:1502–9.
[101] Seiler D, Barrett SL, Dellon AL. Guide to interpretation of neurosensory testing with the pressure-specified sensory device. Baltimore: Sensory Management Services Pub.; 2004.
[102] Dellon ES, Keller KM, Moratz V, Dellon AL. Validation of cutaneous pressure threshold measurements for the evaluation of hand function. Ann Plast Surg 1997;38:485–92.
[103] Buchthal F, Rosenthalk A, Trojaborg W. Electrophysiological findings in entrapment of the median nerve at the wrist and elbow. J Neurol Neurosurg Psych 1974;37:340–60.
[104] Johnson RK, Spinner M, Shrewsbury MM. Median nerve entrapment syndrome in the proximal forearm. J Hand Surg 1979;4:48–51.
[105] Hartz CR, Linscheid RL, Gramse RR, Daube JR. The pronator syndrome: compressive neuropathy of the median nerve. J Bone Joint Surg 1981;63A:885–90.
[106] Breidenbach WC, Tsai T, Manstein C. Ipsilateral pronator teres and carpal tunnel compression of the median nerve [proc abstr]. J Hand Surg 1985;10:432.
[107] Olehnik WK, Manske PR, Szerzinski J. Median nerve compression in the proximal forearm. J Hand Surg 1994; 19A:121–6.
[108] Borud LJ, Lin J, Beasely RW. Compression of proximal median nerve in the forearm. Presented at American Association of Plastic Surgery Meeting, Columbia, South Carolina, May 2000.
[109] Seddon HJ. Peripheral nerve injury. Medical Research Council Special Report Series 282. London: Her Majesty's Stationery Office; 1954.

ELSEVIER
SAUNDERS

Atlas Hand Clin 10 (2005) 33–63

Atlas of the
HAND
CLINICS

Electrodiagnostic Testing in Hand Surgery

David J. Slutsky, MD, FRCS(C)

Private Practice, South Bay Hand Surgery Center, 3475 Torrance Boulevard, Suite F, Torrance, CA 90503, USA

The treatment of nerve disorders of the upper extremity has become a highly specialized area. There has been an evolution in the electrodiagnostic (EDX) approach for evaluating patients who have these disorders. Differential latency testing can aid in the diagnosis of dynamic nerve entrapment disorders such as radial tunnel syndrome. Comparative latency testing increases the test sensitivity in the diagnosis of carpal tunnel syndrome, cubital tunnel, and ulnar tunnel syndrome. Digital nerve conduction testing can detect isolated digital nerve lesions and can be used to monitor the adequacy of reinnervation following a nerve repair [1]. Nerve conduction studies are not a panacea, however, especially in recurrent carpal tunnel syndrome [2].

The EDX evaluation consists of nerve conduction studies (NCS) and electromyography (EMG). Although these studies are invaluable extensions of the physical examination, many physicians are unable to interpret the study results, and so they base their operative decisions on electromyographers' impressions. Techniques for recording the electrophysiologic events in nerve and muscle carry with them several potential pitfalls. This may lead to falsely positive or falsely negative results that in turn lead to erroneous conclusions [3]. A systematic approach to the interpretation of the NCS/EMG allows surgeons to determine the nature and location of lesions and the degree of involvement and the viability of the affected nerve and muscles [4]. The foundation for this understanding can be gained through an understanding of the electrophysiology of nerve and muscle and the methodology underlying the EDX test [5].

Nerve electrophysiology

The nerve cell membrane is composed of a lipid bilayer that has a hydrophilic (water loving) and a hydrophobic end. When placed in an aqueous medium the phospholipids arrange themselves so that the hydrophilic ends are facing outward and the hydrophobic ends are inside. This leads to an ionic separation across the nerve axon that results in a charge separation. Although there are several charged proteins, the electrical gradients are caused mostly by the difference in concentrations between sodium (Na^+) and potassium (K^+) ions. Minute changes in these concentrations lead to a change in the membrane potential even though there is little actual ion flow.

Various membrane channels consist of proteins embedded in the phospholipid bilayer that have a neutral charge and allow the passive flow of charged ions. There are separate channels for Na^+, K^+, and calcium (Ca^{+2}) ions. The interior of the axon has a charge of approximately −90 millivolts (mv) with a greater concentration of K^+ ions with respect to the outside. There is a passive leak of K^+ ions out and Na^+ ions in, which causes the interior of the axon to become less negative relative to the outside. There is an ATP-dependent Na^+/K^+ pump that imports K^+ and exports Na^+ in a ratio of 2 K^+ for every 3 Na^+. This maintains the normal resting membrane potential and prevents spontaneous depolarization. Because maintaining the ionic charge separation across the membrane requires energy, this mechanism stops when the energy

E-mail address: d-slutsky@msn.com

doi:10.1016/j.ahc.2004.08.003

supply is interrupted. In other words, local nerve ischemia prevents depolarization. This is one of the mechanisms for the conduction block that occurs with nerve compression.

When the resting membrane potential reaches −50 mv, the membrane depolarizes. This generates an action potential, which is the electrical wave caused by the flow of ions. The Na^+ channels open in response to depolarization, allowing an influx of Na^+ ions down their concentration gradient. The Na^+ channels then close and become refractory to opening for a finite period of time. The Na^+/K^+ pump then pumps out the Na^+ in exchange for K^+ ions, restoring the membrane potential. The K^+ channels open after the Na^+ channels and remain open longer. This continued efflux of K^+ leads to transient hyperpolarization of the axon interior. An inward K^+ leak ultimately restores the baseline potential.

Nerve anatomy

Schwann cells are specialized satellite cells that separate the axon from the endoneurial fluid. They provide trophic support and aid in maintaining the periaxonal environment. In unmyelinated nerves a single Schwann cell incorporates multiple axons into longitudinal invaginations of its cytoplasm. In myelinated nerves a single Schwann cell surrounds one axon and lays down sphingomyelin. The myelin acts as a capacitor in that it is an insulator that has a high resistance to the flow of electrons. This allows a charge separation to develop on either side of the axonal membrane. The Schwann cells are arranged longitudinally along the axolemma. Each Schwann cell territory delineates an internode. At the junction between adjacent Schwann cells the axon is exposed at a gap called the node of Ranvier. Local currents exit only at the nodes, where the myelin sheath thins down and disappears. A conductive material called gap substance coats the axon membrane and facilitates the flow of ions. There is also a higher concentration of Na^+ channels at the nodes and a relative paucity in the membrane underneath the myelin. In this way there is increased resistance to the flow of ions (current) except at the nodes.

Depolarization—unmyelinated nerves

Depolarization is an all or none phenomenon and cannot be stopped once it starts. The membrane does not allow ion flow except in areas with Na^+ channels. In unmyelinated nerves the Na^+ channels are spread out along the membrane and signal conduction is uniform and successive. Once an action potential (AP) is generated, there is sequential depolarization along the membrane. As the AP propagates down the axon each section of the membrane must be depolarized in turn. This not only takes time, but also diminishes the residual amount of current available to spread down the interior of the axon, which becomes attenuated faster. This leads to slow conduction velocities in the range of 10 to 15 milliseconds.

Depolarization—myelinated nerves

In myelinated nerves the resistance of the axon interior to current flow is much less than the myelinated membrane, which results in preferential ionic flow down the axon. There is also a relative paucity of Na^+ channels except at the internodes. The current flows down the axon, stopping only at the nodes of Ranvier. The Na^+ channels open, allowing the node to depolarize. The depolarizing current then flows down the axon interior to the next node. Depolarization thus jumps from node to node (saltatory conduction) rather than sequentially depolarizing each section of the membrane. This markedly speeds up the conduction velocities, which are in the range of 90 to 100 milliseconds.

Speed of conduction

The electrical resistance to current flow varies inversely with diameter. Larger nerves conduct faster than smaller nerves. To survive, organisms must be able to react quickly to their environment; hence, nerve conduction must be fast. In complex organisms with billions of axons, increasing the nerve diameter is not a viable option. Myelination solves this problem by increasing impulse conduction without the need to increase the fiber diameter. The result of myelination is a 50-times decrease in nerve diameter with a 4-times increase in the conduction velocity [6].

Waveform generation

Recording electrodes detect the small voltage changes associated with a nerve or muscle AP and convey them to an amplifier. Following amplification, the signal is filtered to remove extraneous electrical activity that can distort the waveform. Newer machines change the analog signal into a binary signal (digital) through a convertor. By convention, a deflection that is upward from the baseline is negative. An active electrode (E-1) is placed in an active region of the electrical field. In motor recordings a reference electrode (E-2) is situated where the current flow is low, such as over a tendon insertion. In sensory recordings the electrodes are separated by 3–4 cm so that the wave has passed E-1 completely before it is picked up by E-2. In sensory and motor recordings the signal from the reference electrode is inverted and electronically summated with the signal from E-1 (Fig. 1*A–D*). The net result is an amplification of the differences detected from each electrode and the elimination of like signals.

Methodology

The NCS involves stimulating motor and sensory nerves at specific sites, then recording the time it takes for the stimulus to be sensed by the recording electrodes. E-1 is placed over the mid portion of a muscle belly to record the distal motor latency (DML). The recording electrode is

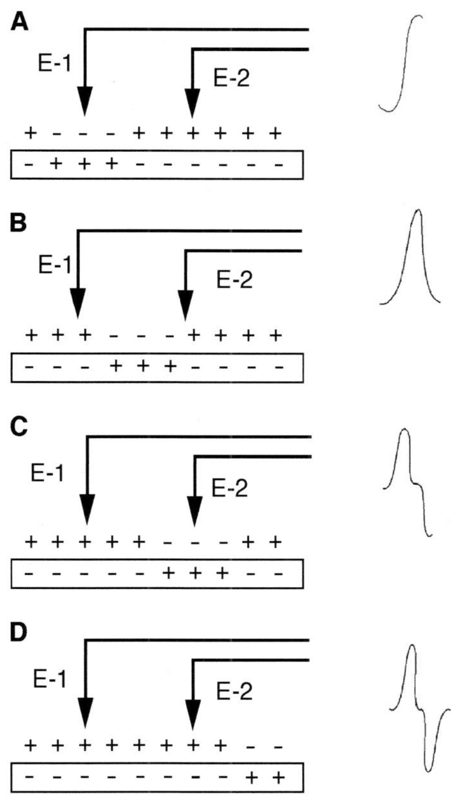

Fig. 1. The electrodes record the change in the electrical charge. (*A*) As the depolarization front approaches, the E-1 electrode records the advancing negative wavefront as an upward deflection. (*B*) When the depolarization passes E-1, the tracing returns to the baseline as the membrane potential reverts back to positive. (*C*) The E-2 senses the negative front in a similar fashion, but the deflection is electrically inverted to give a downward sloping waveform. (*D*) As the negative front passes E-2, the tracing again returns to the baseline. (*From* Slutsky D. Nerve conduction studies in hand surgery. J Am Soc Surg Hand 2003;3:155; with permission.)

placed directly over the nerve to record the sensory nerve action potential (SNAP). The initial stimulus is applied just proximal to the wrist. The subsequent stimuli must be at least 10–12 cm apart, otherwise wave cancellation caused by temporal dispersion results in an erroneously prolonged latency and lower amplitudes (see section on pitfalls). The distances from the recording electrode to the stimulation site are standardized so that the latencies can be compared with tables of normal values. The nerve conduction report must list the distances used and the normal values for the patient group to determine if there is any abnormal prolongation.

The nerve conduction velocity (NCV) is calculated by measuring the distance between stimulation sites and then dividing by the latency difference (NCV = distance/proximal – distal latency). The nerve conduction values are affected by several variables, including height, gender, and age (Table 1). In general the NCV slows by 10 milliseconds for every decade over age 60 years [7]. If this is not factored in, the test results in older patients may be interpreted falsely. Because the conduction velocity must be measured above and below any suspected site of nerve injury or entrapment, the NCS cannot evaluate directly nerve conduction in the neck and does not aid in the diagnosis of cervical nerve root compression. Specialized tests such as F-wave conduction, which is a type of nerve reflex, can be used to infer that proximal nerve conduction may be slower. This test can be fraught with error, however, and may be difficult to evaluate.

Motor recordings

E-1 is placed over the motor endplate, which usually corresponds to the midportion of the muscle belly. There is usually only one motor endplate per muscle except for long muscles, such as the sartorius. The compound motor action potential (CMAP) is a large waveform. A depolarization that starts directly under the recording electrode results in an upward or negative deflection. The time from the stimulation to this deflection is termed the onset latency, which is usually easy to distinguish from the baseline. If there is a preceding positive wave the electrode should be moved or the onset calculated at the point of the initial negative takeoff, otherwise the onset latency may be under calculated.

Sensory recordings

The SNAP is the summation of thousands of individual fibers. Antidromic potentials are measured against the direction of physiologic nerve transmission, whereas orthodromic potentials are measured in the same direction. The height of the negative wave is termed the peak latency. This peak historically was measured because of the small amplitude of the SNAP (50 μv) versus the CMAP, which is 1000 times larger (5000 μv). This makes it difficult to determine the onset of the SNAP from the baseline electrical noise. With newer digital machines this is not as difficult, but peak latencies still are often used by convention.

Stimulation

Any given nerve is composed of faster and slower conducting axons. The measured AP actually consists of a mixture of both. It is important to stimulate the nerve supramaximally so

Table 1
Variables affecting the nerve conduction test

Physiologic factors	Instrumentation
Age	Electrode separation
Gender	Filter settings
Digit circumference	Stimulus spread
Height	Distance measurement
Temperature	Limb position
Anomalous innervation	Anatomic nerve course
Martin Gruber anastomosis	
Riche–Cannieu	

From Slutsky DJ. Nerve conduction studies in hand surgery. J Am Soc Surg Hand 2003;3(3):155; with permission.

that all of the fibers are depolarized, otherwise some of the faster fibers may fail to fire. An insufficient stimulus intensity would lead to an artificially low amplitude, which might lead to the wrong conclusion of axonal loss or conduction block. A two-pronged stimulator is placed over the nerve that is being tested, at a standardized distance from the recording electrode. A square wave current of 50 to 100 milliseconds duration is increased gradually in intensity until there is no further decrease in the AP latency or increase in the amplitude. If the stimulus is too large, costimulation of adjacent nerves occurs, which would result in a spread of the waveform from the adjacent nerve or its muscle (Figs. 2 and 3).

Amplitude

The amplitude is measured from the baseline to the height of the AP. The amplitude of the AP is a rough estimate of the number of axons. This is more reliable for the CMAP, which is usually >4000 μv. Because of the wide variation in the sensory action potentials, it is difficult to know if changes in the sensory amplitude are pathologic, but they are usually >10 μv.

Nerve compression and nerve conduction studies

Nerve fibers show varying susceptibility to compression. The large fibers are more vulnerable to compression and ischemia [8]. The neurophysiology of electrical recording is such that the recording electrode detects activity in the largest myelinated fibers first, because these fibers conduct at the fastest rates and have a lower depolarization threshold than the small unmyelinated nerves. Latency and conduction velocity depend on the time that transpires from stimulation of the nerve to the first recording. If only a fraction of the large, thickly myelinated fibers remain and transmit impulses, the recorded latency and conduction velocity remains normal, because the E-1 electrode mostly detects the fastest fibers [9,10]. The electrical conduction in smaller, thinly myelinated or nonmyelinated nerves is much slower and hence usually is not detected in a routine NCS.

In early nerve compression the symptoms are of a vascular nature. The initial changes occur at the blood–nerve barrier. Fluid shifts that occur with limb position result in endoneurial edema. There is no lymphatic drainage of the endoneurial space; hence, endoneurial edema clears slowly. The edema cuts off the blood supply by pinching off the arterioles that course through the perineurium obliquely [11,12]. This impairs the Na^+/K^+ exchange pump, which is ATP dependent. This ultimately results in a reversible metabolic conduction block that leads to paresthesiae [13].

With early compression the symptoms are intermittent and the edema is reversible. When there are constant symptoms there is usually myelin damage or chronic endoneurial edema. This demyelination is responsible for the slowing of nerve conduction. If the compression continues some of the axons die. If there are fewer nerve fibers the size of the electrical charge is smaller,

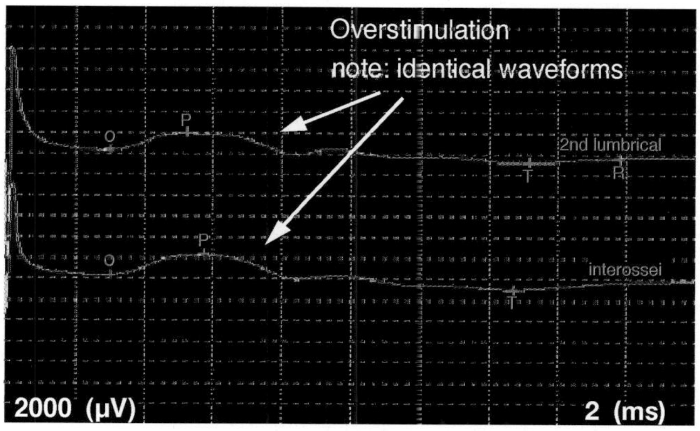

Fig. 2. Lumbrical–interosseous recording in severe CTS. Median nerve overstimulation also depolarizes the ulnar nerve. The 2nd palmar interosseous CMAP replaces the 2nd lumbrical response. The result is identical waveforms. (*From* Slutsky D. Nerve conduction studies in hand surgery. J Am Soc Surg Hand 2003;3:156; with permission.)

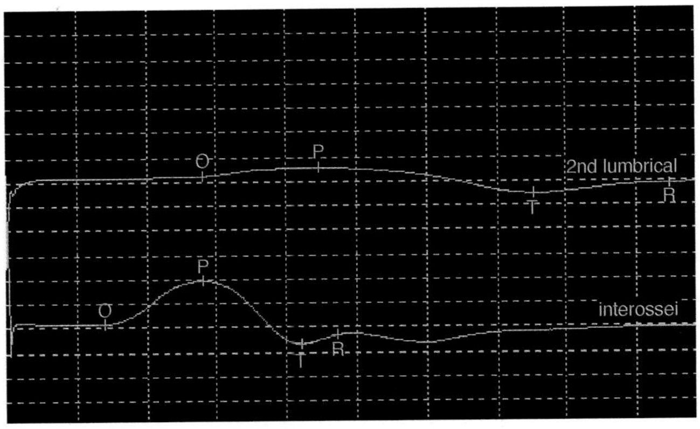

Fig. 3. Lumbrical–interosseous recording in severe CTS. As the median nerve stimulus is decreased, a delayed and low amplitude 2nd lumbrical response is unmasked. Note the difference in the waveform morphology. (*From* Slutsky D. Nerve conduction studies in hand surgery. J Am Soc Surg Hand 2003;3:157; with permission.)

leading to smaller amplitudes. When there is sensory or motor loss, there is usually degeneration of nerve fibers. Despite the restoration of neural blood flow following nerve decompression, remyelination of the axon is often incomplete, which accounts for persistently abnormal nerve conduction even though the patient may be without symptoms [14].

Specific tests

Median nerve motor studies

The recording electrode is placed at the midpoint of the abductor pollicis brevis (APB), and the reference electrode is placed over the APB insertion at the thumb metacarpophalangeal (MP) joint. A ground plate is applied to the dorsum of the hand. The first stimulus (S1) is applied 8 cm proximal to the recording electrode (E-1). Across-elbow conduction is performed by stimulating the median nerve in the antecubital fossa above the elbow (S2). If conduction in the arm is desired, a third stimulus site (S3) is applied in the axilla, 10 to 12 cm proximal to S2. Typical normal values include a DML >4.2 milliseconds, amplitude >4.0 mv, and forearm NCV >48 milliseconds. (Normal values may vary according to the laboratory.)

Median nerve sensory studies

Antidromic studies are popular, because the digital nerves are closer to the skin, which results in larger waveforms than orthodromic studies. Ring electrodes placed 3–4 cm apart are applied to the thumb, index, middle, and ring fingers. The median nerve is stimulated at the wrist, 10 cm proximally for the thumb and 14 cm for the digits.

Comparative latencies have become more prevalent because different sensory nerves can be compared in the same digit under the same conditions of temperature, digit circumference, and skin conductivity. This tends to minimize recording pitfalls. Comparative latencies are taken from radial sensory nerve recordings from the thumb and from the ulnar digital nerve to the ring. Normal values include peak latencies ≤3.5 milliseconds, with <0.5 milliseconds between radial–median and median–ulnar comparative latency differences [15,16]. Because the NCV is calculated over the length of the nerve, focal conduction defects tend to be normalized. Measuring the transcarpal latency directly can aid in the detection of this focal conduction slowing. A direct recording of the conduction across the transverse carpal ligament prevents any slowing in this area from being normalized by the faster conduction of the median nerve proximal to the transverse carpal ligament [17]. The transcarpal conduction reflects the median nerve conduction directly underneath the transcarpal ligament. The median nerve is stimulated 14 cm from the ring electrode and the latency is recorded. The median nerve then is stimulated 7 or 8 cm proximal to the ring electrode and the latencies are subtracted. When a distance of 7 cm is used, a normal latency is ≤1.7 milliseconds. With an 8-cm distance the latency should be ≤2.2 milliseconds.

A median midpalmar orthodromic latency can provide the same information. This is performed by stimulating the median nerve in the second interspace and recording the mixed nerve response at the wrist 8 cm proximally. Normal values are ≤2.2 milliseconds [18]. Segmental stimulation in 1-cm increments across the carpal canal has been reported also [19]. Normal values should be <0.46 milliseconds of slowing per increment.

Ulnar nerve motor studies

Ulnar motor studies are more popular than ulnar sensory studies. The DML is determined by recording from an electrode placed over the midpoint of the abductor digiti minimi (ADM) while stimulating the ulnar nerve 8 cm proximally (S1). Normal values include a DML ≤3.6 milliseconds and amplitude >4.0 mv. Alternatively the latencies can be measured from the first dorsal interosseous (FDI), which then assesses conduction through the deep motor branch of the ulnar nerve. The FDI to ADM latency should not exceed 2.0 milliseconds [20]. The ulnar nerve then is stimulated 4 cm distal to the medial epicondyle (S2). By subtracting the latency for S1 from S2 and measuring the intervening distance, the forearm conduction velocity is obtained. Ulnar nerve conduction across the cubital tunnel is calculated by stimulating the nerve at S3, which is 12 cm proximal to S2, and subtracting the latencies. Most laboratories measure conduction with the elbow flexed between 90° and 135°. Normal forearm NCV is >48 milliseconds. Across the cubital tunnel the NCV should be >45 milliseconds. More than 10 milliseconds of slowing between the above- and below-elbow NCV is abnormal. Amplitude decreases of >20% are a more sensitive indicator of conduction block or axonal loss [21].

Ulnar nerve sensory studies

Ring electrodes are placed on the small finger and the ulnar nerve is stimulated 14 cm proximally. Recordings also are taken from the ring finger after stimulation of the ulnar and median nerves. This allows for comparison of the ulnar to the median SNAPs. Normal peak sensory latencies are ≤3.5 milliseconds and <0.5 milliseconds median–ulnar difference. Mixed palmar orthodromic studies can be elicited by stimulating the ulnar nerve in the fourth webspace and recording over the ulnar nerve at the wrist 8 cm proximally. This measures the sensory nerve conduction through the Guyon canal. Normal values are <2.2 milliseconds [22].

Radial nerve motor studies

E-1 is placed over the extensor indicis proprius (EIP) muscle 4 cm proximal to the ulnar styloid. S1 is applied over the posterior interosseous nerve, 10–12 cm proximal to E-1. S2 is applied over the radial nerve 10 cm proximal to this, above the elbow. S3 is in the axilla. Normal values include a DML of <3.4 milliseconds with amplitudes >4.0 mV. Across-elbow conduction should be >52 milliseconds, and axilla to elbow, >58 milliseconds [23].

Radial nerve sensory studies

Ring electrodes are placed on the thumb and the radial nerve is stimulated 10 cm proximally. Alternatively the recording electrodes can be placed over the extensor pollicis longus. Normal values consist of a peak latency of ≤2.6 milliseconds. The median nerve also is stimulated 10 cm proximal to the ring electrodes. Comparative radial–median latencies should be <0.5 milliseconds [24].

Specialized studies applicable to hand surgery

Standard NCS often fall short in the assessment of many of the nerve disorders seen in a typical hand surgical practice. There are, however, several specific techniques that have special application for hand surgeons [3].

Carpal tunnel syndrome

The standard NCS should include sensory latencies to the thumb, index, and middle fingers, with comparative latencies to the radial sensory and ulnar sensory nerves [18]. The thumb is a more sensitive indicator for carpal tunnel compression, followed by the middle finger and then the index [25]. In mild carpal tunnel syndrome (CTS) the only test abnormality may include a prolongation of the transcarpal latency or an abnormal comparative latency. The incidence of type I errors (false positive) increases with multiple sensitive tests [26]. This had led some investigators to devise a comparative sensory index (CSI) [27]. This consists of the sum of the thumb median–radial difference, the ring median–ulnar difference, and the median–ulnar midpalmar orthodromic difference. A normal value is <1.0 millisecond. The CSI is more sensitive and more specific, because it hinges on three parameters, which diminishes the technical error associated with making the diagnosis on one specific test [28]. The CSI is also temperature independent, because all of the nerves are examined under identical local condition of conductivity, temperature, and digit circumference.

There are some caveats for NCS in CTS. First, sensory abnormalities usually occur before motor abnormalities. In other words, the distal sensory latencies often slow before the DML. This is not surprising, because 94% of the axons in the median nerve at the wrist level are sensory [29]. The sensory nerve axons are larger than the motor axons and hence more susceptible to compression. If the DML is abnormal in the presence of normal SNAPs, extra care must be taken to rule out anterior horn cell disease or a C8 radiculopathy. Isolated recurrent motor branch compression, however, has been reported. Second, the NCS may not return to normal following decompression because of retrograde fiber degeneration or incomplete remyelination, even in the presence of a full clinical recovery.

Large myelinated and small unmyelinated fibers can be affected differently. Connective tissue changes follow with focal nerve fiber changes. The large myelinated nerves undergo segmental demyelination, whereas the small unmyelinated nerves undergo degeneration and regeneration. Normal fascicles are adjacent to abnormal fascicles. The NCS only tests the faster conducting fibers. This explains the seeming paradox of the patient with established CTS with normal EDX studies. It is the worst fascicles that produce symptoms, but it is the best fascicles that account for the normal NCS [10].

Recurrent carpal tunnel syndrome

EDX studies are not a gold standard in recurrent CTS, because they may remain abnormal for many months following surgery. They are most useful when performed by the same examiner pre- and postoperatively. They are used to document the presence or absence of significant changes and to rule out other sites of compression [30]. Traction neuropathy may be the cause of recurrent CTS symptoms rather than compression [31]. In these cases the NCS is normal. Provocative maneuvers to place traction on the nerve while measuring distal median motor latencies may increase the diagnostic yield [32,33]. Inching techniques also may be useful in localizing an area of focal nerve compression [19].

Lumbrical—interosseous latency differences

E-1 is placed over the second palmar interspace at the distal palmar crease. This roughly corresponds to the motor end plates for the second lumbrical (L2) and the second palmar interosseous (P2). By stimulating the median nerve, a lumbrical response is obtained. Ulnar nerve stimulation elicits an interosseous response. The L2–P2 latency difference should not exceed >0.4 milliseconds [34]. This test is especially useful with a coexistent polyneuropathy in which localization at the wrist is otherwise difficult. In severe CTS or CTS with an associated neuropathy, absence of the median DML or sensory latencies is of no localizing value. The lumbrical conduction is preserved compared with the APB; hence, a response may be obtained even when other responses are absent. Prolongation of the latency difference caused by a delayed L2 hence can lead to the diagnosis of an associated median nerve compression. Alternatively if the P2 response is delayed, the latency difference also is prolonged but in a reversed manner. This can lead to the diagnosis of deep ulnar motor nerve compression (see Example 3) [35].

Digital nerve conduction studies

Antidromic and orthodromic techniques have been described [36–38]. Measuring individual digital nerve APs can aid in the diagnosis of isolated digital nerve injuries. Errors caused by volume conduction from an intact digital nerve on the opposite side must be watched for [39]. Occasionally it is necessary to perform a digital nerve block of the unaffected side to prevent contamination of the response in the nerve under consideration. This technique is useful for monitoring the recovery of a digital nerve repair proximal to the proximal interphalangeal joint. With more distal repairs, conduction still can be measured. As the distance between E-1 and E-2 becomes smaller, however, the amplitude of the response diminishes accordingly. This makes it difficult to observe the digital SNAP above the baseline electrical noise. In the author's experience of 24 patients who underwent digital nerve repairs, the author found the presence of a digital nerve AP to be a good predictor of clinical recovery.

Example 1: digital nerve injury [1]

A 56-year-old man presented with a knife laceration to his right hand (Fig. 4*A*). He had no flexor tendon function to his index and middle fingers. He had no active abduction of the FDI, but a CMAP was recordable with ulnar nerve stimulation. He had normal two-point discrimination to the radial side of the index, but >25 mm for the ulnar side. Digital nerve conduction revealed a normal radial digital SNAP but an absent ulnar digital SNAP (Figs. 4*B* and 5). At time of surgery, the common digital nerve to the second webspace was noted to have a partial laceration, accounting for the physical findings (Fig. 4*C,D*).

Proximal ulnar nerve compression

The ulnar nerve is comprised of one large fascicle and two to three small fascicles at the elbow. The fascicles within a nerve are not affected uniformly by compression. Those on the periphery of the nerve sustain greater injury than centrally placed fascicles [40]. The usual sites of compression in cubital tunnel syndrome are superficial to the nerve (Osborne bands, arcuate ligament, arcade of Struthers). The internal topography of the ulnar nerve at the elbow explains the relative sparing of the flexor carpi ulnaris and flexor digitorum profundus, because their motor fibers lay deep within the nerve [41]. The intrinsics often are uninvolved until the late stages of compression for similar reasons, whereas the superficially located sensory fibers are more susceptible to early compression.

Conduction velocities can be misleading if the surface measurement of the nerve is off, even by 1 cm. Testing inaccuracies also occur following ulnar nerve transposition, because the nerve no longer follows its anatomic course [42]. With longer conduction distances an area of focal block may be missed, because it tends to be averaged out. Segmental stimulation of the ulnar nerve skirts these pitfalls and is a sensitive method for determining focal conduction abnormalities. Measurement errors are minimized, because the nerve is localized at each stimulation site. If the nerve is stimulated in 1-cm segments, a >0.40 millisecond jump in NCV indicates a focal abnormality. If the nerve is stimulated in 1-inch increments, a >0.75 millisecond jump is abnormal [43]. There is a poor correlation between the area of focal conduction block and the site of entrapment at time of surgery. This is likely, given that if there is a partial conduction block it is necessary to turn up the gain on the stimulation to obtain a response. With increasing current, the current flow tends to arc ahead of the stimulation, resulting in depolarization ahead of the applied stimulus site (Table 2) [44].

Across-elbow sensory nerve studies also have been described [45]. The above and below-elbow stimulation sites are the same as S2 and S3 for the motor studies, but in this case the SNAPs are recorded from ring electrodes placed on the small finger. Normal NCV values are >50 milliseconds. Combining ulnar motor and sensory techniques adds useful information in complex cases in which clinical examination fails to localize the lesion. Conduction to the dorsal

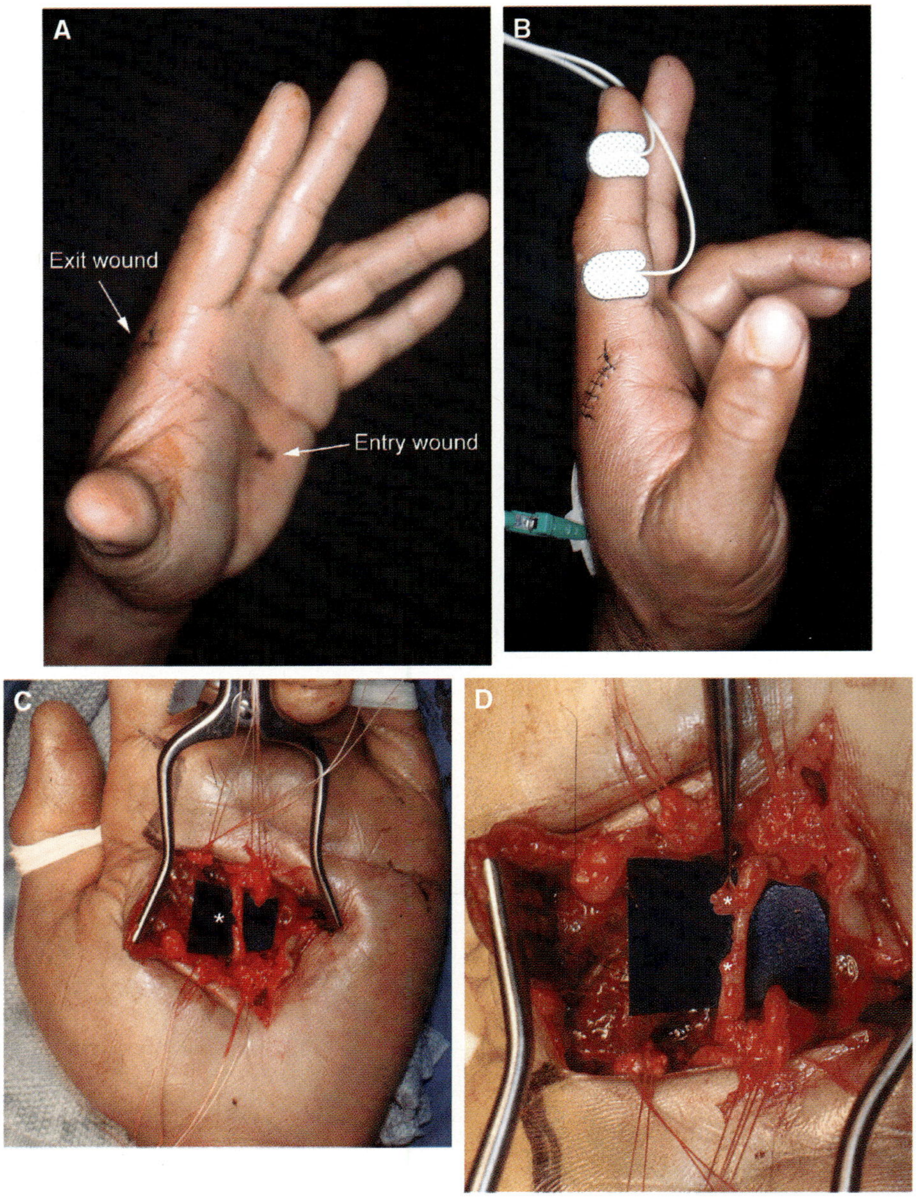

Fig. 4. Partial common digital nerve laceration. (*A*) Knife laceration to left hand. Note the entrance wound in mid-palm and exit wound over first webspace. (*B*) Radial digital nerve recording. (*C*) Common digital nerve to the 2nd webspace. Note the partial laceration (*asterisk*). (*D*) Close-up of the proximal and distal ends of the partial common digital nerve laceration (*asterisk*). (*From* Slutsky D. Nerve conduction studies in hand surgery. J Am Soc Surg Hand 2003;3:161; with permission.)

cutaneous branch of the ulnar nerve can be measured [46]. This test is insensitive for detecting proximal ulnar nerve compression, because it is abnormal in only 55% of patients who have cubital tunnel syndrome [47]. As in carpal tunnel syndrome, the patient's clinical findings and response to conservative measures should be a major determinant in the surgical decision making. Patients who have paresthesiae only, with no motor or sensory abnormalities (McGowan stage I), still can benefit from an in situ release of the ulnar nerve, even if the NCS are normal [48].

Example 2: proximal ulnar neuropathy

A 47-year-old male grocery clerk presented with a past history of bilateral submuscular ulnar nerve transpositions 2 years previously [1]. He complained of a 1-year history of recurrent tingling of the small and ring fingers bilaterally, exacerbated by use of a bottom scanner at work.

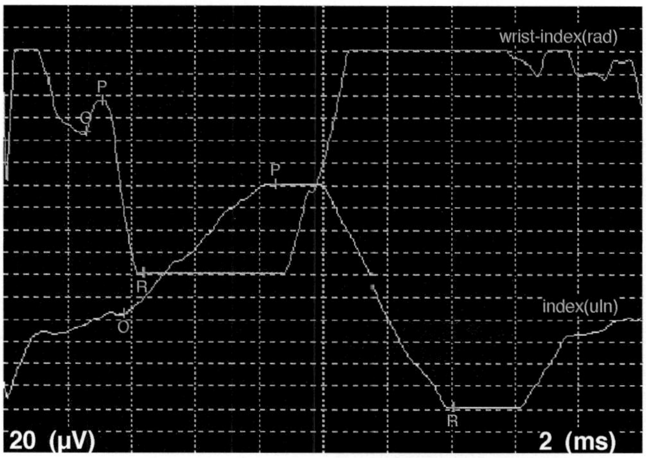

Fig. 5. Index digital nerve recording. (*Upper trace*) Normal appearing radial digital SNAP: peak 3.1 milliseconds, amplitude 155 μV. (*Lower trace*) Absent ulnar digital SNAP. (*From* Slutsky D. Nerve conduction studies in hand surgery. J Am Soc Surg Hand 2003;3:162; with permission.)

He had a normal ulnar motor and sensory examination. He had a positive Tinel sign over the ulnar nerves bilaterally. His elbow flexion test was equivocal. The referring neurologist's report indicated that the NCS were normal, yet there was a >40% decrease in amplitude across the cubital tunnel bilaterally. Incremental stimulation of the ulnar nerves across the elbow localized the exact course of the nerve, reducing any measurement errors. There was no focal conduction slowing (ie, <0.40 milliseconds) or any significant amplitude decreases on either side (Table 2).

Across-elbow sensory conduction velocities were normal bilaterally. Lumbrical interosseous latency testing and NCV differences from the ADM to the FDI were also normal. Based on this testing, continued conservative treatment with activity modification was recommended, rather than repeat surgery.

Distal ulnar nerve compression

The usual NCS are inadequate at assessing ulnar nerve entrapment in the palm. The standard teaching divides the Guyon canal into three zones. In zone I, nerve compression leads to mixed motor and sensory symptoms. In zone II, symptoms are purely sensory, and in zone III, symptoms are purely motor and restricted to muscles innervated by the deep ulnar motor branch [49]. Two sites of entrapment distal to the ADM also have been described [50]. Short segment incremental studies (SSIS) are a sensitive and specific way to assess the deep motor branch, because focal conduction abnormalities also tend to be normalized over the distance between the ADM and the FDI [51]. The ulnar nerve is stimulated in 1-cm increments from

Table 2
Incremental ulnar nerve stimulation at the elbow

	Onset (ms)	Amplitude (mv)	Δ - O (ms)
Site (right/left)			
−2 cm	7.03/7.11	5.75/7.50	—
−1 cm	7.19/7.27	5.79/7.39	0.16/0.16
Epicondyle	7.42/7.58	5.43/7.28	0.23/0.31
+1 cm	**7.81**/7.66	5.58/7.31	0.39/0.08
+2 cm	**7.81/7.81**	5.66/7.33	**0.00**/0.16
+3 cm	7.89/**7.81**	5.56/7.32	0.08/**0.00**
+4 cm	8.20/8.13	5.38/7.25	0.31/0.31

The identical latencies difference between 1–2 cm proximal to the epicondyle on the right and 2–3 cm on the left (in bold) most likely represent arcing of the current with depolarization proximal to the actual site of stimulation.

Δ - O = difference in onset.

Used with permission from Slutsky DJ. Nerve conduction studies in hand surgery. J Am Soc Surg Hand 2003;3(3):162.

3–4 cm proximal and distal to the wrist crease. Abnormal values include a >0.5 millisecond jump or a >120% decrease in amplitude. When this is combined with FDI conduction and interosseous-latency differences the diagnostic yield increases.

Example 3: distal ulnar neuropathy

A 31-year-old male emergency department resident presented with a 4-month history of right hand weakness but no sensory symptoms [1]. He had a remote past history of plate fixation of a fifth metacarpal base fracture. His clinical examination demonstrated clawing of his small and ring fingers and 5+ power of the ADM but weak to absent intrinsic muscle power distal to this (Fig. 6*A*). He had normal two-point discrimination. An ultrasound demonstrated no ulnar artery aneurysm, screw protrusion, or tumors in the Guyon canal. Standard NCS testing

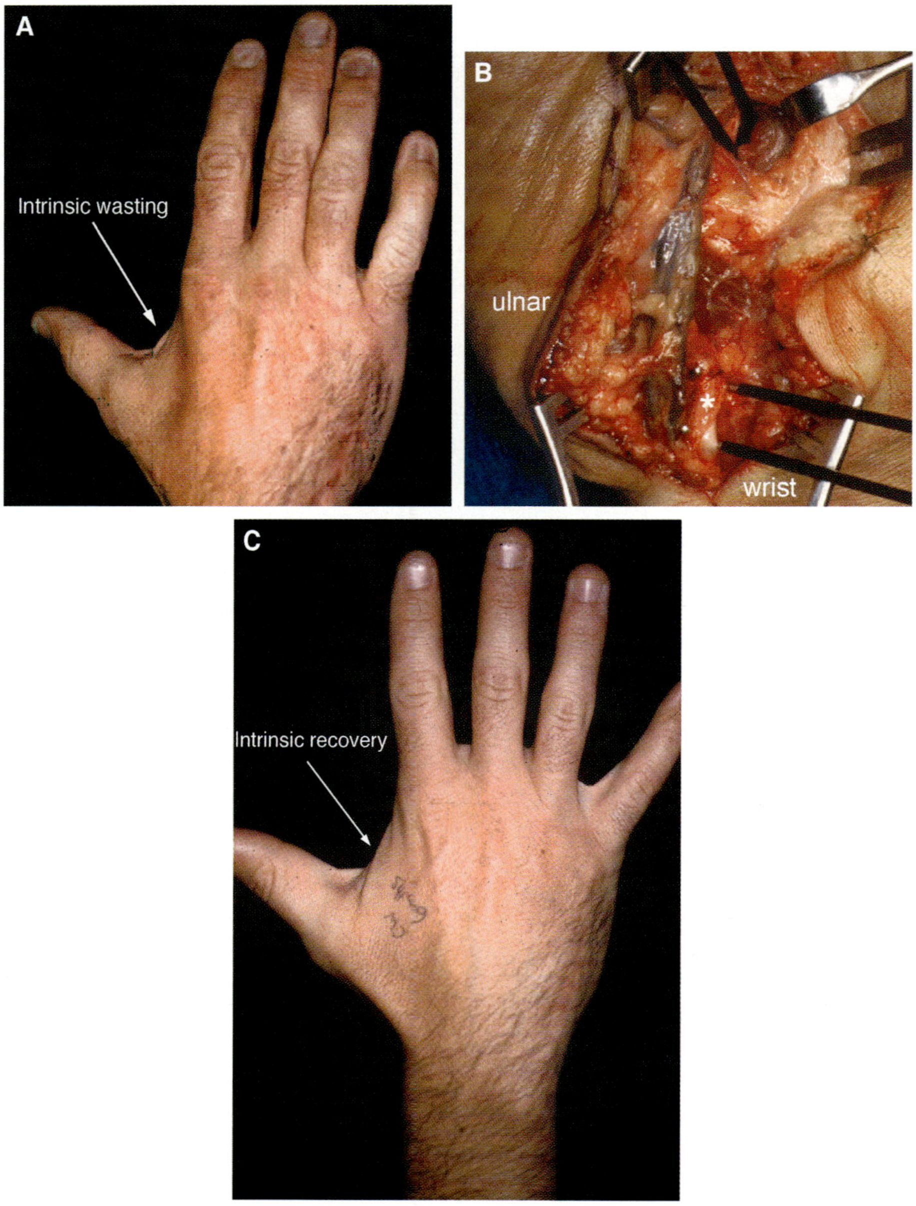

Fig. 6. (*A*) Distal ulnar neuropathy. Preoperative photograph of attempted index finger abduction. Note the marked wasting of the 1st, 2nd, and 3rd dorsal interossei, but the normal bulk of the abductor digiti minimi. (*B*) Intraoperative nerve conduction of the deep motor branch of the ulnar nerve (*asterisk*). (*C*) Six months after operation. Note the normal bulk of the dorsal interossei and the active index finger abduction. (*From* Slutsky D. Nerve conduction studies in hand surgery. J Am Soc Surg Hand 2003;3:163; with permission.)

showed normal latencies with a <2.0 milliseconds difference between the ADM and FDI but a markedly reduced FDI amplitude (Table 3). Lumbrical–interosseous latency testing showed a marked delay in P2 with a decrease in amplitude (Table 4, Figs. 7 and 8). SSIS revealed a conduction block 4 cm distal to the wrist (Table 5, Figs. 9 and 10). Intraoperative nerve conduction testing following decompression of the deep motor branch revealed a small nerve AP and a definite CMAP response of the FDI (see Fig. 6*B*). At 6 months the patient had normal clinical function (see Fig. 6*C*), but the NCS were still mildly abnormal.

Radial tunnel syndrome

Classically the NCS is normal in radial tunnel syndrome. Some investigators have postulated that this syndrome reflects a dynamic entrapment of the posterior interosseous nerve. Differential latency testing is based on this premise [52]. Across-elbow radial motor nerve conduction is performed with the elbow extended and the forearm in neutral, pronation, and supination for 30 seconds. The testing then is repeated. An abnormal latency difference of >0.30 milliseconds indicates radial tunnel entrapment.

Example 4: radial tunnel syndrome

A 50-year-old woman presented with a 3-year history of right proximal forearm pain [1]. A lateral epicondylectomy 1 year previously failed to relieve her symptoms. She was tender over the distal border of the supinator and the lateral epicondyle. She had a positive middle finger extension test and pain with wrist flexion, pronation, and ulnar deviation. A local anesthetic block of the posterior interosseous nerve on two separate occasions relieved her pain completely. Standard NCS revealed normal radial motor conduction velocities. EMG testing of radial innervated muscles was normal. The results of differential latency testing revealed an abnormal latency difference in the first trial (Table 6). Based on the clinical examination and this testing, a radial tunnel decompression was recommended.

Nerve conduction study pitfalls

There are several factors that affect the NCS. Certain potential pitfalls must be looked for, such as volume conduction. Placing an electrode on the skin over a specific muscle does not ensure that the only response detected arises from the desired tissue [53]. If the nerve in question has a partial or complete block, it is usual to turn up the gain (current). At some point an adjacent nerve is stimulated that can lead to a false waveform (see traces 1 and 2). Often the only clue is the morphology of the waveform plus a high index of suspicion. Error also may arise when the onset marker is positioned erroneously, as often occurs with the double peaked ulnar CMAP. This leads to falsely prolonged distal motor latencies and lower amplitudes. The newer digital machines set the markers automatically, so it is good practice to review the waveforms quickly before looking at the data.

Falsely low amplitudes may result from temporal dispersion [7]. Any given nerve is composed of faster and slower conducting axons. The nerve AP is the summation of thousands of individual fibers. When there is a longer distance between the site of nerve stimulation and the

Table 3
Distal ulnar neuropathy

	Latency (ms)	Amplitude (μv)
ADM	2.86	5000
FDI	3.42	240[a]
$SNAP_L$	3.30	30.8

[a] Note the low amplitude of the FDI motor potential.

FDI, first dorsal interosseous; ADM, abductor digiti minimi; $SNAP_L$, sensory nerve action potential, little finger.

From Slutsky DJ. Nerve conduction studies in hand surgery. J Am Soc Sur Hand 2003;3(3):163; with permission.

Table 4
Lumbrical–Interosseous latency testing, distal ulnar neuropathy

	Right		Left	
	Latency (ms)	Amplitude (MV)	Latency (ms)	Amplitude (MV)
Second lumbrical	2.78	3.10	3.03	3.57
Second palmar interosseous	5.38[a]	2.57[a]	2.84	6.10

[a] Note the delayed latency and loss of amplitude of the second lumbrical response on the right as compared with the normal left hand.

Used with permission from Slutsky DJ. Nerve conduction studies in hand surgery. J Am Soc Surg Hand 2003;3(3):152–69.

recording electrodes, such as with above-elbow stimulation, there is less synchronous arrival of APs because of a marked variation in conduction velocities between the individual nerve fibers. Less in-phase summation of similar waveform aspects leads to phase cancellation and amplitude reduction. This leads to a wave with a longer duration. This occurs more with sensory than with motor nerves because of their faster conduction velocity, and this can lead to falsely low amplitudes that may be interpreted as axonal loss. This can be suspected by calculating the area under the waveform, which is normal in temporal dispersion and reduced with axonal loss.

Temperature can affect the values considerably; hence, it is important to measure the hand temperature during testing. The conduction velocity changes 5% for each 1 °C change [54]. The distal latencies may increase and conduction velocities may decrease when the hand is cool [55]. In general the hand should be at least 30 °C. The need for rewarming also should be indicated on the report.

Essential components of the electrodiagnostic report

One study of 100 reports revealed widespread inadequacies [56]. To be able to interpret the test results adequately, several parameters must be included in the report. These include the distances between the recording electrodes and the stimulation sites (because reference values are based on standardized distances), the amplitude of the waveform, conduction velocities, limb temperature, and normal reference values.

Electromyography

EMG involves the insertion of a needle electrode into muscle tissue with the intent of recording normal and abnormal spontaneous activity and voluntary motor unit APs. Some investigators consider this to be the most sensitive means for demonstrating axonal loss [53]. The EMG differs from the NCS in that it incorporates the amplified sounds of the electrical activity of muscle to aid the examination. A knowledge of muscle anatomy and physiology is requisite to understanding the methodology behind the examination.

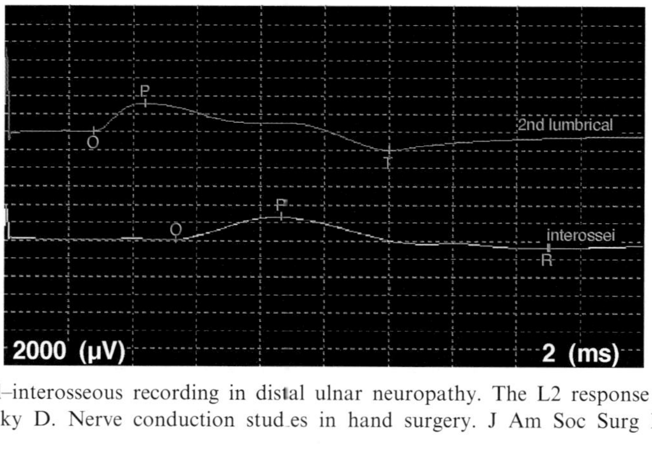

Fig. 7. Right lumbrical–interosseous recording in distal ulnar neuropathy. The L2 response is delayed and of low amplitude. (*From* Slutsky D. Nerve conduction studies in hand surgery. J Am Soc Surg Hand 2003;3:165; with permission.)

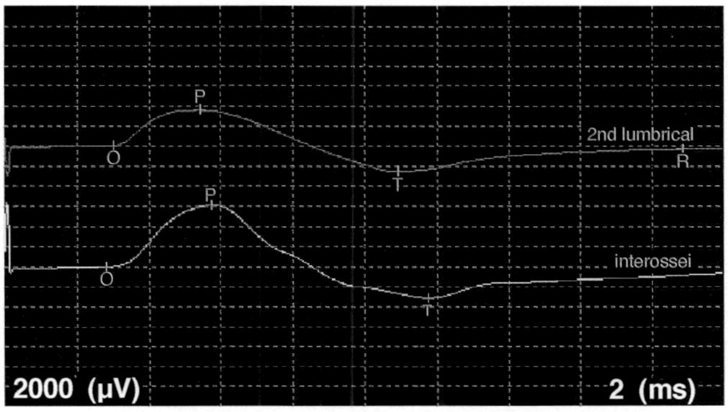

Fig. 8. Left lumbrical–interosseous recording, normal hand. Comparison study of the left hand. Note the normal onset and amplitude of the P2 response. (*From* Slutsky D. Nerve conduction studies in hand surgery. J Am Soc Surg Hand 2003;3:166; with permission.)

Muscle fiber anatomy

Any given muscle is composed of thousands of individual fibers or sarcomeres. A single sarcomere is a multinucleated cell surrounded by a 50-nm thick basement membrane, the sarcolemma. This membrane is similar to the nerve cell membrane in that it also consists of a lipid bilayer with hydrophobic tails forming the interior and hydrophilic heads facing outward. Transmembrane ions embedded in this bilayer serve as voltage gated channels for the passage of sodium (Na^+) and potassium (K^+) ions. The sarcolemma differs from the axonal membrane by forming an intricate intramuscular system of transverse extensions (T-tubules) that allow extracellular fluid to extend across the muscle interior.

The sarcomere contains myofibrils composed of actin and myosin filaments. The myofibrils are contractile elements that slide past one another on exposure to calcium (Ca^{+2}) ions. This energy-dependent process requires ATP, which explains the paralysis that accompanies muscle ischemia. The myofibrils are bathed in an ion rich intracellular fluid (sarcoplasm). They are surrounded by a series of longitudinal channels (sarcoplasmic reticulum) that end in a large terminal cisterna. The T-tubules, although not connected directly, are sandwiched between the cisterna at each end of the sarcomere.

Muscle electrophysiology

The sarcolemma is a semipermeable membrane that restricts the passage of Na^+ but not K^+ or chloride ions (Cl^-). The relative concentrations of these ions results in a resting membrane potential of −90 mv, similar to the nerve axon. An AP that arrives at the terminal axon is transmitted chemically across the neuromuscular junction through the release of acetylcholine (ACh). If the voltage decrease exceeds the sarcolemma threshold (15 mV), the membrane is depolarized, initiating a propagating muscle AP. The inward flow of Na^+ spreads longitudinally

Table 5
Short segment incremental studies

Distance (cm)	Latency (ms)	Amplitude (MV)
−1	5.78	2.60
Wrist crease	7.89	1.80
1	5.31	2.21
2	5.31	2.03
3	3.05	1.51
4	NR	NR

The right deep ulnar motor branch response is universally delayed in onset (left side ≤3.2 ms) and of low amplitude (left side ≥6.5 mv).

NR, no response.

Used with permission from Slutsky DJ. Nerve conduction studies in hand surgery. J Am Soc Surg Hand 2003;3(3): 166.

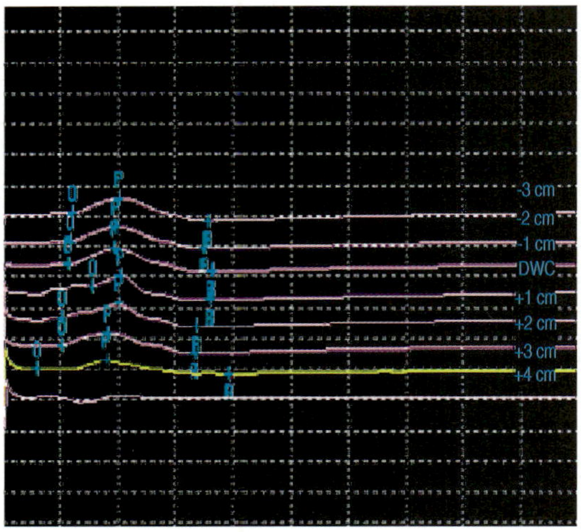

Fig. 9. Short-segment incremental studies in distal ulnar neuropathy. Note the gradual loss of amplitude of the waveform. (*From* Slutsky D. Nerve conduction studies in hand surgery. J Am Soc Surg Hand 2003;3:167; with permission.)

down the muscle fiber, sequentially depolarizing each segment of the muscle membrane, similar to unmyelinated nerve. Because of the increased surface area of the T-tubules, however, it takes much longer to depolarize the sarcolemma than it does a comparably sized unmyelinated nerve. Conduction velocities are in the range of 3 to 5 milliseconds versus 25–30 milliseconds, and the AP duration is five times as long.

As the AP spreads down the T-tubule system, Ca^{+2} is released from the sarcoplasmic reticulum of the terminal cisterna. The Ca^{+2} floods the myofibrils, resulting in a contraction lasting approximately 1/30 of a second. An energy-dependent pump rapidly sequesters the Ca^{+2} back into the sarcoplasmic reticulum, ending the contraction. If the pump fails, the contraction is maintained indefinitely (rigor mortis).

Motor unit anatomy

The motor unit is composed of the anterior horn cell, its peripheral nerve, and multiple terminal axons, each innervating many individual muscle fibers. A skeletal muscle fascicle consists of 20–60 fibers surrounded by a connective tissue sheath. A single muscle fiber is innervated by only one motor unit, but there may be 2–3 motor units within a fascicle [57]. The

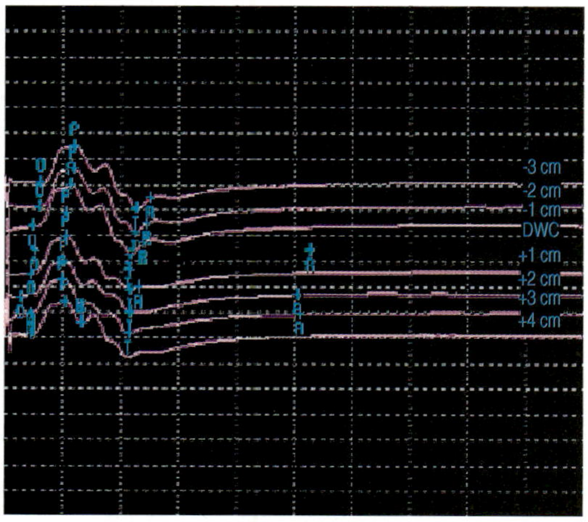

Fig. 10. Short-segment incremental studies, normal hand. Comparison study. Note the faster onset and preservation of amplitude. (*From* Slutsky D. Nerve conduction studies in hand surgery. J Am Soc Surg Hand 2003;3:167; with permission.)

Table 6
Differential latency testing of the radial nerve

	Trial 1 (ms)	Trial 2 (ms)	Trial 3(ms)
AE NCV in neutral	5.16	4.77	4.53
AE NCV in pronation	4.92	4.61	4.61
AE NCV in supination	4.69	4.61	4.50
Δ	**0.55**	0.16	0.08

Note the abnormal latency difference between the AE NCV in neutral versus supination.

AE, above elbow; NCV, nerve conduction velocity; Δ, difference in latency.

Used with permission from Slutsky DJ. Nerve conduction studies in hand surgery. J. Am Soc Surg Hand 2003;3(3): 168.

muscle fibers of one motor unit may be distributed over 100 fascicles. They are not contiguous, but are distributed randomly over a 4–6-mm circumference, extending 30 mm longitudinally along the muscle itself [58]. When the anterior horn cell fires, all of these muscle fibers depolarize. Their electrical activity summates to produce a motor unit action potential (MUAP). Up to 10 motor units may share the same oval territory. As will be seen, this has implications with respect to the recording of denervation potentials (see section on MUAP pathology).

Neuromuscular junction transmission

The axon becomes smaller and loses its myelin sheath as it approaches the muscle endplate. This results in a slowing of the nerve conduction velocities from 50 milliseconds to 10–20 milliseconds [59]. Depolarization of the terminal axon opens voltage-sensitive Ca^{+2} gates, which results in release of ACh. The ACh diffuses across the synaptic cleft, which takes approximately 1.0 millisecond. ACh binding to receptors on the muscle membrane results in Na^{+} channel activation and subsequent muscle depolarization, which adds an additional 0.1 milliseconds. The end result is an additional 1.1 millisecond delay in the generation of the CMAP [53]. Because of this the conduction velocity for the distal segment of a motor nerve should not be calculated because it would include the time for the chemical transmission of ACh across the neuromuscular junction. Because of the AP slowing across the muscle endplate, the measured motor NCV is much slower than sensory NCV. The conduction velocity for the distal segment of a sensory nerve can be calculated, because the nerve APs are recorded directly from the nerve.

Muscle conduction

Muscle fibers conduct APs similar to unmyelinated nerves. They do not possess myelin and must rely on sequential discharge of each muscle segment to depolarize adjacent regions. Muscle fibers also have a larger surface area than the nerve axolemma because of the increased surface area of the T-tubules. A muscle fiber of comparable size to an unmyelinated nerve thus has a slower conduction velocity (3–5 milliseconds) and the AP duration is five times as long. This affects the waveform during EMG if muscle to muscle conduction has replaced nerve to muscle conduction of the electrical impulse. In NCS, a volume conducted muscle response from costimulation of an adjacent nerve can be picked up by the recording electrode and appear as a delayed waveform, which may be misinterpreted as a prolongation of the nerve latency.

Instrumentation

The EMG equipment includes various recording, reference and grounding electrodes, a cathode ray tube (or laptop computer), and audio speakers. Typically E-1 consists of a needle recording electrode (monopolar or concentric) that is inserted directly into the muscle tissue, although a surface electrode may be used (surface EMG). The needle shaft is insulated with Teflon. The exposed needle tip (17 mm^2) records the electrical activity within a 1.0–2.5-mm radius. It is therefore crucial to position the needle tip close to the muscle fibers to be examined to avoid recording artificially abnormal MUAP (see section on pitfalls). Needle placement is guided by the MUAP morphology and the sound. As the needle tip moves closer to the contracting muscle fiber, the sound of the MUAP changes from dull and muffled to crisp and loud. The amplitude, duration, and morphology of the recorded MUAP are influenced by the type of electrode, which should be specified in the EMG report.

A concentric (coaxial) needle electrode consists of a steel cannula, which serves as the reference electrode, and a central 0.1-mm platinum or silver wire. Bipolar concentric needles have two central wires. A monopolar electrode consists of a solid, Teflon-coated, 25-gauge steel needle. A separate surface electrode is required. When recording with monopolar electrodes the MUAPs have larger amplitudes and more turns and phases, but similar durations as compared with concentric needles. The type of electrode should remain constant throughout the testing for these reasons.

Motor unit action potential morphology

During minimal voluntary contraction of a muscle, a correctly placed needle electrode can record the spatial summation of the electrical activity of single muscle fibers innervated by one anterior horn cell (ie, the MUAP). A depolarization wave that propagates (ie, is moving toward the electrode) initially produces a positive deflection. As it passes under E-1 a negative deflection occurs. As the wave continues past E-1 a positive deflection is produced. A propagating wave thus appears as an initially positive, triphasic waveform. A depolarization that is directly under the electrode and does not propagate results in a monophasic negative waveform. An AP traveling toward and past the recording electrode produces a bi- or triphasic potential (Fig. 11).

MUAP are large (300–3000 μV), with three to four phases and a duration of $\leq$12 milliseconds. The summated voltage from all of the single muscle fibers often leads to small serrations (turns) or multiple baseline crossings (phases) in the observed waveform. MUAP with >5 phases are termed polyphasic potentials (Fig. 12). Up to 30% of polyphasic MUAP (recorded with a monopolar electrode) may be normal [60]. The MUAP duration increases with an increase in the number of phases and turns, because it is a function of the synchrony of firing of the individual muscle fibers. The amplitude declines exponentially from the source. There is more than a 50% reduction in the amplitude at 200 μm. It is believed that the MUAP amplitude may arise from only 20 fibers within a 1.0-mm radius of the electrode tip [9]. Fibers that are further away contribute less and may be out of phase [61]. Denervation potentials found in only one region of the muscle therefore may have questionable significance (see section on fibrillation potentials).

Motor unit action potential pathology

A disorder that affects any component of the motor unit (ie, the anterior horn cell, its peripheral nerve, or the muscle fiber) alters the MUAP morphology. Denervation of a muscle

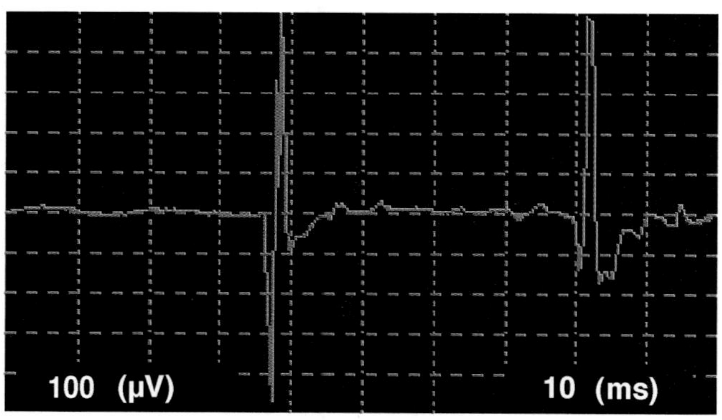

Fig. 11. Normal MUAPs. Each grid moving from left to right represents 10 milliseconds. Each grid from top to bottom represents 100 μV. The first MUAP has a duration of approximately 5 milliseconds and an amplitude of 900 μV. (*From* Slutsky D. Electromyography in hand surgery. J Am Soc Surg Hand 2004;4(3):178; with permission.)

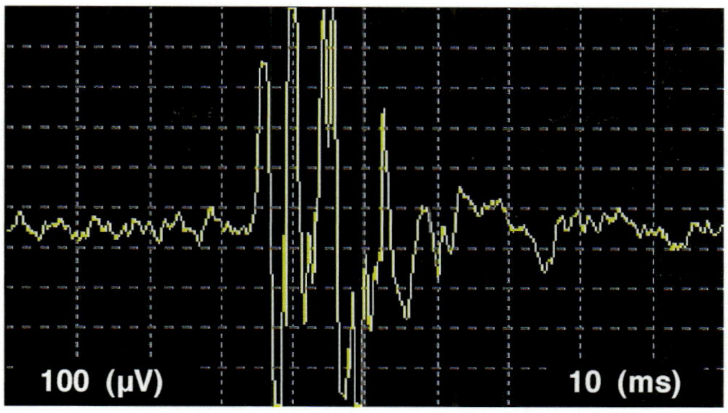

Fig. 12. Polyphasic MUAP. (*From* Slutsky D. Electromyography in hand surgery. J Am Soc Surg Hand 2004;4(3):185; with permission.)

fiber induces axon sprouting from adjacent nerve terminals or distal nodes of Ranvier. The axon sprout reinnervates the orphaned muscle fiber, which now comes under the control of a different motor unit. Axon sprouting following nerve injury has been demonstrated as early as 4 days [62]. In animal studies a single motor unit is capable of increasing the number of fibers it supplies by as much as five times [63]. The new axon sprouts initially are poorly myelinated and slower conducting, which results in a longer duration MUAP. There is also an increased spatial separation of the newly added endplates, which prevents all of the muscle fibers from depolarizing at the same time. This asynchronous summation of the AP results in more phases, which increases the MUAP duration. The addition of orphaned muscle fibers combined with atrophy of the intervening denervated fibers leads to an increase in the MUAP amplitude. Reinnervation caused by axon sprouting results in an MUAP that is larger in amplitude (more fibers), longer in duration (slower conduction), and polyphasic (asynchronous summation).

As reinnervation progresses over time the axonal sprouts become myelinated. They conduct faster and depolarize synchronously. The large MUAP become less polyphasic. Clinically, muscle strength returns but fine motor control does not. Following reinnervation, there is a net loss of motor units even though some muscle fibers have been recaptured. In general, highly dexterous muscles, such as the first lumbrical, have more neurons dedicated to the control of the available muscle fibers (108 muscle fibers/motor unit) as compared with large, less dexterous muscles, such as the gastrocnemius (1934 fibers/motor unit) [64].

Normal electrical potentials in muscle

Spontaneous activity

In a normal muscle at rest, the isoelectric line should be silent except when the electrode is close to a neuromuscular junction. There are two types of spontaneous potentials that can be recorded from the endplate. When the tip of the needle rests near a muscle endplate, mechanical irritation of the nerve terminals provokes miniature endplate potentials (MEPPs). These are nonpropagating, irregular, mono- or biphasic negative waveforms of 10–50 μV that last 1–3 milliseconds. They sound like a dull roar (distant ocean waves). Endplate potentials (EPP) are believed to be caused by needle tip impalement of the endplate. They also originate from the neuromuscular junction but are larger than MEPP (Fig. 13). They are initially negative, irregular/continuous, biphasic potentials of 100–300 μV, lasting 2 to 4 milliseconds. They have a high pitched *rat-a-tat-tat* similar to a fibrillation.

Endplate spikes (EPS) are short (3–5 milliseconds), irregularly firing, biphasic, initially positive waves of 100–200 μV that are believed to be subthreshold endplate APs from a single muscle fiber. They may be confused with positive sharp waves (which are regular and have an initial positive deflection). They also may be triphasic, initially positive waves and may be mistaken for fibrillation potentials [65]. They most likely occur when the needle tip touches one of the small terminal branches of an intramuscular nerve near the neuromuscular junction, which

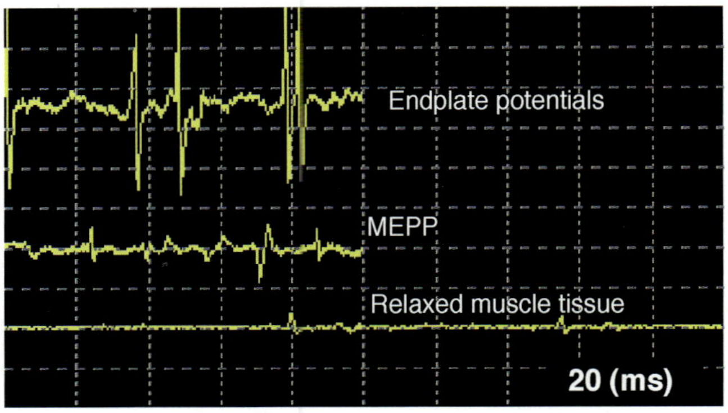

Fig. 13. Spontaneous potentials. MEPP, mini-endplate potential. (*From* Slutsky D. Electromyography in hand surgery. J Am Soc Surg Hand 2004;4(3):179; with permission.)

then leads to the subsequent contraction of a muscle fiber. Because the needle usually is recording from the muscle fiber and not the neuromuscular junction, the waveform is initially positive.

MUAP are distinguished from spontaneous potentials in that they are more regular and have slower rates. The MUAP disappears when the needle is moved slightly or the antagonist muscle is contracted. EPP and EPS do not disappear, but their rate may slow if the needle is not moved. In a suspected denervated muscle when the electromyographer is unable to record muscle activity or a compound motor nerve action, spontaneous endplate activity would indicate that some axons are intact. In other words, MEPP, EPP, and EPS are not detected following denervation. If a patient is feigning paralysis and MEPP or EPP are detected, the patient is malingering.

Abnormal spontaneous potentials in muscle

Fibrillation potentials

Denervation results in muscle membrane instability, which may lead to spontaneous depolarization. The instability of the muscle fiber membrane is theorized to result from oscillations of the membrane potential, which becomes less negative until threshold is reached. Once threshold is reached, a propagating AP is induced, which is referred to as a fibrillation potential [66]. These are spontaneous depolarizations of a single muscle fiber. This process regularly repeats on a time interval that depends on the depolarization to threshold turnaround time [67]. They also may be precipitated by needle movement when introduced into denervated or myopathic muscle. The regularly occurring fibrillation potentials fire in a cyclic pattern with periods of quiescence. Fibrillations may be seen after direct muscle injury. This can make it difficult to localize a coexisting nerve lesion, such as a radial nerve palsy after a humeral fracture [68].

Fibrillation potentials are regular, biphasic (occasionally triphasic) waveforms with a positive wave and negative phase. They have a duration of 1–5 milliseconds and an amplitude ranging from 20–1000 μV [69]. Fibrillation potentials also may fire irregularly up to 50% of the time. They fire at rates of 1–50 times per second (cycles/second = hertz [Hz]) and have a high-pitched, manual typewriter sound. They usually are associated with axonal denervation, but they also may occur in upper motor neuron lesions and myopathies. Fibrillations decrease as muscle tissue becomes fibrotic, wherein all electrical activity stops. Clinically it is not possible to determine the extent of damage solely based on the number of fibrillations. Fibrillation potentials can be differentiated from EPP in that they are usually regular and the rate of firing (1–30 Hz) is usually slower than EPP or EPS (2–100 Hz).

Fibrillation potentials and positive sharp waves are graded on a 1–4 scale (see Table 2) [28]. This is an ordinal (density) scale rather than a ratio scale. In other words, 4+ fibrillations are not twice as bad as 2+ fibrillations [29]. The presence of 4+ fibrillation potentials does not by itself indicate that the entire muscle is denervated, but rather only a specific region of the muscle surrounding the needle electrode. One must look for MUAP and examine multiple areas of the muscle before concluding that it is completely denervated. In addition, comparison of fibrillation numbers from one examination to another is not reliable [70]. Axon loss is better evaluated by a loss of recruitment and a decrease in the distal CMAP.

Positive sharp waves

This potential consists of a primary initial positive monophasic wave although there may be a small negative phase (biphasic). They have a duration of 2–100 milliseconds with amplitudes of 100–1000 μV and a regular firing rate of 1–50 Hz [71]. The origin of positive sharp waves (PSW) and their relationship to fibrillation potentials has not been identified clearly. PSWs are believed to have the same significance as fibrillation potentials but often appear a few days earlier. They may be seen in distal muscles of normal subjects and have no clinical significance. They also may occur after local muscle trauma [69].

Muscle relaxation or contraction abolishes MUAP but does not have any effect on the spontaneous potentials. The time necessary for membrane instability is length dependent. The greater the distance between the lesion and the muscle, the longer it takes. Nerve lacerations close to the endplate region may require only a few days for the onset of fibrillations/PSWs versus cervical lesions that may take weeks. This is the rationale behind waiting 10 days or more following injury to distinguish between neurapraxia versus axonotmesis/neurotmesis. Other abnormal spontaneous potentials that may be seen include complex repetitive discharges, myokymic potential, myotonic discharges, and fasciculation potentials (see Table 1).

The electromyography examination

The EMG examination has three parts: (1) observing the muscle at rest, (2) insertional activity, and (3) analyzing the morphology and the recruitment of motor units at minimal to moderate voluntary muscle contraction.

Muscle at rest

The examination starts with an observation of the muscle at rest, looking for any spontaneous electrical activity not under voluntary control. Healthy muscle is electrically silent.

Insertional activity

A needle is advanced sequentially into the muscle to three successive depths. The needle then is withdrawn and redirected along a different line at four regions of the muscle for a total of 12 sampling sites. Insertion of a needle electrode mechanically depolarizes muscle tissue. With normal insertional activity the muscle produces brief bursts (<300 milliseconds) of high frequency positive and negative spikes that sound somewhat like static [72]. The activity stops after cessation of needle movement. Increased insertional activity is present if the potentials persist for more than 50 milliseconds. The needle also may provoke transient or sustained fibrillation potentials or PSWs before they are seen at rest. This is often but not invariably a sign of membrane instability. Decreased insertional activity occurs in myopathies and when muscle tissue is ischemic or has undergone fibrosis and is no longer capable of electrical activity.

Minimal to moderate voluntary contraction

This is done to observe the MUAP morphology. Because MUAP amplitude varies with respect to the distance between the recording electrode and the muscle fiber, the MUAP should be analyzed only when the needle electrode is close to the muscle fiber under examination. A nearby MUAP sounds crisp and loud and has a short rise time, whereas a distant MUAP sounds like a muffled thud and has a long rise time. In general 20 different MUAP are analyzed for amplitude, duration, and phases.

Recruitment is the successive activation of motor units with increasing strength of muscle contraction. Minimal muscular effort results in the repetitive firing of one to two motor units, which are low amplitude, slow twitch (type I) muscle fibers [73]. With stronger effort the already activated motor units must fire more rapidly to maintain the strength of contraction. New high amplitude, fast twitch motor units (type II) then are recruited (Fig. 14). With maximum contraction, many rapidly firing motor units ultimately run together, interfering with the recognition of individual MUAP (ie, a full interference pattern [Fig. 15]). Generally after one MUAP fires at a rate of 10 times per second, a second MUAP is recruited. The recruitment ratio is the frequency of the fastest firing MUAP divided by the number of different MUAP seen. A normal recruitment ratio is close to five [74]. For example, if the fastest MUAP is firing 15 times per second, there should be three different MUAP on the screen (see Fig. 14*B*).

In neurogenic disorders there are fewer viable motor units, but there is no change in the number of muscle fibers. The remaining motor units must fire faster in an attempt to maintain the force of contraction. One observes too few MUAP firing rapidly, leading to decreased recruitment (Fig. 16). In myopathies the number of motor units is unchanged, but each motor unit contains fewer muscle fibers. Because the patient feels weaker, they try to compensate by stimulating the remaining motor units to fire earlier and faster. One observes more MUAP firing at a faster rate, resulting in increased recruitment.

Classification of nerve injury

Physiologic conduction block

Lundborg described a physiologic conduction block that is caused by intraneural ischemia or a metabolic (ionic) conduction block, with little or no fiber pathology [13]. Intraneural ischemia would impair the ATP-dependent Na^+/K^+ pump, which would stop any nerve impulse transmission. An example of this would be the reversible compression of the sciatic nerve that

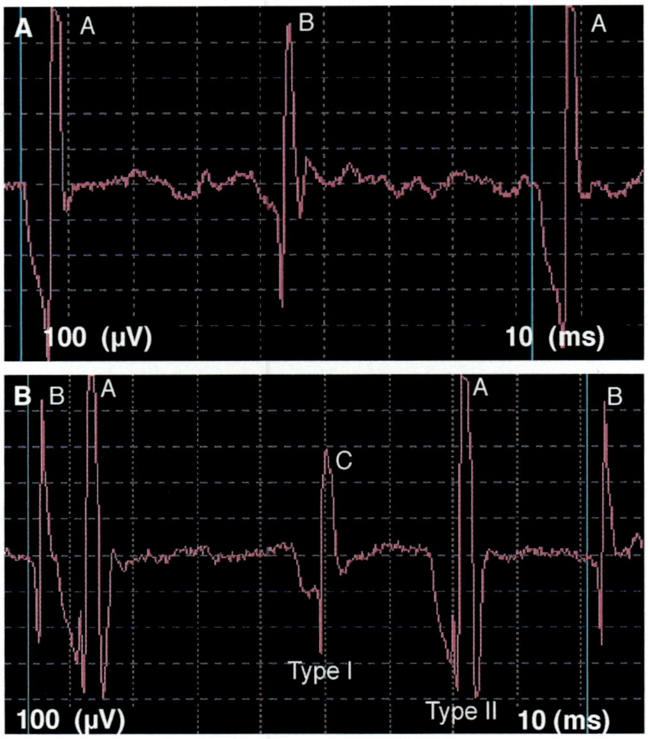

Fig. 14. Normal recruitment. (*A*) MUAP A fires every 80 milliseconds (8 grids at 10 ms/grid). The firing rate is thus 1000/80 = 12.5 cycles/s (Hz). As MUAP A starts firing at more than 10 Hz, a second MUAP (MUAP B) is recruited. The recruitment ratio is 12.5/2 = 6.25. (*B*) The recruitment ratio for the fastest-firing MUAP (MUAP A) is 1000/60 = 16.6 Hz. According to the rule of 5's there should be three different MUAPs on the screen. Both Type I and Type II MUAPs are firing. The recruitment ratio is 5.5. (*From* Slutsky D. Electromyography in hand surgery. J Am Soc Surg Hand 2004;4(3):182; with permission.)

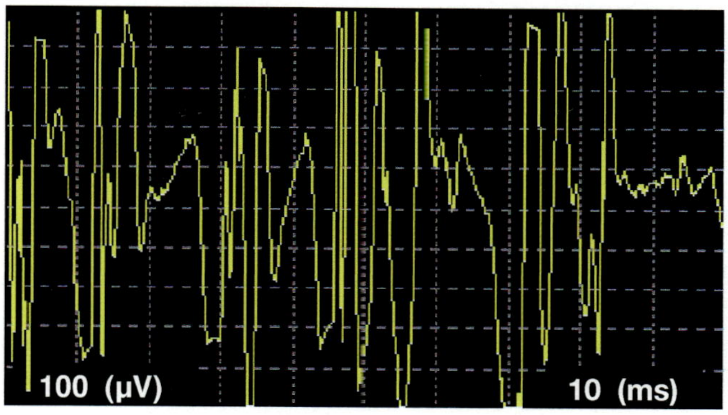

Fig. 15. Full interference pattern. The baseline is completely obliterated by the MUAPs. (*From* Slutsky D. Electromyography in hand surgery. J Am Soc Surg Hand 2004;4(3):183; with permission.)

one may experience with prolonged sitting at a movie theater. Sensory and motor conduction across the compressed segment is blocked by this loss of circulation but immediately recovers once the compression is released. With more prolonged ischemia, intraneural edema develops; hence, recovery occurs over days or weeks. Axonal transport is also energy dependent; hence, extended ischemia may affect the nerve cell body function and viability [75]. Irreversible nerve fiber damage does occur if the ischemia lasts more than 6 to 8 hours [11].

Neurapraxia

Initial phase

The nerve connective tissue remains intact, but there is focal demyelination that allows current leakage. The time for the AP to reach threshold at successive nodes consequently is prolonged. Partial lesions demonstrate slowing caused by the loss of faster conducting fibers or demyelination of surviving fibers. The more protracted the compression, the slower the NCV caused by repeated episodes of demyelination and subsequent remyelination. More extensive demyelination results in complete conduction block. The blocked nerve conduction prevents muscle fiber depolarization, which simulates axonal loss. Amplitude decreases of more than 20% over a distance of 25 cm or less are abnormal. With stimulation proximal to the lesion, the potential is smaller or absent. Although there may be a sensory and motor loss, nerve conduction distal to the lesion is always normal. There is no axonal loss and no Wallerian degeneration has occurred.

The most apparent finding on the EMG is reduced recruitment caused by a reduced number of motor unit potentials firing more rapidly than normal. The clinical correlate is that of muscle weakness without denervation, but fibrillation potentials occasionally may be seen (Fig. 17) [76].

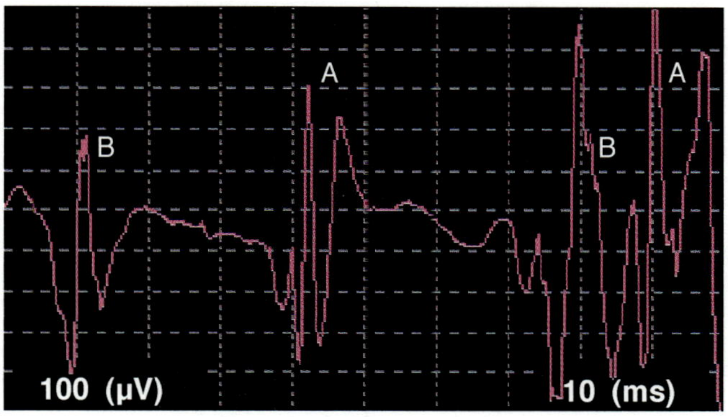

Fig. 16. Decreased recruitment. MUAP A is firing at 16.6 Hz. There should be three different MUAPs on the screen, but there are only two. The recruitment ratio is 8.3. (*From* Slutsky D. Electromyography in hand surgery. J Am Soc Surg Hand 2004;4(3):183; with permission.)

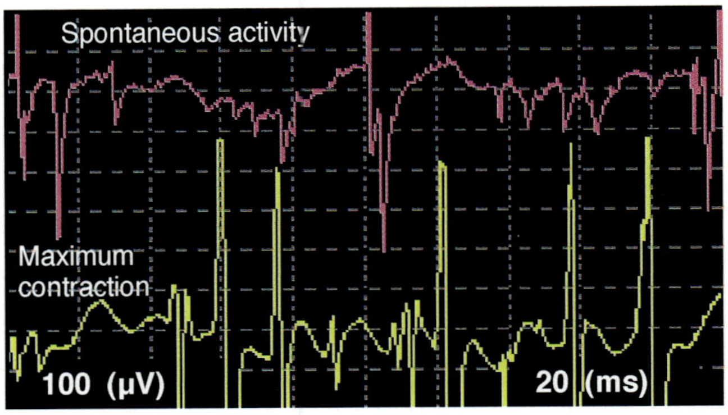

Fig. 17. Partial ulnar nerve injury at 3 months. The top tracing shows trains of PSWs obliterating the baseline. The bottom tracing shows only one rapidly firing MUAP at maximum contraction, which reflects a loss of motor units. There is no polyphasia, indicating an absence of axonal sprouting (reinnervation). (*From* Slutsky D. Electromyography in hand surgery. J Am Soc Surg Hand 2004;4(3):184; with permission.)

Recovery phase

Clinical recovery may occur in a patchy fashion rather than proximal to distal. The nerve conduction ultimately should revert to normal if myelination is complete.

Axonotmesis

Initial phase

The axons are disrupted but the surrounding stroma is intact. Initially the nerve segments distal to the lesion remain excitable and demonstrate normal conduction, but this ultimately wanes. Amplitude decreases by more than 50% within the first few days are suggestive of an axonal injury [53]. Axonotmesis cannot be distinguished from complete severance of the nerve (neurotmesis) until sufficient time has passed for Wallerian degeneration to occur. Proximal stimulation results in an absent or small response from distal muscles.

Recovery phase

The conduction velocity of the nerve proximal to the lesion returns to normal after 200 days if the target organ is reinnervated. The NCV distal to the nerve lesion only reaches 60% to 90% of its preinjury value (see section on neurotmesis) [77].

Partial lesions usually represent axonotmesis, in which recovery depends on axonal sprouting and nerve fiber regeneration. With an incomplete axonal injury, loss of motor units results in reduced recruitment. As axonal sprouting occurs, innervation of noncontiguous muscle fibers results in increased waveform duration, polyphasia, and an increased MUAP amplitude. With time the polyphasia diminishes but the increased amplitudes remain (see section on pathology). There may be a biphasic pattern of recovery caused by early axonal sprouting followed by late end organ reinnervation.

Neurotmesis

Initial phase

The nerve is no longer in continuity, but the myelin remains intact until the axon degenerates. There is a preservation of the fastest conducting fibers until complete failure of the nerve AP. The latency and NCV remain unchanged until the end. Neuromuscular junction (NMJ) transmission fails before nerve excitability because the motor endplate degenerates before Wallerian degeneration is complete. As a consequence one sees a disappearance of the CMAP by 3 to 5 days following nerve transection [78]. The SNAP amplitude is preserved until days 5 to 7, and sensory nerve conduction persists until day 11 [79].

Although it depends on the length of the distal nerve stump, Wallerian degeneration typically occurs by 10 to 14 days [79]. Membrane instability is manifested by the appearance of fibrillation potentials and PSWs. The appearance of the PSWs, however, may predate fibrillation potentials by 2 to 3 days [69]. Fibrillations decrease in number as muscle reinnervation progresses. This also occurs in the absence of reinnervation because of a loss of viable muscle fibers 2° to fibrosis. The amplitude of the fibrillation potentials can be used to estimate the duration of the pathology, because it decreases with time. They may be 1000 μV in acute conditions, but it is rare to find any larger than 100 μV after 12 months (Fig. 18) [80].

Recovery phase

When the nerve is divided completely, recovery depends solely on axonal regeneration. The conduction velocity of the nerve proximal to the lesion remains at 60% to 70% if nerve continuity is not re-established [77]. This is in part because the axon relies on retrograde transport of neurotrophic factors for maximal conductivity. Following nerve regeneration remyelination is incomplete. The regenerating Schwann cells revert back to their shorter embryonic internodal length, which is a 2:1 to 3:1 ratio as compared with normal nerve. The regenerated nerve diameter slowly decreases distal to the lesion because of a failure to reexpand the endoneurial tube completely. These factors explain why the NCV distal to the nerve lesion only reaches 60% to 90% of preinjury value even though there may be full clinical recovery.

The EMG is initially silent, followed by the appearance of small, long duration, unstable, and polyphasic nascent potentials (Fig. 19). They usually precede the onset of clinically evident voluntary movement [70]. It is prudent to wait 2 to 4 months and then look for evidence of reinnervation in previously completely denervated muscles [81]. As a general rule nerve regrowth occurs at approximately 1 inch per month [82]. Motor endplates degrade at approximately 1% per week; hence, the maximum length that a nerve can grow to restore motor function is approximately 13 to 18 inches. Lesions that have spontaneous recovery are treated nonoperatively, whereas those without recovery are explored. Repairs at the brachial plexus level rarely result in the recovery of any intrinsic muscle function. Sensory end organs, however, remain viable and can be reinnervated even after many years [83].

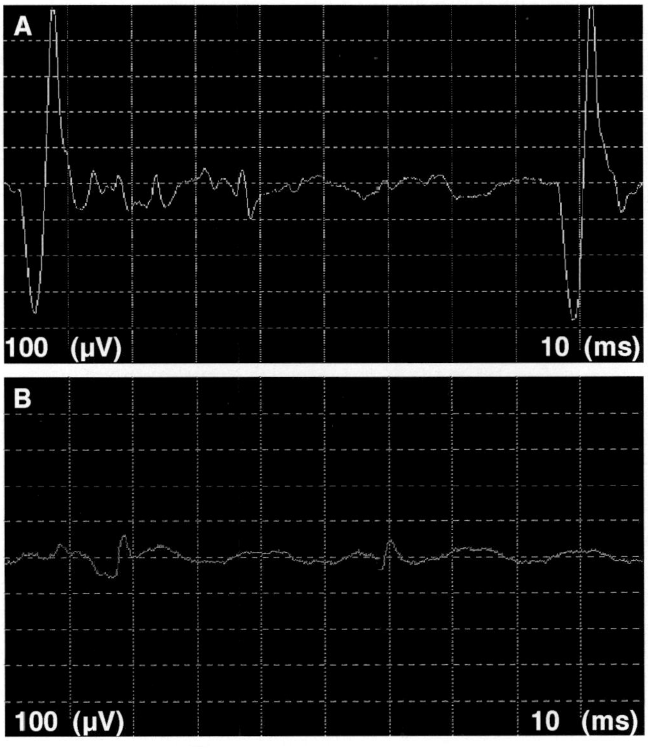

Fig. 18. (*A*) Recent denervation. The fibrillation potentials are of large amplitude. (*B*) Chronic denervation. Note the small-amplitude fibrillation potentials. (*From* Slutsky D. Electromyography in hand surgery. J Am Soc Surg Hand 2004;4(3):181; with permission.)

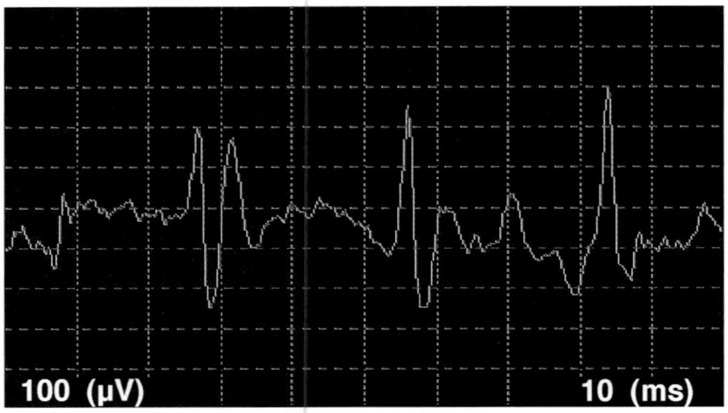

Fig. 19. Early reinnervation of first dorsal interosseous following nerve repair. (*From* Slutsky D. Electromyography in hand surgery. J Am Soc Surg Hand 2004;4(3):185; with permission.)

Radiculopathy

A myotome consists of all the muscles of a limb that are innervated by a specific nerve root level. Because of the multilevel innervation of limb muscles, each muscle belongs to more than one myotome. Anterior (efferent) and posterior (afferent) nerve roots arising from the spinal cord fuse to form the spinal nerve, which in turn divide into the anterior and posterior primary rami. Efferent motor fibers from the anterior cervical rami fuse to form the brachial plexus. Afferent sensory fibers from the posterior root fuse to form the dorsal root ganglion outside the neural foramen where the sensory nerve cell bodies reside. Nerve root compression may result in subjective sensory abnormalities, though the SNAP remain normal. This is because the distal sensory nerve axons remain connected to healthy cell bodies in the dorsal root ganglion, which are distal to the lesion at the foraminal level. Cell bodies of the motor fibers are located in the ventral horn of the spinal cord. Radicular lesions thus lead to a loss of motor axons and Wallerian degeneration, with the subsequent appearance of fibrillation potentials and PSWs (see Table 3).

It is necessary to examine at least two to three muscles per myotome in the anterior and posterior primary rami distribution. In a C6 lesion, for example, denervation potentials may be seen in the biceps, extensor carpi radialis, and pronator teres, but not the triceps, APB, or FDI muscles. For uncertain reasons, EMG abnormalities may be seen occasionally in only one to two limb muscles. It is not uncommon for patients to have a C6–C7 cervical radiculopathy and carpal tunnel compression or a C8–T1 radiculopathy and cubital tunnel syndrome. An NCS likewise should be performed.

Paraspinal electromyography

If abnormalities are noted in the paraspinal muscles and the upper limb, the lesion must be as far proximal as the root level, because the anterior and posterior 1° rami are affected. Approximately 25%–40% of patients who have a radiculopathy may demonstrate fibrillation potentials only in the paraspinal muscles [7]. Radiculopathies are one possible cause of paraspinal abnormalities, but any disorder of the anterior horn cell, posterior rami, or the muscle fibers themselves can produce membrane instability, such as motor neuron disease, myopathies, diabetes, and so on.

Brachial plexus lesions

An axonal lesion distal to the origin of the posterior primary ramus, such as a brachial plexus lesion, should not affect the paraspinals. Because the plexus is distal to the dorsal root ganglion, the SNAP amplitudes should be decreased because of the loss of afferent sensory fibers. The EMG findings reflect the loss of motor axons as discussed previously.

Electromyography pitfalls

False positive

Insufficient muscles examined

Radicular injuries are diagnosed not only by documenting abnormalities in a particular myotome, but by demonstrating a distinct lack of abnormalities in other myotomes, especially of the opposite limb.

Misidentification of normal potentials

EPS that fire irregularly at high rates may be mistaken for fibrillation potentials, which fire regularly at slower rates.

Overinterpretation of normal variants

Trains of PSWs may last longer than anticipated after needle insertion or movement, which is a normal variant and is not diagnostic of any nerve or muscle disorder [84].

Motor unit action potential overlap

MUAPs that run together may appear polyphasic and of increased duration (Fig. 20). This can be minimized by using a trigger and delay line on the EMG trace to ensure that the same MUAP is being examined.

False negative

Time of study

Generally the peak of fibrillations and PSWs is 2 to 4 weeks. An examination performed within the first 7 to 10 days may be falsely negative.

Temperature

Decreased temperature suppresses the firing rates and the number of fibrillations and PSWs.

Instrumentation defects

Defective EMG needles may lead to faulty recordings.

Motor unit action potential parameters

MUAP amplitude varies with respect to the distance between the recording electrode and the muscle fiber. An MUAP should be analyzed only when the distance between the needle electrode and the muscle tissue is optimal so that the needle is close to the fiber that it is recording. The MUAP sound should be crisp and loud, otherwise error may be introduced in measuring the amplitude, duration, and phases.

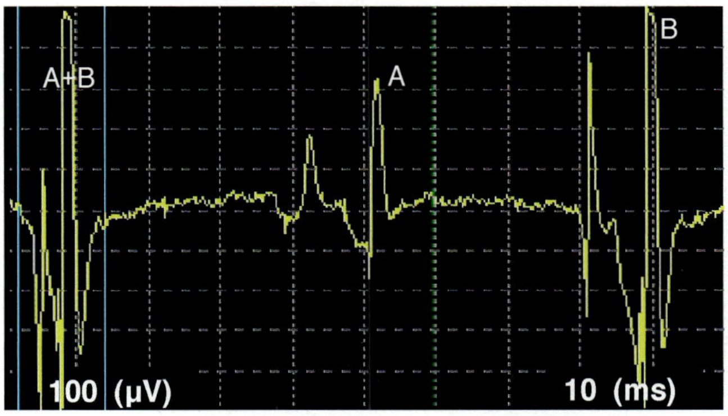

Fig. 20. Pseudopolyphasia. MUAP A and B run together, producing an artificially polyphasic MUAP. (*From* Slutsky D. Electromyography in hand surgery. J Am Soc Surg Hand 2004;4(3):187; with permission.)

Polyphasia

Polyphasic potentials are of diagnostic value only when quantified with a trigger line by examining at least 20 individual MUAP, then calculating the percent of polyphasic potentials. An increase in polyphasic potentials only implies that at some point the motor unit has undergone remodeling. This is not by itself diagnostic of any specific disease or time of occurrence. All persons have some degree of polyphasic potentials.

Recruitment

Recruitment abnormalities are not especially sensitive and rarely aid in the diagnosis unless accompanied by fibrillation potentials, PSWs, and MUAP duration changes. It can be difficult for some patients to recruit only a single motor unit even during minimal voluntary contraction. Distal muscles are more prone to false positive results.

Interference pattern

An interference pattern is not equivalent to recruitment. It rarely provides any information and can be the subject of false positive results because of lack of patient cooperation, pain, or needle placement too distant from the muscle tissue.

Age

It is believed that there is a gradual loss of anterior horn cells with age [85]. This subclinical muscle denervation induces collateral sprouting to remodel the remaining motor units. The increase in the number of muscle fibers per motor unit results in an increase of the MUAP duration and amplitude with age, which can be interpreted falsely as a neurogenic lesion.

Summary

Combined with a detailed medical history and a thorough upper extremity examination, the nerve conduction test can yield useful information. The test results, however, cannot be taken out of context. It is not uncommon for a patient to be totally asymptomatic yet an NCS is reported as showing mild slowing of the conduction velocities and latencies if the hand is cold or if the electrode is making poor contact. The NCS findings may be of subclinical or no clinical significance. More so than NCS, EMG is an art form honed through practice and experience. The EMG examination can provide useful information as to the normal and abnormal electrophysiology of muscle and its nerve. The various potentials described, however, do not point to a specific diagnosis.

Most hand surgeons intuitively understand, however, that the indication for surgery still hinges on reproducible physical findings combined with the appropriate clinical symptoms rather than on a test abnormality. Through an understanding of the methodology and principles of testing, the clinician is better suited to recognize when the report conclusions do not match the EMG data or when to request further testing in cases in which insufficient data compromise one's ability to draw definitive conclusions.

References

[1] Slutsky D. Nerve conduction studies in hand surgery. J Am Soc Surg Hand 2003;3(3):152–69.
[2] Slutsky D. Recurrent carpal tunnel syndrome: pathophysiology and diagnosis. Programs and abstracts of the 59th annual meeting of the American Society for Surgery of the Hand. New York, NY, September 11, 2004.
[3] Slutsky D. Nerve conduction studies in the office and operating room. Programs and abstracts of the 57th annual meeting of the American Society for Surgery of the Hand. Phoenix, AZ, October 3, 2002.
[4] Slutsky D. Electromyography in hand surgery. J Am Soc Surg Hand 2004;4(3):176–86.
[5] Slutsky D. Electrophysiology in nerve injury. Programs and abstracts of the 58th annual meeting of the American Society for Surgery of the Hand. Chicago, IL, September 18, 2003.
[6] Waxman SG. Determinants of conduction velocity in myelinated nerve fibers. Muscle Nerve 1980;3:141.
[7] Johnson EW, Melvin JL. Value of electromyography in lumbar radiculopathy. Arch Phys Med Rehabil 1971;52: 239.

[8] Dahlin LB, Shyu BC, Danielsen N, et al. Effects of nerve compression or ischaemia on conduction properties of myelinated and non-myelinated nerve fibres. An experimental study in the rabbit common peroneal nerve. Acta Physiol Scand 1989;136:97.
[9] Brumback RA, Bobele GB, Rayan GM. Electrodiagnosis of compressive nerve lesions. Hand Clin 1992;8:241.
[10] Dellon A. Pitfalls in interpretation of electrophysiological testing. In: Gelberman RH, editor. Operative nerve repair and reconstruction. Vol. 1. Philadelphia: JB Lippincott Co.; 1991; vol. 1. p. 185–96.
[11] Lundborg G. Ischemic nerve injury. Experimental studies on intraneural microvascular pathophysiology and nerve function in a limb subjected to temporary circulatory arrest. Scand J Plast Reconstr Surg Suppl 1970;6:3.
[12] Rydevik B, Lundborg G. Permeability of intraneural microvessels and perineurium following acute, graded experimental nerve compression. Scand J Plast Reconstr Surg 1977;11:179.
[13] Lundborg G, Dahlin LB. The pathophysiology of nerve compression. Hand Clin 1992;8:215.
[14] Eversmann WW Jr, Ritsick JA. Intraoperative changes in motor nerve conduction latency in carpal tunnel syndrome. J Hand Surg [Am] 1978;3:77.
[15] Felsenthal G. Median and ulnar distal motor and sensory latencies in the same normal subject. Arch Phys Med Rehabil 1977;58:297.
[16] Johnson EW, Kukla RD, Wongsam PE, et al. Sensory latencies to the ring finger: normal values and relation to carpal tunnel syndrome. Arch Phys Med Rehabil 1981;62:206.
[17] Wongsam PE, Johnson EW, Weinerman JD. Carpal tunnel syndrome: use of palmar stimulation of sensory fibers. Arch Phys Med Rehabil 1983;64:16.
[18] Stevens JC. AAEM minimonograph #26: the electrodiagnosis of carpal tunnel syndrome. Muscle Nerve 1997;20: 1477.
[19] Kimura J. The carpal tunnel syndrome: localization of conduction abnormalities within the distal segment of the median nerve. Brain 1979;102:619.
[20] Olney RK, Wilbourn AJ. Ulnar nerve conduction study of the first dorsal interosseous muscle. Arch Phys Med Rehabil 1985;66:16.
[21] Eisen A. Early diagnosis of ulnar nerve palsy. An electrophysiologic study. Neurology 1974;24:256.
[22] Buschbacher RM. Ulnar 14-cm and 7-cm antidromic sensory studies to the fifth digit: reference values derived from a large population of normal subjects. Am J Phys Med Rehabil 1999;78:S63.
[23] Trojaborg W, Sindrup EH. Motor and sensory conduction in different segments of the radial nerve in normal subjects. J Neurol Neurosurg Psychiatr 1969;32:354.
[24] Ma DM, Kim SH, Spielholz N, et al. Sensory conduction study of distal radial nerve. Arch Phys Med Rehabil 1981; 62:562.
[25] Kothari MJ, Rutkove SB, Caress JB, et al. Comparison of digital sensory studies in patients with carpal tunnel syndrome. Muscle Nerve 1995;18:1272.
[26] Redmond MD, Rivner MH. False positive electrodiagnostic tests in carpal tunnel syndrome. Muscle Nerve 1988;11: 511.
[27] Robinson LR, Micklesen PJ, Wang L. Optimizing the number of tests for carpal tunnel syndrome. Muscle Nerve 2000;23:1880.
[28] Robinson LR, Micklesen PJ, Wang L. Strategies for analyzing nerve conduction data: superiority of a summary index over single tests. Muscle Nerve 1998;21:1166.
[29] Lundborg G, Gelberman RH, Minteer-Convery M, et al. Median nerve compression in the carpal tunnel—functional response to experimentally induced controlled pressure. J Hand Surg [Am] 1982;7:252.
[30] Steyers CM. Recurrent carpal tunnel syndrome. Hand Clin 2002;18:339.
[31] Hunter JM. Recurrent carpal tunnel syndrome, epineural fibrous fixation, and traction neuropathy. Hand Clin 1991;7:491.
[32] Bronson J, Beck J, Gillet J. Provocative motor nerve conduction testing in presumptive carpal tunnel syndrome unconfirmed by traditional electrodiagnostic testing. J Hand Surg [Am] 1997;22:1041.
[33] Read RL. Stress testing in nerve compression. Hand Clin 1991;7:521.
[34] Preston DC, Logigian EL. Lumbrical and interossei recording in carpal tunnel syndrome. Muscle Nerve 1992;15: 1253.
[35] Kothari MJ, Preston DC, Logigian EL. Lumbrical-interossei motor studies localize ulnar neuropathy at the wrist. Muscle Nerve 1996;19:170.
[36] Nasr JT, Kaufman MA. Electrophysiologic findings in two patients with digital neuropathy of the thumb. Electromyogr Clin Neurophysiol 2001;41:353.
[37] Spaans F. Neurographic assessment of lesions of single proper digital nerves. Clin Neurophysiol 2001;112:2113.
[38] Terai Y, Senda M, Hashizume H, et al. Selective measurement of digital nerve conduction velocity. J Orthop Sci 2001;6:123.
[39] King JC, Dumitru D, Wertsch JJ. Digit distribution of proper digital nerve action potential. Muscle Nerve 2001;24: 1489.
[40] Spinner M, Spencer PS. Nerve compression lesions of the upper extremity. A clinical and experimental review. Clin Orthop 1974 Oct;0(104):46–67.
[41] Campbell WW, Pridgeon RM, Riaz G, et al. Sparing of the flexor carpi ulnaris in ulnar neuropathy at the elbow. Muscle Nerve 1989;12:965.
[42] Dellon AL, Schlegel RW, Mackinnon SE. Validity of nerve conduction velocity studies after anterior transposition of the ulnar nerve. J Hand Surg [Am] 1987;12:700.
[43] Campbell WW, Pridgeon RM, Sahni KS. Short segment incremental studies in the evaluation of ulnar neuropathy at the elbow. Muscle Nerve 1992;15:1050.

[44] Campbell WW, Sahni SK, Pridgeon RM, et al. Intraoperative electroneurography: management of ulnar neuropathy at the elbow. Muscle Nerve 1988;11 75.
[45] Felsenthal G, Freed MJ, Kalafut R, et al. Across-elbow ulnar nerve sensory conduction technique. Arch Phys Med Rehabil 1989;70:668.
[46] Jabre JF. Ulnar nerve lesions at the wrist: new technique for recording from the sensory dorsal branch of the ulnar nerve. Neurology 1980;30:873.
[47] Venkatesh S, Kothari MJ, Preston DC. The limitations of the dorsal ulnar cutaneous sensory response in patients with ulnar neuropathy at the elbow. Muscle Nerve 1995;18:345.
[48] Tomaino MM, Brach PJ, Vansickle DP. The rationale for and efficacy of surgical intervention for electrodiagnostic-negative cubital tunnel syndrome. J Hand Surg [Am] 2001;26:1077.
[49] Shea JD, McClain EJ. Ulnar-nerve compression syndromes at and below the wrist. J Bone Joint Surg [Am] 1969;51: 1095.
[50] Wu JS, Morris JD, Hogan GR. Ulnar neuropathy at the wrist: case report and review of literature. Arch Phys Med Rehabil 1985;66:785.
[51] McIntosh KA, Preston DC, Logigian EL. Short-segment incremental studies to localize ulnar nerve entrapment at the wrist. Neurology 1998;50:303.
[52] Kupfer DM, Bronson J, Lee GW, et al. Differential latency testing: a more sensitive test for radial tunnel syndrome. J Hand Surg [Am] 1998;23:859.
[53] Dumitru D. Electrodiagnostic medicine. In: Vol. I. Philadelphia: Hanley and Belfus, Inc.; 1995. p. 47.
[54] Halar EM, DeLisa JA, Soine TL. Nerve conduction studies in upper extremities: skin temperature corrections. Arch Phys Med Rehabil 1983;64:412.
[55] Denys EH. AAEM minimonograph #14. The influence of temperature in clinical neurophysiology. Muscle Nerve 1991;14:795.
[56] Corwin HM, Kasdan ML. Electrodiagnostic reports of median neuropathy at the wrist. J Hand Surg [Am] 1998; 23:55.
[57] Buchthal F, Schmalbruch H. Motor unit of mammalian muscle. Physiol Rev 1980;60:90.
[58] Buchthal F, Erminio F, Rosenfalck P. Motor unit territory in different human muscles. Acta Physiol Scand 1959; 45:72.
[59] Katz B, Miledi R. Propagation of electric activity in motor nerve terminals. Proc R Soc Lond B Biol Sci 1965;161: 453.
[60] Chu J, Bruyninckx F, Chan RC. Significance of motor unit action potential parameters in normal and neurogenic situations. Electromyogr Clin Neurophysiol 1986 26:465.
[61] Thiele B, Bohle A. Number of spike-components contributing to the motor unit potential (author's transl). EEG EMG Z Elektroenzephalogr Elektromyogr Verwandte Geb 1978;9:125.
[62] Miller RG. AAEE minimonograph #28: injury to peripheral motor nerves. Muscle Nerve 1987;10:698.
[63] Brown MC, Ironton R. Sprouting and regression of neuromuscular synapses in partially denervated mammalian muscles. J Physiol 1978;278:325.
[64] Feinstein B, Lindegard B, Nyman E, et al. Morphologic studies of motor units in normal human muscles. Acta Anat (Basel) 1955;23:127.
[65] Dumitru D, King JC, Stegeman DF. Endplate spike morphology: a clinical and simulation study. Arch Phys Med Rehabil 1998;79:634.
[66] Buchthal F, Rosenfalck P. Spontaneous electrical activity of human muscle. Electroencephalogr Clin Neurophysiol 1966;20:321.
[67] Thesleff S, Ward MR. Studies on the mechanism of fibrillation potentials in denervated muscle. J Physiol 1975;244: 313.
[68] Partanen JV, Danner R. Fibrillation potentials after muscle injury in humans. Muscle Nerve 1982;5: S70.
[69] Kraft GH. Are fibrillation potentials and positive sharp waves the same? No. Muscle Nerve 1996;19:216.
[70] Dorfman LJ. Quantitative clinical electrophysiology in the evaluation of nerve injury and regeneration. Muscle Nerve 1990;13:822.
[71] Nandedkar SD, Barkhaus PE, Sanders DB, et al. Some observations on fibrillations and positive sharp waves. Muscle Nerve 2000;23:888.
[72] Wiechers D, Stow R, Johnson EW. Electromyographic insertional activity mechanically provoked in the biceps brachii. Arch Phys Med Rehabil 1977;58:573.
[73] Warmolts JR, Engel WK. Open-biopsy electromyography. I. Correlation of motor unit behavior with histochemical muscle fiber type in human limb muscle. Arch Neurol 1972;27:512.
[74] Petajan JH. AAEM minimonograph #3: motor unit recruitment. Muscle Nerve 1991;14:489.
[75] Dahlin LB, Lundborg G. The neurone and its response to peripheral nerve compression. J Hand Surg [Br] 1990; 15:5.
[76] Trojaborg W. Early electrophysiologic changes in conduction block. Muscle Nerve 1978;1:400.
[77] Kiraly JK, Krnjevic K. Some retrograde changes in function of nerves after peripheral section. Q J Exp Physiol Cogn Med Sci 1959;44:244.
[78] Landau WM. The duration of neuromuscular function after nerve section in man. J Neurosurg 1953;10:64.
[79] Chaudhry V, Cornblath DR. Wallerian degeneration in human nerves: serial electrophysiological studies. Muscle Nerve 1992;15:687.
[80] Kraft GH. Fibrillation potential amplitude and muscle atrophy following peripheral nerve injury. Muscle Nerve 1990;13:814.
[81] Kline DG. Surgical repair of peripheral nerve injury. Muscle Nerve 1990;13:843.

[82] Trojaborg W, Sindrup E. Radial nerve palsies; clinical and electrophysiological aspects. Electroencephalogr Clin Neurophysiol 1969;26:342.
[83] Terzis JK, Michelow BJ. Sensory receptors. In: Gelberman RH, editor. Operative nerve repair and reconstruction. Vol. 1. Philadelphia: JB Lippincott; 1991. p. 85.
[84] Wiechers DO. Mechanically provoked insertional activity before and after nerve section in rats. Arch Phys Med Rehabil 1977;58:402.
[85] Brown WF. Functional compensation of human motor units in health and disease. J Neurol Sci 1973;20:199.

ELSEVIER
SAUNDERS

Atlas Hand Clin 10 (2005) 65–72

Atlas of the
HAND
CLINICS

Methods of Primary Nerve Repair

Edward Diao, MD[a,*], Mark Ashkan[b]

[a]Department of Orthopaedic Surgery and Neurosurgery, Division of Hand, Upper Extremity and Microvascular Surgery, University of California–San Francisco/Mount Zion Orthopaedic Faculty Practice, 500 Parnassus Avenue, Mu-320-W, San Francisco, CA 94143, USA

[b]University of California–Berkeley/University of California–San Francisco, 3700 Dean Drive, Unit 2308, Ventura, CA 93003, USA

Nerves are the essential part of the human nervous system and their proper working is absolutely critical. Nerve injury recognition and techniques for repairing injured nerves date back to the works of Galen (130–200 AD). Throughout the years these techniques have been improved on and enhanced. These methods are still undergoing further perfection. In addition, new sutureless methods, such as repair using fibrin glue, tubulation and conduits, and lasers are emerging. These sutureless methods are still in their preliminary stages, however, and until these methods are refined, tested, and tested again, standard suture microsurgical techniques remain the standard for clinical care. This article focuses on the surgical principles of primary nerve repair by suture repair.

Rationale and basic science pertinent to the procedure

Anatomy

Peripheral nerves provide a protected region within which neurons operate. A peripheral nerve is composed of three elements—motor, sensory, and sympathetic fibers. Each neuron has a cell body that contains the nucleus, an axon to carry impulses away, and dendrites to receive impulses from other neurons. A motor nerve's cell body is located in the anterior horn of the spinal cord and its axon ends in the muscle (Fig. 1). A sensory nerve's cell body is located in the dorsal root ganglion and its dendrites are located in the skin, either as special receptors or free nerve endings (Fig. 1).

The nerves comprising the sympathetic part of the peripheral nervous system consist of a two-neuron chain of presynaptic and postsynaptic fibers. The cell bodies of the presynaptic fibers are located in the lateral horn of the thoracolumbar spinal cord. Their axons synapse with a postsynaptic fiber in one of the many ganglia in the paired sympathetic chain or paravertebral ganglion. From there, the axons of the postsynaptic fibers innervate their respective organs, which include muscles and glands.

Axons of peripheral nerves can be myelinated or unmyelinated. Myelinated axons have supportive Schwann cells surrounding them, whereas unmyelinated axons do not. Both types of nerve fibers are found in motor and sensory nerves in a 4:1 ratio of slower conducting unmyelinated to faster conducting myelinated fibers [1]. Interruptions in myelinated neurons are referred to as nodes of Ranvier. With the nodes of Ranvier, the depolarization of the axon and the exchange of ions (sodium and potassium) only occur at these points. As a result, nodes of Ranvier allow for jumping of impulses from node to node and this is faster and more

* Corresponding author.
E-mail address: diaoe@orthosurg.ucsf.edu (E. Diao).

1082-3131/05/$ - see front matter
doi:10.1016/j.ahc.2004.08.001

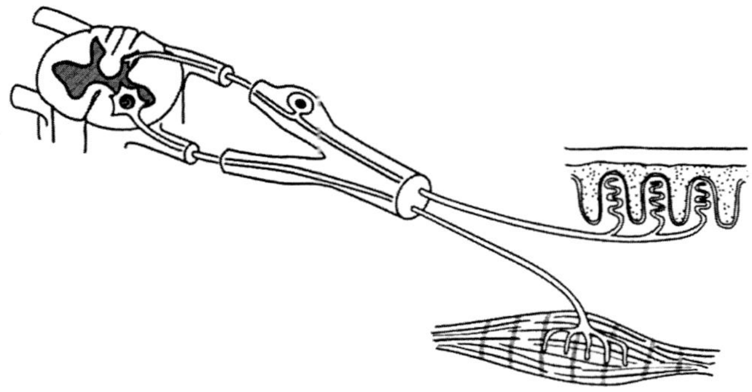

Fig. 1. A schematic of a peripheral nerve. Peripheral nerve origin is within the spinal cord with motor sensory components and their respective end organs. *Used with permission from* Diao E, Vannuyen T. Techniques for primary nerve repair. Hand Clin 2000;16(1):54.

energetically favorable than continuous conduction. This type of conduction in myelinated axons is referred to as saltatory conduction (Fig. 2).

A peripheral nerve is composed of many fascicles (Fig. 3). Each fascicle is associated with supporting Schwann cells that form a basement membrane. Outside this membrane is the endoneurium, which is a thin collagen tissue (Fig. 3). The endoneurium together with the Schwann cell basement membrane form a cylindric structure called the endoneurial or Schwann cell tube. This cylindric structure plays an important role in nerve degeneration and regeneration after injury. The number of fascicles differs among individuals and throughout a nerve's course, ranging from 3–36 in the median nerve [2]. Each fascicle is bounded by perineurium (Fig. 3), a connective tissue layer of multiple concentric lamellae of perineurial cells. This is a strong layer that resists longitudinal stress and retains the nerve's elasticity during elongation. Furthermore, because this layer is a continuation of the pia-arachnoid mater of the CNS, it serves as a blood–brain barrier. The perineurium is vital to the functioning of the nerve and its removal or interruption results in the cessation of nerve function. A fascicle is thus a group of nerve axons each surrounded within its endoneurium and encased within the perineurium (Fig. 3).

There are three fascicular patterns: monofascicular, with one large fascicle; oligofascicular, with few fascicles; and polyfascicular, with multiple fascicles of various sizes (Fig. 3). Fascicles also can be found in groups of three to six, surrounded by the inner or internal epineurium, which is composed of collagen fibers that fill the space between each individual fascicle. A dense layer of connective tissue termed the external epineurium surrounds these groups of fascicles and the entire nerve. The epineurium is primarily a protective layer and in contrast to the perineurium, it can be removed surgically with few physiologic sequelae.

The outermost tissue is the mesoneurium. It is a loose areolar tissue layer that is continuous with the epineurium and extends to the adjacent tissues. The mesoneurium is important because the blood supply enters the nerve through this layer. The mesoneurium facilitates nerve gliding

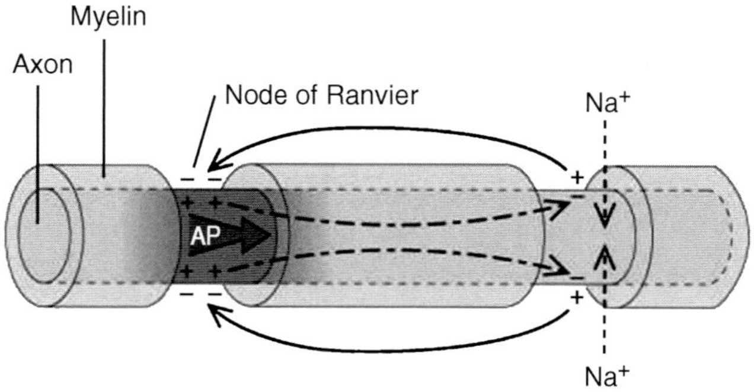

Fig. 2. The nodes of Ranvier allow for saltatory conduction of action potentials through an axon. *Used with permission from* Delcomyn, Fred. Foundations of neurobiology. New York: WH Freeman; 1998.

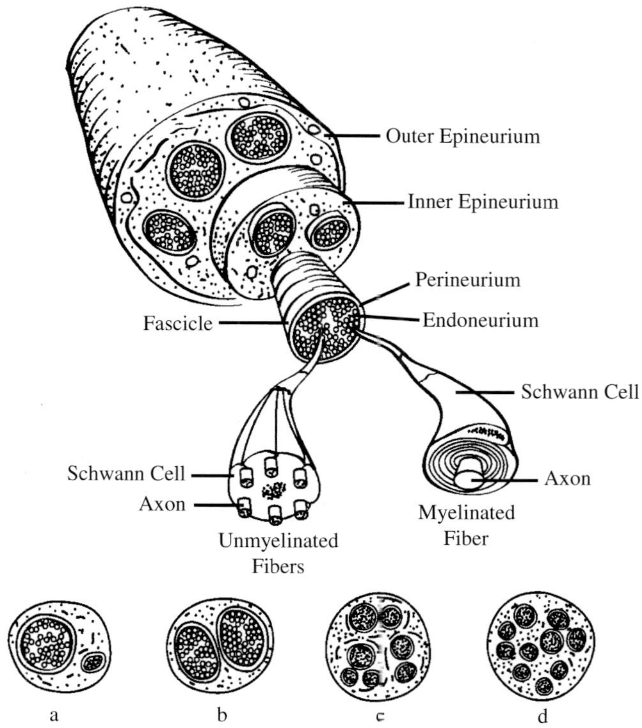

Fig. 3. A peripheral nerve demonstrating the classification, respective connective tissue layers, and cross-sectional anatomy. (*A*) Monofascicular. (*B*) Oligofascicular. (*C*) Polyfascicular. (*D*) No identifiable group patterns. *Used with permission from* Diao E, Vannuyen T. Techniques for primary nerve repair. Hand Clin 2000;16(1):55.

throughout the full range of motion of extremity, thus maintaining longitudinal nerve excursion [3].

Problem

A nerve injury is a defect that results in the inability of the nerve to transmit an action potential. Classification of nerve injury was well established by Seddon in 1943, expanded by Sunderland in 1951 [2], and refined by Mackinnon [4] (Table 1). Seddon's classifications include three types: neurapraxia, axonotmesis, and neurotmesis. Sunderland's classifications include first- through fifth-degree injuries. Mackinnon's classification added a sixth degree, signifying a combination of the other degrees of injury in one patient.

Neurapraxia or first-degree injury is the mildest form of injury. It involves a demyelination of a segment of the axon resulting in a local conduction block with paralysis in the absence of peripheral degeneration. The nerve fibers are intact and no Wallerian degeneration occurs. (Wallerian degeneration refers to changes in the distal nerve segments of myelinated nerves. The processes, however, are similar proximally and distally.) Furthermore, a Tinel sign is not present at the site of injury. Full recovery is expected and can vary from minutes to several weeks.

Axonotmesis is a nerve injury with damage to the axon resulting in Wallerian degeneration distally; regeneration produces axonal sprouting proximally. The endoneurium and perineurium

Table 1

Seddon	Sunderland	Mackinnon	Description	Tinel sign	Progress distally	Spontaneous recovery pattern	Surgery
Neuropraxia	1°		Second paragraph	−	Fast	Complete (fast)	None
Axonotmesis	2°		Third paragraph	+	+	Complete (slow)	None
	3°		Fourth paragraph	+	+	Varies (slow)	Varies
	4°		Fifth paragraph	+	−	None	Yes
Neurotmesis	5°		Sixth paragraph	+	−	None	Yes
		6°	Seventh paragraph	Varies depending on the injuries			

are still intact and regeneration is directed along the proper path by these supporting sheaths. A Tinel sign can be elicited at the injury level and advances distally as the nerve regenerates. The Schwann cell basement membrane also is not damaged. Full nerve recovery thus is expected and occurs at a rate of 1 inch per month or 1.5 mm/day.

In Sunderland's third-degree nerve injury, endoneurial damage and scarring are seen while perineurium and epineurium remain intact. This impedes some fibers from eventually reaching their end organs or receptors, thus rendering regeneration incomplete. Although the fascicles remain in continuity, their internal structure is disorganized. Furthermore, mismatching of fibers and receptors is possible because of the destruction of basal lamina of the Schwann cells and the endoneurial tubes. Because the perineurium remains intact, however, the fibers within it have the capacity to reorganize and regenerate appropriately. There is an advancing Tinel sign and incomplete recovery occurs at the same rate as in a second-degree injury. The level of recovery depends on the level of injury. Whether the fascicles are mixed or pure and the extent of the scar tissue are also factors determining the amount of regeneration. Recovery is variable and can range from nearly complete recovery to minimal recovery.

Fourth-degree injury is the worst form of closed nerve damage and is described by Sunderland as one that leaves internal structure of the nerve completely disorganized and nonfunctional but physically in continuity. The fascicles are not intact and the nerve is only continuous through intercalated scar tissue; the nerve trunk itself, however, is intact. Wallerian degeneration occurs distally. Tinel sign is present at the injury level because regeneration is prevented by scar tissue, but the Tinel sign does not advance distally. Furthermore, proximal regeneration cannot occur. In this instance, because the conduction of impulses down the axon is not possible, these injuries never gain any motor or sensory recovery. Only surgical intervention is able to restore some degree of nerve recovery by ensuring physical proximity. Fourth-degree nerve injury, however, is diagnosed clinically after no evidence of recovery has been seen for a period of 3 months.

Neurotmesis or fifth-degree injury is the most severe type of injury and is applied to the complete transaction of the nerve trunk. This type of injury is easy to diagnose because it is an open injury with associated peripheral nerve deficit. Surgical repair is required to restore function.

The sixth-degree injury described by Mackinnon is a combination of all or several of Sunderland's injuries occurring within the same zone of injury [1,4]. This is demonstrated by the neuroma-in-continuity injury. In this case, the patterns of injury and regeneration are mixed among various fascicles. In this case, the surgeon is responsible for the careful preoperative functional assessment to determine which lesions are likely to require operative intervention. This is most relevant when there is a plexus of nerves, as in the brachial plexus.

Indications and contraindications

Operative nerve repair of a peripheral nerve performed within the first week after injury is referred to as primary nerve repair. Surgery performed after the first 3 or 4 days after injury generally is considered a delayed primary repair. Surgeries performed a week or more after the injury are referred to as secondary repairs. Primary nerve repair of nerve injuries has been shown superior to secondary nerve repair in several animal [5–7] and clinical studies [8–11].

Several conditions are required for primary nerve repair to be successful; these are discussed in the following sections.

Characteristics of the wound

The wound should be free of gross contamination. The nerve laceration should be a sharp transaction rather than a crush or avulsion. With a sharp transaction, the zone of injury is small and coaptation of nerve ends is easy during surgery. If there is a significant crush component or length of avulsion injury is present, it is more difficult to determine the true extent of the zone of injury. As a result, repair may be improved by delay so that the zone of injury can be determined and all damaged nerve excised. Furthermore, there should not be significant debris mixed with the soft tissue such as one might see from blast injury or large mutilating lacerations/contusions. The injured nerve ideally should be surrounded by normal soft tissue, fat, or muscle.

Overall condition of patient

The absence of associated injuries is obviously preferable. If there are other injuries to the limb in which the peripheral nerve resides, they should be of the type that can be remedied easily at the time of nerve repair. The patient should be metabolically stable enough to warrant the time for elective treatment as opposed to life-saving treatment. Furthermore, the patient must have the ability to give appropriate consent for elective surgery. They should not have an altered metabolic or emotional state, such as that caused by psychiatric problems or drug and alcohol consumption.

Appropriate setting for optimal medical treatment

Nerve repair should be performed with the appropriate microsurgical techniques and personnel trained in these techniques. An operating microscope, microsurgical instruments and sutures, and the ability to perform a tension-free primary repair with accurate coaptation are necessities. If achieving this goal is not possible at the time of primary repair, then the proximal and distal ends of the separate nerves should be tagged to prevent retraction and to allow for easy identification of the injured nerve at the time of reopening.

Surgical technique

Primary nerve repair

Primary nerve repair with suture can be performed as an epineural repair, group fascicular repair, fascicular repair, or a mixture of these (Fig. 4). The initial task of the surgeon is to cut back nerve ends until all visible signs of damage have been débrided and the remaining nerve is normal in appearance and normal to gentle palpation. Palpation of the end of the injured nerve with microforceps often allows for the determination of the swelled or thickened region of the nerve. This procedure can be performed with a number 11 scalpel blade for large nerves and an ophthalmic knife for small nerves. It usually is performed against a wooden disposable sterile tongue depressor. Appropriate preparation of the nerve leads to the visibility of the bands of Fontana and the visibility of individual fascicles at the end.

To properly align the nerve, longitudinal blood vessels in the nerve tissue should be noted. Furthermore, if there is more than one fascicle, an assessment of the arrangement of the fascicles should be made.

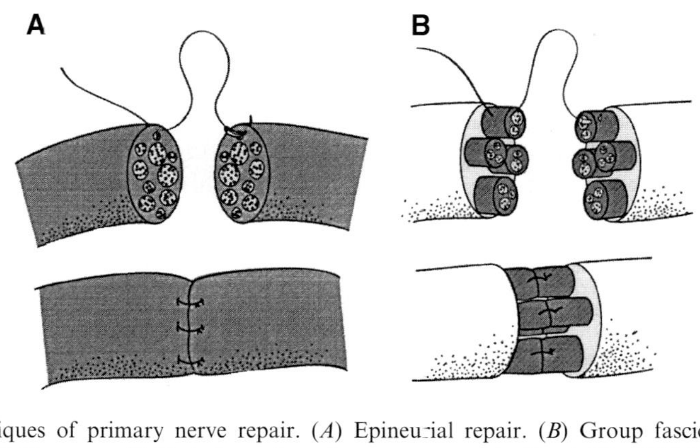

Fig. 4. Various techniques of primary nerve repair. (*A*) Epineurial repair. (*B*) Group fascicular repair. *Used with permission from* Diao E, Vannuyen T. Techniques for primary nerve repair. Hand Clin 2000;16(1):63.

Nonabsorbable sutures should be used for the neurorrhaphy. Depending on the caliber of the nerve, the finest caliber suture that prevents nerve retraction should be used. In the digital nerve, 9-0 or 10-0 nylon usually is used and in the large nerves 8-0 is used.

Epineurial repair

Epineurial repair is the most traditional method of nerve repair. This method is ideal for sharp nerve lacerations with no loss of nerve substance and for partial nerve lacerations when the proper alignment of the nerve is established already (Hurst et al., 1991). In this method, it is the external epineurium surrounding the entire nerve that receives the sutures. If the number of fascicles is limited to one or a few, then epineural repair can be used to coapt the epineurium that surrounds the fascicle. Otherwise individual fascicles are not handled at the level of the repair itself.

Epineurial repair depends on the accurate placement of the suture in the epineurium but not in the nerve fascicle itself. The appropriate tension is the tension at which the underlying fascicles are coapted but not so tightly that there is a misalignment among them. The elasticity of the epineurium determines the amount of closure of the epineurium and the tension of coaptation. As a result, a suture that is applied somewhat loosely can be at the appropriate tension for the nerve tissue in question.

The number of sutures placed depends on the size of the nerve. For a small digital nerve, two or three interrupted simple sutures often provide the appropriate coaptation for a proper repair. Suture caliber can be 6-0, 7-0, or 8-0 for a larger nerve, and 10–12 sutures may be required. Sutures should be placed in an orderly manner. They often are placed with 180° placement of the second suture and then halving sequentially the distance. The backside of the nerve also should be repaired in a similar manner, by rotating the nerve gently with forceps. Suture tails can help facilitate gentle manipulation of the nerve during the repair process.

At completion of a successful epineurial repair, the epineurium should be closed and there should not be any herniation of fascicular tissue between the sutures.

Group fascicular repair

Group fascicular repair is most appropriate for a large nerve with multiple fascicles. This method is also useful when there is a crush component to the injury or when the repair requires the trimming of the nerve ends because of delay. This method consists of grouping the fascicles together and repairing these groups separately. Suturing the fascicular groups optimizes the alignment of the nerve without requiring an excess number of sutures. Too many sutures may contribute to scarring at the site of nerve repair and to foreign body response [12].

Before placing sutures, the fascicular groups must be identified and placed in groups. Groups of fascicles then would be joined together by interfascicular epineural sutures. These sutures generally would be of finer caliber than those used for epineural repair alone. Matching of the groups is based on the preservation of fascicular groups in the proximal and distal nerve stumps. This type of repair is suitable for nerves in which the known topography does not have fascicular crossover. Examples include those in the distal ulnar or median nerves or the radial nerve at the elbow [2,13–15].

Individual fascicular repair

Repair of individual fascicles is at times possible and preferred by the surgeon. Dissection is performed the same way as outlined previously for this method. There are, however, additional steps necessary for the isolation of the individual internal epineurium separating individual fascicles. The repair is done after trimming the appropriate segments of the nerve, if this has not been done before, and joining the fascicular stumps. This type of repair therefore must be performed with minimal tension. Number 10-0 sutures are used; larger caliber sutures could interfere significantly with nerve regeneration. Larger sutures also could cause deleterious scarring. In the case in which tension is present, the tension could be relieved by the placement of epineurial sutures that can be placed first and then the individual fascicular 10-0 sutures.

Fascicle matching techniques

Several techniques enhance the surgeon's ability to match fascicles in the proximal and distal nerve stumps after nerve injury. These techniques work best by separating the sensory and motor fascicles in a mixed nerve.

In the patient who is awake and comfortable with participation in the refining process, intraoperative nerve stimulation is used. The surgery must be performed under local anesthesia. The wound then is débrided and the fascicles are isolated. At this point the tourniquet is deflated for 15 minutes to reverse nerve ischemia and local anesthesia is used at the level of the wound. Before stimulating the nerve it is best to inform the patient of the feeling of the stimulation. Afterward a stimulus of 0.2–0.5 mA is delivered to the proximal nerve fascicles using a nerve stimulator. The stimulation of a motor in the proximal nerve segments would lead to no response at low intensities and vague responses of pain at high intensities. The stimulation of a proximal sensory fascicle, however, leads to a sensation that is localized to a portion of the hand or upper extremity. The patient's verbalization of the anatomic area in which the sensation appeared and the elicitation of the sensations can lead to the creation of a sensory map of the nerves. The appropriate distal nerve also needs to be identified to ensure optimal nerve coaptation.

When the motor nerve is stimulated, the stimulation of the distal nerve produces a motor contraction. This motor contraction only occurs in the first few days after injury, however. Intraoperative nerve stimulation therefore is used in positively identifying proximal sensory fascicles and, in ideal circumstances, distal motor fascicles. It is ideal if the surgeon can appropriately match nerve fascicles: motor proximal to motor distal and sensory proximal to sensory distal, which leads to the best eventual reconstitution of neurophysiology.

Besides intraoperative nerve stimulation, a histochemical technique also exists for the identification of motor and sensory fibers. This technique includes the detection of acetylcholinesterase and carbonic anhydrase through histochemical means. Acetylcholine esterase is a neurotransmitter involved at motor endplates. As a result, it is present in myelinated motor axons but not in myelinated sensory axons. Carbonic anhydrase is found in myelin and axoplasm of myelinated sensory axons but not in myelinated motor axons.

Small samples from proximal and distal cut ends of the nerve are needed for histochemical identification. The process (which usually takes 1–2 hours) can be used to determine which cross-sectional fascicles are predominantly sensory or motor. A gross determination of the nature of the nerve, sensory or motor, therefore can be made at the level of the nerve injury. Having this information allows the surgeon to line up the gross anatomy of the various fascicles to enhance the appropriate maximal coaptation of like fascicles. Because of the logistical issues surrounding the methods discussed, however, the vast majority of surgeons still rely on the traditional methods of dissection and magnification to perform their primary nerve repair.

References

[1] MacKinnon SE, Dellon AL. Anatomy and physiology of the peripheral nerve. In: MacKinnon SE, Dellon AL, editors. Surgery of the peripheral nerve. New York: Thieme Medical Publishers; 1988. p. 1–33.

[2] Sunderland S. Nerves and nerve injuries. New York: Churchill Livingstone; 1978.

[3] Millesi H. The nerve gap. Theory and clinical practice. Hand Clin 1986;2:651–63.

[4] MacKinnon SE, Dellon AL. Classification of nerve injuries as the basis for treatment. In: MacKinnon SE, Dellon AL, editors. Surgery of the peripheral nerve. New York: Thieme Medical Publishers; 1988. p. 35–63.

[5] Bolesta MJ, Garrett WE Jr, et al. Immediate and delayed neurorrhaphy in a rabbit model: a functional, histologic, and biochemical comparison. J Hand Surg [Am] 1988;13:352–7.

[6] Grabb WC. Median and ulnar nerve suture. An experimental study comparing primary and secondary repair in monkeys. J Bone Joint Surg [Am] 1968;50:964–72.

[7] Van Beek A, Glover JL, et al. Primary versus delayed primary neurorrhaphy in rat sciatic nerve. J Surg Res 1975;18: 335–9.

[8] Birch R, Raji AR. Repair of median and ulnar nerves. Primary suture is best. J Bone Joint Surg [Br] 1991;73:154–7.

[9] Marsh D, Barton N. Does the use of the operative microscope improve the results of peripheral nerve suture? J Bone Joint Surg [Br] 1987;69:625–30.

[10] Merle M, Amend P, et al. Microsurgical repair of peripheral nerve lesions. Periph Nerve RepRegen 1986;2:17–26.

[11] Vastamäki M, Kallio PK, et al. The results of secondary microsurgical repair of ulnar nerve injury. J Hand Surg [Br] 1993;18:323–6.

[12] Trumble TE, McCallister WV. Physiology and repair of peripheral nerves. In: Trumble TE, editor. Principles of hand surgery and therapy. Philadelphia: WB Saunders; 2000. p. 279–96.

[13] Chow JA, Van Beek AL, et al. Surgical significance of the motor fascicular group of the ulnar nerve in the forearm. J Hand Surg [Am] 1985;10(6 Pt 1):867–72.

[14] Chow JA, Van Beek AL, et al. Anatomical basis for repair of ulnar and median nerves in the distal part of the forearm by group fascicular suture and nerve grafting. J Bone Joint Surg [Am] 1986;68:273–80.

[15] Jabaley ME, Wallace WH, et al. Internal topography of major nerves of the forearm and hand: a current view. J Hand Surg [Am] 1976;1:119–30.

ELSEVIER
SAUNDERS

Atlas Hand Clin 10 (2005) 73–92

Atlas of the
HAND
CLINICS

A Practical Approach to Nerve Grafting in the Upper Extremity

David J. Slutsky, MD, FRCS(C)

Private Practice, South Bay Hand Surgery Center, 3475 Torrance Boulevard, Suite F, Torrance, CA 90503, USA

In this era of tissue bioengineering an autogenous nerve graft may be considered the ultimate biocompatible, resorbable nerve conduit, with a basil lamina, preformed guidance channels, a reserve of viable Schwann cells, and nerve growth factors. In addition, it is capable of developing an intrinsic circulation. The nerve graft provides a regenerating axon with a means for passage to the distal nerve stump, while protecting it from the surrounding environment. There is no foreign body reaction and no graft-versus-host response. An enterprising biotechnology company undoubtedly would have no difficulty marketing this product. The results obtained with nerve autografts constitute the gold standard by which nerve conduits are designed and measured. Despite this seemingly utopian picture, the donor site morbidity and the limitations of nerve grafting have led to a search for alternate methods. This search has been addressed eloquently by Strauch and Chui and their coauthors elsewhere in this issue. This article focuses on the ways in which the nerve responds to injury and how it regenerates, followed by some practical considerations for autologous nerve grafting.

Nerve response to injury

Cell body

The neuron consists of a central cell body, located within the central nervous system, and a peripheral axon. The axon represents a tremendously elongated process attached to the nerve cell body. Thousands of axons make up the substance of a peripheral nerve. The axon contains 90% of the axoplasmic volume. When a nerve is severed, one immediate consequence is loss of this vital fluid [1]. The normal retrograde transport of neurotrophic factors from the target organ ceases. The cell body undergoes chromatolysis, which includes mitochondrial swelling, migration of the nucleus to the periphery, and dispersal of Nissl substance. The more proximal the site of transection, the more intense the reaction, which peaks by 2 to 3 weeks. The cell body may die and is lost from the neuron pool. If it survives, however, the cell body shifts its resources toward replacing the axoplasm and rebuilding the axon.

Distal axon

The distal axon cannot survive without its connection to the cell body and disintegrates (ie, wallerian degeneration). Endoneurial edema occurs within a few hours [2]. The microtubules and neurofilaments of the distal axon, which are responsible for axoplasmic transport, undergo proteolysis by a calcium-activated neutral protease [3]. At 72 hours, the Schwann cells can be seen digesting the myelin sheath and axonal subcomponents [4]. Endoneurial collagen

E-mail address: d-slutsky@msn.com

1082-3131/05/$ - see front matter
doi:10.1016/j.ahc.2004.09.005

production from Schwann cells and fibroblasts increases, causing progressive shrinkage of the distal tubules [5]. The Schwann cells rapidly proliferate, forming columns (the bands of Büngner) that appear to stimulate the direction and magnitude of axonal growth.

Proximal axon

After transection, there is demyelination of the distal stump. The axons degenerate to one or more proximal internodes. The distance varies with the severity of injury, ranging from a few millimeters with mild trauma to several centimeters with severe injury [6]. The endoneurial tube lies empty, consisting mostly of the Schwann cell basal lamina.

Axon regeneration

Nerve regeneration does not involve mitosis and multiplication of nerve cells. Instead the cell body restores nerve continuity by growing a new axon. Axon sprouting has been shown 24 hours after nerve transection. One axon sends out multiple unmyelinated axon sprouts from the tip of the remaining axon or collateral sprouts from a nearby proximal node of Ranvier. The distal sprout contains the growth cone; this sends out filopodia [7], which adhere to sticky glycoprotein molecules in the basil lamina of Schwann cells, such as laminin and fibronectin (neurite-promoting factors) [8]. The filopodia contain actin, which aids in pulling the growth cone distally [9]. The basil lamina of two abutting Schwann cells forms a potential endoneurial tube into which the regenerating axon grows. These axons deteriorate if a connection with a target organ is not reached. There are 50 advancing sprouts from one axon. Initially, there are many more nerve fibers crossing a nerve repair than in the parent nerve [10]. Although more than one axon may enter the same endoneurial tube, there is eventual resorption of the multiple sprouts, leaving one dominant axon.

Axons grow 1 to 2 mm/day [11]. The normal 16-day turnover rate of acetylcholine receptors is shortened in denervated muscle to about 4 days [12]. For practical purposes, the maximum length that a nerve can grow to restore motor function is approximately 35 cm. This fact in part accounts for the poor motor recovery when grafting nerve defects proximal to the elbow in adults. Sensory end organs remain viable because there is no end plate and retain the potential for reinnervation [13]. Nerve grafting a digital nerve defect may provide protective sensation even after many years.

Role of the Schwann cell

The importance of maintaining Schwann cell viability in the nerve graft is evident. After nerve transection, the Schwann cell removes the axonal and myelin debris in the severed nerve ends and the nerve graft. Schwann cells produce an immediate source of nerve growth factor, which helps to support the proximal stump [14,15]. The Schwann cell expresses nerve growth factor receptors, which aid in directing the advancing growth cone [16]. It also increases its production of other neurotrophic factors, including ciliary neurotrophic factor, brain-derived neurotrophic factor, and fibroblast growth factor, which promote axonal growth [17]. The laminin and fibronectin in the Schwann cell basil lamina act as a rail for the advanced axon sprouts to grow down. The Schwann cell produces a myelin sheath for the immature axon sprout. Cell biologists have attempted to mimic these functions by incorporating Schwann cells, laminin, fibronectin, and nerve growth factors into synthetically engineered nerve conduits.

Role of the nerve graft

The nerve graft acts to provide a source of empty endoneurial tubes through which the regenerating axons can be directed. Any tissue that contains a basil lamina, such as freeze-dried muscle or tendon, can be substituted [18], but only the autogenous nerve graft also provides a source of viable Schwann cells. To be effective, the graft must acquire a blood supply. If the nerve graft survives, the Schwann cells also survive [19].

Graft incorporation

When separated from its blood supply, the graft undergoes wallerian degeneration. Schwann cells can survive 7 days, depending purely on diffusion [19a]. By 3 days after implantation, there is invasion of the nerve graft by endothelial buds from the surrounding tissue bed, with evidence of high nerve blood flows by 1 week [20,21]. This segmental vascular sprouting from extraneural vessels is not limited by the length of the graft [22,23]. The length of the graft is, within certain limits, of no significance to the end result, provided that there is a tension-free anastomosis [24]. The ingrowth of vessels from the ends of the graft (inosculation) does not seem to be of major importance, unless the recipient bed is poorly vascularized [23]. The late phase of nerve graft incorporation shows migration of Schwann cells from the proximal nerve end into the graft and from the graft into both host nerve ends [25].

Graft diameter

Small-diameter grafts spontaneously revascularize, but large-diameter grafts do so incompletely [26]. Thick grafts undergo central necrosis with subsequent endoneurial fibrosis. This fibrosis ultimately impedes the advancement of any ingrowing axon sprouts. Cable nerve grafts are similar to thick grafts. They consist of numerous nerve grafts that are sutured or glued together to match the caliber of the recipient nerve. Because a large percentage of the surface is in contact with another graft and not in contact with the recipient bed, the central portions may not revascularize. With large-diameter recipient nerves, it is preferable to use multiple smaller caliber grafts to bridge fascicular groups in the proximal and distal stumps to increase the surface area that is in contact with the recipient bed.

Nerve biomechanics

A normal nerve has longitudinal excursion, which subjects it to a certain amount of stress and strain in situ. Peripheral nerve is initially easily extensible. It rapidly becomes stiff with further elongation as a result of the stretching of the connective tissue within the nerve [27]. Chronically injured nerves become even stiffer [28]. Elasticity decreases by 50% in the delayed repair of nerves in which wallerian degeneration has occurred [29]. Experimentally, blood flow is reduced by 50% when the nerve is stretched 8% beyond its in vivo length. Complete ischemia occurs at 15% [30]. Suture pullout does not occur until a 17% increase in length; this suggests that ischemia and not disruption of the anastomosis is the limiting factor in acute nerve repairs [31]. This observation also is applicable to nerve grafting.

Nerve is a viscoelastic tissue in that when low loading in tension is applied over time, the nerve elongates, without a deterioration in nerve conduction velocities. Stress relaxation results in recovery of blood flow within 30 minutes at 8% elongation [29]. Intriguing experimental work has been done with gradual nerve elongation to overcome nerve gaps using tissue expansion [32] and external fixation [33], but this cannot be considered an accepted standard of treatment as yet.

A normal nerve can compensate for the change in length with limb flexion and extension because it is surrounded by gliding tissue that permits longitudinal movement. The change in length is distributed over the entire nerve so that the elongation of each nerve segment is small. A nerve graft becomes welded to its recipient bed by the adhesions through which it becomes vascularized. As a consequence, the nerve graft is exquisitely sensitive to tension because it has no longitudinal excursion. The harvested length of the graft must be long enough to span the nerve gap without tension while the adjacent joints are extended; this is also the position of temporary immobilization. If the limb or digit is immobilized with joint flexion, the graft becomes fixed in this position. When the limb is mobilized at 8 days, the proximal and distal stumps are subject to tension even though the graft initially was long enough. Early attempts at lengthening the graft lead to disruption of the anastomosis.

Grafting versus primary repair

A tension-free repair is the goal for any nerve anastomosis. When there is a clean transection of the nerve and the gap is caused by elastic retraction, an acute primary repair is indicated. When treatment of a nerve laceration is delayed, fibrosis of the nerve ends prevents approximation, and nerve grafting is indicated even though there is no loss of nerve tissue. As a general rule, primary nerve repair yields superior results to nerve grafting, provided that there is no tension across the anastomotic site [34]. Grafting can obtain similar results to primary repair under ideal conditions [35]. If a nerve is repaired under tension, however, the results are superior with an interpositional graft [36]. Axon sprouts are able to cross two tension-free anastomotic sites more easily than crossing one anastomosis that is under tension [37].

Nerve grafting is indicated to bridge a defect when greater than 10% elongation of the nerve would be necessary to bridge the gap [29]. This is a better indication for grafting than the nerve gap per se, although 4 cm is often used as the critical defect for grafting in the limb [38]. Defects less than this may be overcome by nerve rerouting and transposition in some instances.

Nerve gap

There is a difference between the nerve gap and a nerve defect. A *nerve gap* refers to the distance between the nerve ends, whereas a *nerve defect* refers to the actual amount of nerve tissue that is lost. With simple nerve retraction after division, the fascicular arrangement is similar. As the defect between the proximal and distal stumps increases, there is a greater fascicular mismatch between the stumps, which leads to poorer outcomes. Gaps greater than 5 cm have been reported to affect the result adversely [39].

Considerations for donor nerve grafts

Many conditions must be met for a nerve to be considered as a potential graft. First, the relationship between the surface area and the diameter of the graft must be optimal to allow rapid revascularization. The donor site defect from sacrifice of any given nerve must be acceptable for the patient. The harvested nerve must be long enough to ensure a tension-free anastomosis with the adjacent joints in full extension. Finally, the cross-sectional area and number of fascicles should match those of the recipient nerve at the level of injury as closely as possible. For these reasons, most of the available grafts are cutaneous nerves.

Most donor grafts are imperfect matches of the recipient nerve. The fascicular arrangement of the nerve graft is dissimilar to the nerve being repaired in size, number, and fascicular topography. The branching pattern of the grafts usually changes from an oligofascicular pattern proximally to a polyfascicular pattern distally, which typically corresponds to the branching pattern of the recipient nerve. There may be some loss of axon sprouts owing to growth down peripheral branches that leave the nerve graft. Some authors have recommended inserting the grafts in a retrograde manner for this reason, but others belief this is not warranted [24]. The choice of nerve graft is dictated by the length of the nerve gap, the cross-sectional area of the recipient nerve, the available expendable donor nerves for that particular nerve injury, and the surgeon's preference.

Donor nerve grafts

As a general rule, it is good practice to divide the donor nerve in an intermuscular plane rather than in the subcutaneous tissue to diminish the risk of a painful neuroma. Innovative surgeons continue to provide novel ways in which to bridge nerve gaps, such as using the fascicular group to the third web space as a source of nerve graft material for bridging median nerve gaps [40] and the distal anterior interosseous nerve to reconstruct neuromas of the recurrent motor branch of the median nerve [41]. Some commonly used donor nerves are summarized here.

Upper extremity grafts

Medial antebrachial cutaneous nerve

The medial antebrachial cutaneous nerve (MABCN) arises from either the medial cord or the lower trunk of the brachial plexus. It travels down the arm medial to the brachial artery, then pierces the deep fascia with the basilic vein about the middle of the arm. More than 90% of the time, the MABCN bifurcates into anterior and posterior branches proximal to the medial epicondyle [42], which provide sensation to the medial forearm and posteromedial elbow. It is preferable to use the anterior branch to avoid a bothersome sensory loss over the elbow. The anterior branch crosses the elbow between the medial epicondyle and the biceps tendon usually in front of the cubital vein, then travels superficial to the flexor carpi ulnaris muscle, ending 10 cm from the wrist. It is approached through an anteromedial incision on the proximal forearm. It provides a graft of 20 cm.

Lateral antebrachial cutaneous nerve

The lateral antebrachial cutaneous nerve (LABCN) is the distal continuation of the musculocutaneous nerve. It exits from underneath the biceps tendon, then divides into anterior and posterior branches at the elbow crease. The donor site defect corresponds to the anterolateral forearm, but it also may innervate the volar radial or dorsoradial thumb. For this reason, it is not harvested for grafting a sensory nerve deficit to the thumb [43]. There is a partial or complete overlap of the sensory territory of the superficial radial nerve 75% of the time [44]. The nerve is approached through an anterolateral incision on the proximal forearm, as it passes deep to the cephalic vein (Fig. 1). The LABCN provides a nerve graft of 5 to 8 cm.

Posterior cutaneous nerve of the forearm

The posterior cutaneous nerve of the forearm (PCNF) is a sensory branch of the radial nerve that rarely may be used as a source of graft material. It arises from the radial nerve in the spiral groove and pierces the lateral head of the triceps. It descends the lateral side of the arm, then travels down the dorsal forearm to the wrist, where it communicates with terminal branches of the LABCN. It supplies sensation to the posterolateral forearm. It is identified via a dorsolateral incision at the elbow between the junction of the brachioradialis and the extensor carpi radialis longus. The PCNF provides 2 to 5 cm of graft material [45].

Superficial radial nerve

The superficial radial nerve (SRN) is prone to painful neuroma formation after trauma; it is not a first-line choice of graft. It may be used for proximal radial nerve injuries, where it is excluded from grafting, unless it can be separated from the motor fibers; this is to prevent any regenerating motor nerve fibers from being misdirected to cutaneous reinnervation. The SRN separates from the radial nerve just distal to the elbow in the front of the lateral epicondyle, then descends behind the brachioradialis along the lateral side of the upper forearm. It branches into a major palmar and dorsal branch. The SRN can be identified through a dorsolateral incision approximately 7 cm from the wrist, where it winds around the tendon of the brachioradialis to pierce the deep fascia. The area of hypoesthesia corresponds to the dorsum of the thumb and adjacent sides of the first and second web space. It can provide a nerve graft of 15 to 20 cm.

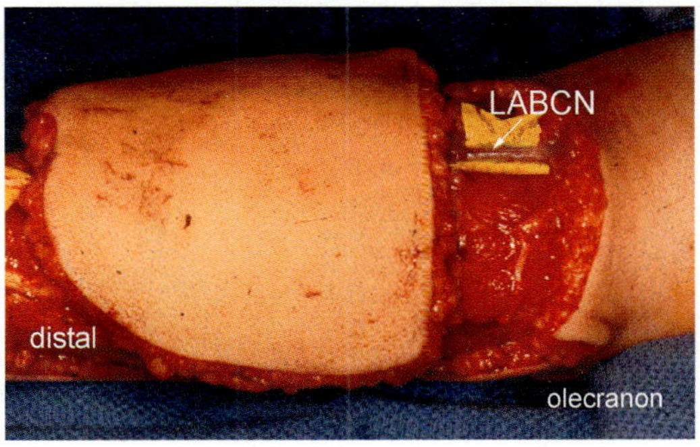

Fig. 1. Isolation of the LABCN while harvesting a radial forearm flap.

Dorsal cutaneous branch of the ulnar nerve

The dorsal cutaneous branch of the ulnar nerve (DCBUN) is an uncommon source of nerve graft that has been employed with clinical success. It is an appropriate size and length for use as a digital nerve graft. It can be identified at its takeoff from the main ulnar nerve, 5 cm proximal to the wrist. It passes distally under cover of the flexor carpi ulnaris (FCU), then perforates the deep fascia. It runs along the dorsomedial aspect of the wrist and hand before dividing into two to three dorsal digital branches. The area of sensory loss corresponds to the dorsal ulnar aspect of the carpus and proximal parts of the ring and small fingers. Painful neuroma formation or loss of hand function related to the use of this nerve is not typical [46]. The nerve can be approached through a dorsomedial incision centered over the distal radioulnar joint. The DCBUN provides a graft of 4 to 6 cm (see Fig. 2).

Posterior interosseous nerve

The terminal portion of the posterior interosseous nerve (PIN) provides proprioception to the joint capsule. Harvesting the nerve leaves no apparent motor or sensory deficit. The PIN lies adjacent to the posterior interosseous artery on the dorsal surface of the interosseous membrane, deep to the fourth extensor compartment. It ranges from 1 to 5 mm and contains one to five fascicles. It is a good match for grafting digital nerve defects at the distal interphalangeal joint (DIP) [47]. The nerve can be located through a dorsal wrist incision just proximal to Lister's tubercle, developing the plane between the third and fourth extensor compartments. The mean length of the PIN from its terminal expansion at the wrist to its most distal muscular branch (to the extensor pollicus longus) is 6 cm [48].

Anterior interosseous nerve

The terminal portion of the anterior interosseous nerve (AIN) also provides proprioception to the joint capsule. Harvesting the nerve similarly leaves no apparent motor or sensory deficit. The nerve is located adjacent to the anterior interosseous artery on the anterior surface of the interosseous membrane, deep to the pronator quadratus. It also can be approached through a dorsal incision as for the PIN, after excising a window in the interosseous membrane (Fig. 3). The primarily motor fibers of the AIN provide an expendable donor of adequate size and fascicle number suitable for grafting the recurrent motor branch of the median nerve [41] or the deep motor branch of the ulnar nerve at the wrist [49].

Lower extremity grafts

Sural nerve

The sural nerve is a common source of nerve graft material. It is formed from the medial cutaneous sural nerve that originates from the tibial nerve. It descends between the two heads of the gastrocnemius piercing the deep fascia in the upper part of the leg, where it is joined by the

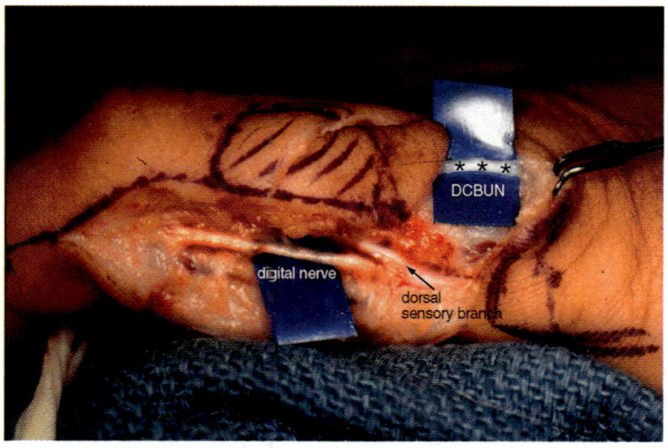

Fig. 2. Dorsal sensory branch arising from the proper digital nerve of the small finger. *Abbreviation:* *(DCBUN), dorsal cutaneous branch of the ulnar nerve.

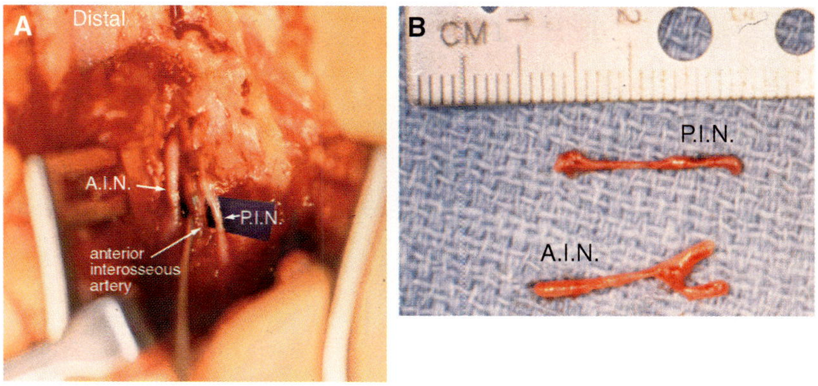

Fig. 3. AIN and PIN grafts. (*A*) Intraoperative photo of PIN. A window in the interosseous membrane allowed isolation of the AIN. (*B*) Typical size of harvested grafts.

lateral sural cutaneous branch off the peroneal nerve. It then passes downward near the lateral margin of the Achilles tendon to the interval between the lateral malleolus and the calcaneus. After giving off a medial calcaneal branch, it runs forward, below the lateral malleolus, and is continued along the lateral side of the foot. It supplies the skin of the lateral and posterior part of the lower one third of the leg. To harvest the nerve, the patient is positioned supine on the operating table, with a sandbag placed at midcalf level. The leg is flexed with the foot on the sandbag to maintain the flexed knee position. The nerve is located via a longitudinal incision that is 1 cm posterior and superior to the lateral malleolus, where it often is accompanied by the lesser saphenous vein. Traction is placed on the nerve until it can be palpated 3 cm proximally, then a second transverse incision is made. In this manner, the nerve is followed as high as the popliteal fossa by dividing all of the sural communicating branches. The sural nerve provides graft lengths of 30 to 40 cm (Fig. 4).

Superficial peroneal nerve

The superficial peroneal nerve generally has been overlooked as a potential donor nerve graft. It is the major lateral branch of the common peroneal nerve that innervates the peroneus longus and brevis muscles and provides sensation to the lateral aspect of the lower leg and dorsal foot. It begins at the bifurcation of the common peroneal nerve between the fibula and the proximal peroneus longus. It then descends on the interosseous membrane with the anterior tibial artery to the front of the ankle joint, where it divides into a lateral and medial terminal branch. It can be located through an anterolateral ankle incision, then followed proximally. It provides a consistently long graft, comparable to the sural nerve. It has been used successfully for grafting of the median, radial, and ulnar nerves, including digital nerve defects. It is of particular use when multiple or long nerve grafts are required [50].

Lateral femoral cutaneous nerve

The lateral femoral cutaneous nerve is an independent branch off the lumbosacral plexus that provides sensation to the anterolateral aspect of the thigh. It pierces the fascia lata 2 cm below and medial to the anterior superior iliac spine. It is approached through an incision medial and inferior to the anterior superior spine. The nerve is identified where it becomes subcutaneous, just distal to the sartorius. It provides a graft 10 to 20 cm long.

Saphenous nerve

The saphenous nerve is the largest cutaneous branch of the femoral nerve. It descends on the lateral side of the femoral artery and enters the adductor canal. It descends along the medial side of the knee, then becomes subcutaneous between the tendons of the sartorius and gracilis. It passes down the medial side of the leg next to the saphenous vein. It divides into a medial and lateral branch in the lower one third of the leg, continuing as far as the great toe. The nerve can be identified through a posteromedial incision adjacent to the long saphenous vein, midway between

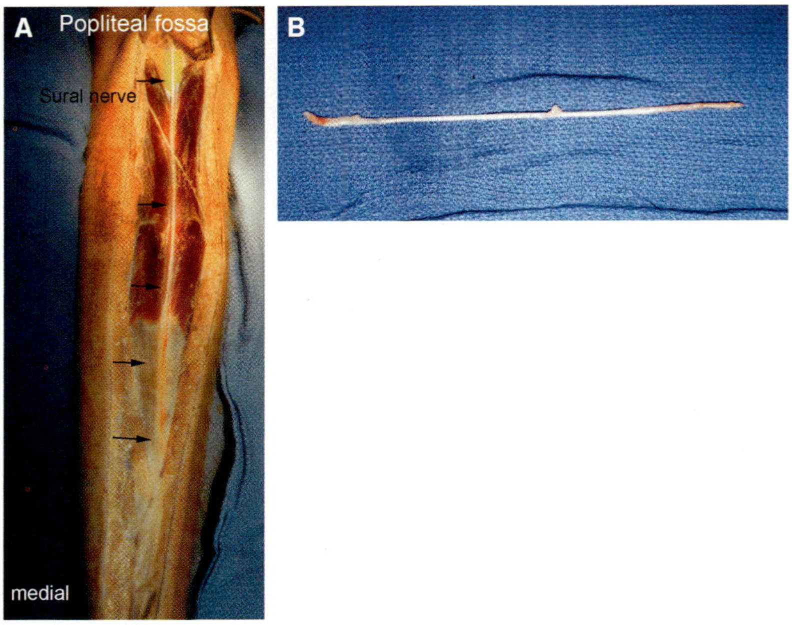

Fig. 4. (*A*) The sural nerve anatomy looking from the posterior aspect of a prone right leg (*arrows*). (*B*) Harvested sural nerve graft.

the medial malleolus and Achilles tendon. It provides a graft of 40 cm in length. It should not be harvested if the sural nerve also is being used because of the large combined donor site defects.

Nerve graft preparation

Millessi [24,51] has written extensively on nerve graft preparation. If the recipient nerve is the approximate diameter of the graft, the two stumps are transected until normal-appearing tissue without fibrosis is seen. The graft is inserted by an epineurial repair. If the recipient nerve is larger than the graft, the fascicular pattern determines the type of preparation. If the nerve contains one to four fascicles, the stump is resected until healthy tissue is encountered. Multiple nerve grafts are used to cover completely the cross-sectional area of each fascicle (ie, 1:2 or 1:3 ratio).

When there are 5 to 12 fascicles that are the size of the nerve graft, each fascicle is grafted individually. When there is a polyfascicular pattern with a group fascicular arrangement, interfascicular dissection is performed to isolate the fascicle groups, which are grafted individually. Millessi recommended sectioning each group of fascicles at different levels to prevent an overlap of the suture lines. If there is no group fascicular arrangement, interfascicular dissection is not performed. Graft insertion is guided by the intraneural topography of the nerve for that specific level of injury.

Motor sensory differentiation

The use of intraoperative motor and sensory nerve differentiation can diminish the risk of fascicular mismatch when grafting a nerve. Available methods are the anatomic method, based on separate identification of groups of fascicles [52–55]; the electrophysiologic method, using awake stimulation [56]; and histochemical methods, which rely on staining for enzymes specific to motor or sensory nerves [57].

Electrical fascicle identification

Awake stimulation requires the cooperation of the anesthesiologist and the patient. It is based on the observation that motor and sensory fascicles can be differentiated by direct stimulation [58]. The median and ulnar nerves in the distal forearm are most amenable to this technique [56]. It is especially useful when there is a nerve defect, owing to the dissimilar fascicular pattern between the proximal and distal nerve ends. The initial nerve dissection is performed under a regional block with tourniquet control. The wound is infiltrated with local anesthetic before release of the tourniquet. After 20 minutes, the patient is awakened. A low-amperage stimulator is applied to the major fascicles of the proximal nerve end in a systematic manner, starting at 0.2 to 0.5 mA. Sensory fascicles elicit pain and may be localized to a specific digit. Motor fascicles elicit no response at lower intensities and poorly localized pain at higher intensities. A cross-sectional sketch of the proximal stump is made (Fig. 5). The sensory fascicles are tagged with 10–0 nylon, and the patient is placed under general anesthesia. The distal stump is stimulated in a similar fashion. The reverse picture is seen, with motor fascicles eliciting a muscle twitch and sensory fascicles being silent. A cross-sectional map is made again and used to match the proximal and distal motor and sensory fascicles.

Use of nerve action potentials

Neuromuscular function in humans, as in other mammals, disappears 3 to 5 days after nerve section [59]. The preservation of nerve action potentials for 10 days after nerve transection can be used in place of the muscle twitch to map the distal stump (unpublished data); this prevents the need to dissect the nerve to its distal motor branch. Nerve action potential recordings after acute nerve transection are characterized by diminishing amplitudes with preserved latencies until the action potential is no longer present. The compound motor action potential (CMAP) disappears at 7 to 9 days versus the sensory nerve action potential (SNAP), which disappears at 10 to 11 days [60].

The initial dissection is performed with nitrous oxide because fentanyl can abolish the response. The nerve stimulation is performed after the tourniquet has been deflated for 20 minutes using a pulse width duration of 0.05 ms and a repeat rate of 1 to 2 per second. Averaging is used for small-amplitude nerve action potentials. CMAPs are recorded from the thenar/hypothenar muscles, and SNAPs are recorded from either the index or small finger using ring electrodes (Fig. 6). A grouped fascicular repair is performed as described previously.

In chronic injuries, the awake stimulation of the proximal stump is unchanged. Because the nerve action potentials are no longer present, it is necessary dissect the distal motor branch, then follow the motor fascicles proximally to the nerve stump (Fig. 7).

Nerve lesions in continuity

Electrical stimulation is useful to determine if there are any intact fascicles in a neuroma in continuity [61]. Bipolar hook electrodes are used with the stimulating and recording electrodes separated by at least 4 cm. The stimulus frequency is two to three times per second with a pulse duration of less than 0.1 ms. The intensity is slowly increased to the range where a response is expected (3–15 V). The recorder sensitivity is increased to a maximum of 20 μV/cm. The nerve is stimulated proximal to, across, and below the lesion. It is estimated that there must be at least 4000 myelinated axons for a recordable nerve action potential to conduct through a neuroma

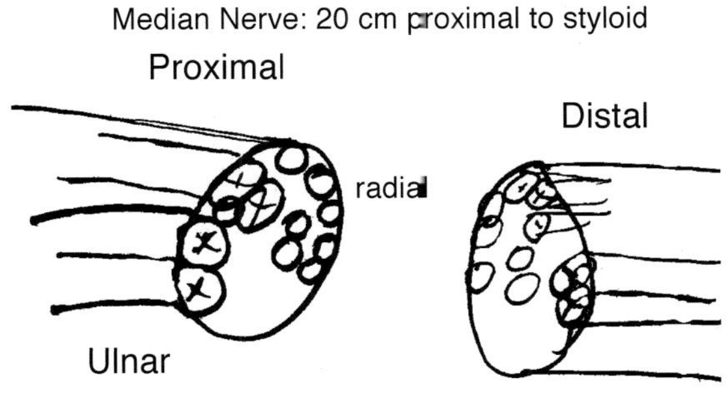

Fig. 5. Intraoperative drawing of fascicular mapping.

(Fig. 8) [62]. A neurolysis is performed to single out any normal-appearing fascicles; this is confirmed electrically. Nonconducting fascicles are excised and grafted.

Grafting specific nerves

Median nerve

Anatomy

The median nerve arises from the medial and lateral cords of the brachial plexus. It contains the nerve root fibers from C6-T1. It provides the motor supply to the pronator teres, the flexor digitorum sublimus, the palmaris longus, the flexor carpi radialis, the thenar muscles, and the radial two lumbricals. Its anterior interosseous branch supplies the flexor pollicus longus, the pronator quadratus, and the flexor digitorum profundus to the index and middle fingers. Its sensory distribution includes the palmar surface of the thumb, index, middle, and radial half of the ring finger. It lies lateral to the axillary artery, but then crosses medial to it at the level of the coracobrachialis. At the elbow, the median nerve travels behind the bicipital aponeurosis but in front of the brachialis. It enters the forearm between the two heads of the pronator teres and is adherent to the undersurface of the flexor digitorum sublimus muscle until it becomes superficial, 5 cm proximal to the wrist. It then passes underneath the carpal transverse ligament, giving off the recurrent motor branch and sensory branches to the thumb and fingers.

Injury at the elbow

The median nerve is located through an S-shaped anteromedial incision at the cubital fossa. The lacertus fibrosus is divided taking care to preserve the LABCN. The median nerve and brachial vein lie medial to the artery. At this level, the motor branches of the median nerve consistently collect into three fascicular groups. There is an anterior group (to the pronator teres and flexor carpi radialis), a middle group (to the flexor digitorum sublimus and hand intrinsics), and a posterior group (to the AIN branch) [63]. These branch groups can be traced proximally without harm, within the main trunk of the median nerve for 2.5 to 10 cm [64].

Injury in the forearm

The median nerve is approached through an S-shaped incision over the volar forearm. The nerve is identified on the undersurface of the sublimus muscle. In the upper third of the forearm, the motor branches usually lie peripherally, typically on the radial and ulnar sides. The motor fascicles from the recurrent motor branch are in a slightly radial position at 100 mm proximal to the radial styloid. The central core of the proximal stump should be connected distally with the motor and sensory components of the hand. Any large identifiable forearm motor branches should be attached about the periphery (Fig. 9).

Injury at the wrist

The median nerve at the wrist has approximately 30 fascicles. The motor recurrent branch often consists of two fascicles, which are situated in a volar position, with the various sensory groups in the radial, ulnar, and dorsal positions. The motor branch can be separated from the main trunk without harm for 100 mm proximal to the thenar muscles [55]. The motor fascicles in the recurrent motor branch are identified where they leave the median nerve trunk, then are followed proximally to the distal nerve end. To maintain motor continuity when there is a median nerve gap at the wrist level, a sural nerve graft should be sutured to the large bifascicular group of fascicles along the volar aspect of the distal stump and connected to a matching radial group of fascicles in the proximal stump (Fig. 10).

Injury in the hand

The median nerve is approached through an extensile carpal tunnel approach, with division of the transverse carpal ligament. The recurrent motor branch most commonly is found distal to the transverse carpal ligament as it enters the thenar muscles (Fig. 11) [65]. The terminal portion of the AIN provides a good-caliber match at this level.

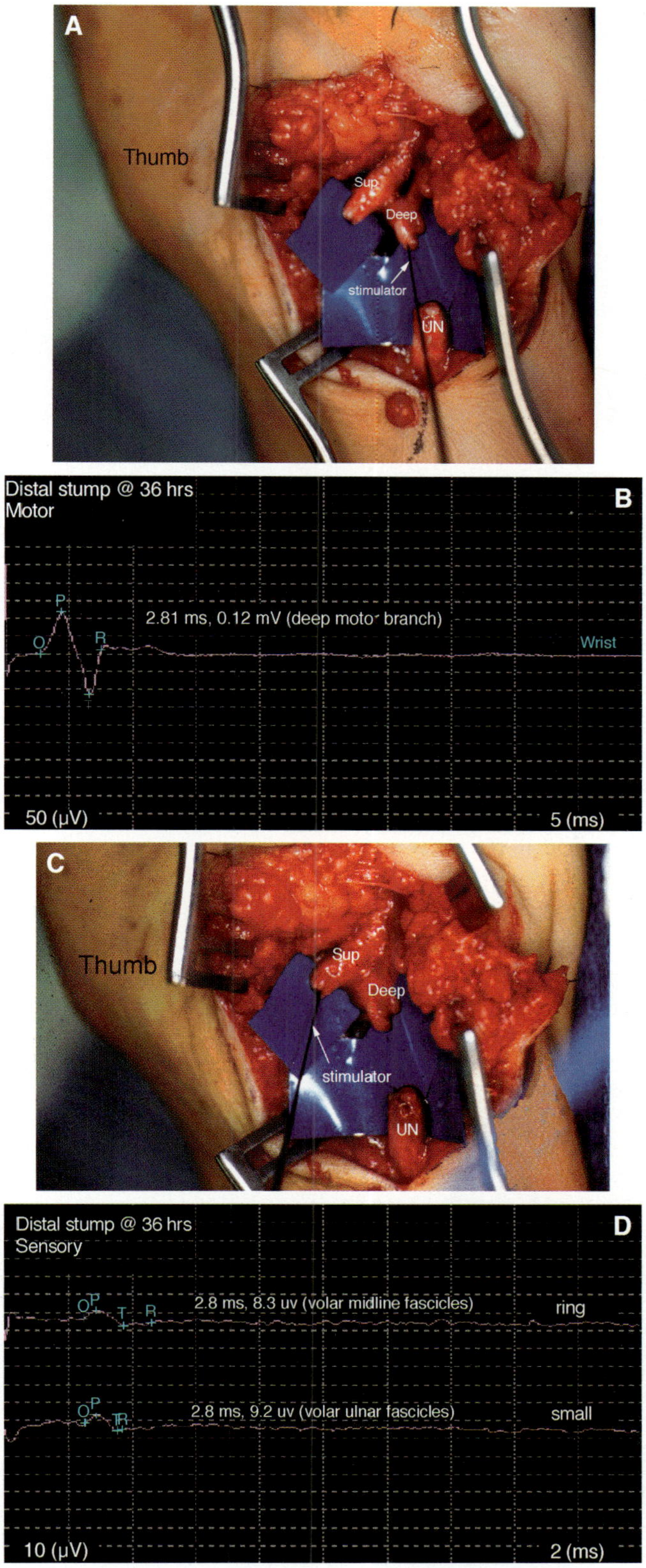

Fig. 6. Intraoperative stimulation of ulnar nerve (UN) at wrist. (*A*) Stimulation of deep motor branch. (*B*) CMAP with normal latency but low amplitude [recorded from abductor digiti minimi (ADM)]. (*C*) Stimulation of superficial (Sup) sensory fascicles. (*D*) SNAPs with normal latencies but low amplitudes (recorded from small and ring fingers).

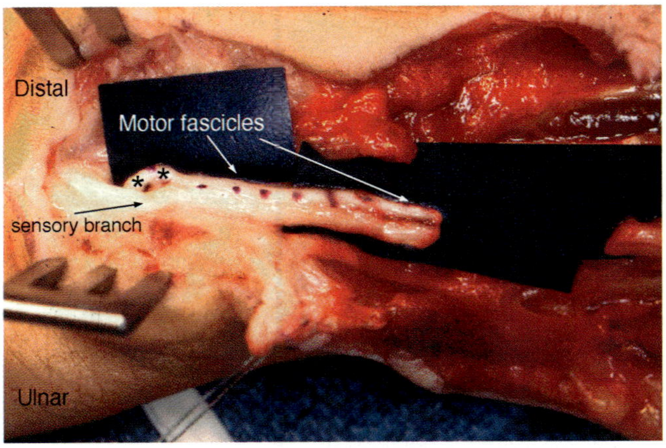

Fig. 7. Ulnar nerve motor fascicles (*arrows*) traced from the distal stump to the deep motor branch in the palm.

The sensory fibers travel within the common digital nerves to the thumb, index finger, and middle finger and the communicating branch to the third web space. The LABCN and MABCN are suitable grafts for nerve gaps at this level (Fig. 12). When the median nerve defect is greater than 5 cm and extends from the wrist to the common digital nerve bifurcation, sural grafts are more appropriate (Fig. 2).

Digits

Many authors recommend nerve grafting when the gap exceeds 1 cm with the wrist and all three finger joints extended [43]. The digital nerves are approached through a midlateral or a volar Brunner incision. The LACBN is a good-caliber match at this level. The dorsal sensory branch that arises from the proper digital nerve also can be used as graft material. This branch most commonly arises proximal to the PIP flexion crease, then crosses superficial or deep to the digital artery to lie just above the extensor mechanism, innervating the dorsum of the middle phalanx [66]. This branch can be provide a 1- to 2-cm nerve graft (see Fig. 2). Distal to the DIP joint, the nerve trifurcates. The terminal PIN is a suitable graft at this level.

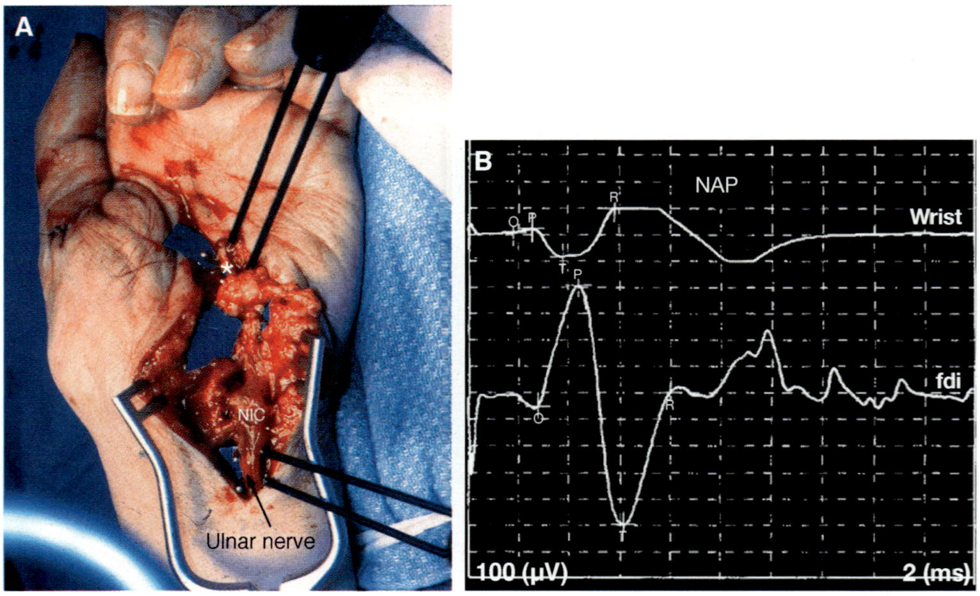

Fig. 8. Neuroma in continuity of ulnar nerve. (*A*) Nerve stimulation with bipolar electrodes proximal to a neuroma-in-continuity (NIC), with recording over a common digital nerve (*). (*B*) Nerve action potential (nerve action potentials) recorded from the common digital nerve (*top tracing*). Nerve stimulation also elicited a CMAP from the first dorsal interosseous (fdi).

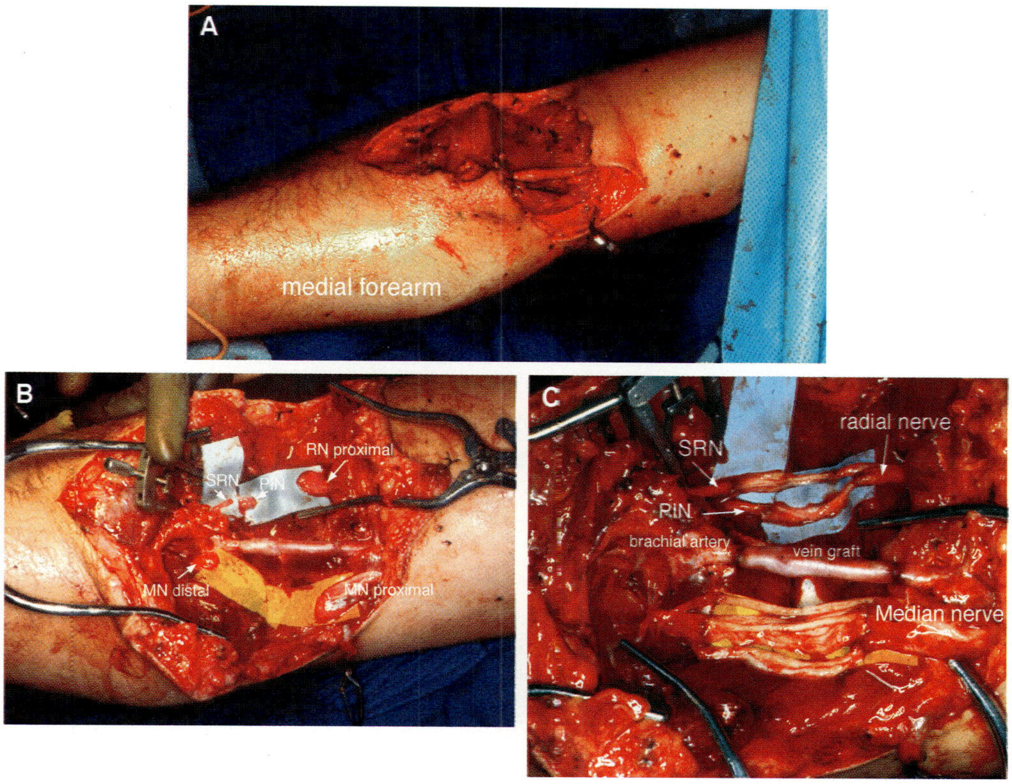

Fig. 9. Proximal median and radial nerve grafts. (*A*) Laceration through antecubital fossa. (*B*) Note median nerve laceration and radial nerve laceration at bifurcation of SRN and PIN. (*C*) Multiple fascicular grafts to median nerve, SRN, and PIN.

Ulnar nerve

Anatomy

The ulnar nerve arises from the medial cord of the brachial plexus. It contains the nerve root fibers from C8-T1. It provides the motor supply to the hypothenar muscles, the ulnar two lumbricals, the interosseous muscles, the adductor pollicis, the FCU, and the profundus to the ring and small fingers. Its sensory distribution includes the palmar surface of the small finger, the ulnar half of the ring finger, and the dorsoulnar carpus. It lies medial to the axillary artery and continues distally to the midarm, where it pierces the medial intermuscular septum. The nerve often is accompanied by the superior ulnar collateral artery. At the elbow, it lies between the medial epicondyle and the olecranon, where it is covered by Osborne's ligament. It enters the forearm between the two heads of the FCU covered by a fibrous aponeurosis (the cubital tunnel). It runs deep to the FCU until the distal forearm. At the wrist, it passes over the transverse carpal ligament, medial to the ulnar artery through Guyon's canal. The deep motor branch is given off at the pisiform and passes underneath a fibrous arch to lie on the palmar surface of the interossei. It crosses the palm deep to the flexor tendons, to terminate in the adductor pollicis and ulnar head of the flexor pollicis brevis.

Injury at the elbow

The ulnar nerve is located through a curved posteromedial incision behind the medial epicondyle. At the elbow, the ulnar nerve contains about 20 fascicles, including the motor branches to the forearm muscles. The motor fascicles to the FCU and the intrinsics are centrally located, whereas the sensory fibers are superficially located. The proximal motor branches to the FCU and flexor digitorum profundus often can be traced for 6 cm before interfascicular connections [54]. It is possible to distinguish between sensory and motor fascicles in the distal nerve end using low-intensity electrical stimulation, if performed within a few days of the injury.

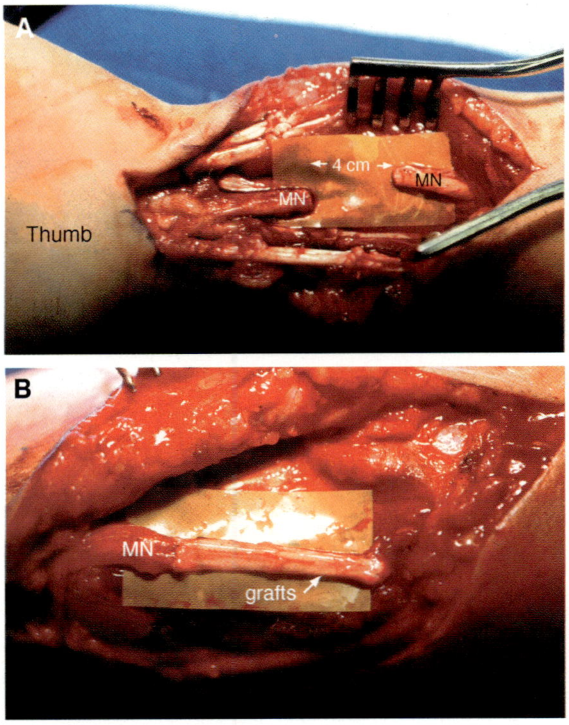

Fig. 10. Median nerve (MN) laceration near wrist. (*A*) A 4-cm defect between MN ends. (*B*) Sural nerve grafts with matching of volar radial fascicle groups.

Occasionally, fascicles innervating the flexor muscles can be separated from fascicles supplying the intrinsic muscles in the hand [67]. The sural nerve commonly is used as graft material at this level (Fig. 13).

Injury in the forearm

The motor fascicles lie dorsal and slightly ulnarly to the sensory fascicles at the wrist level and usually maintain a dorsal relationship as one moves proximally. The motor component remains as a distinct entity 90 mm proximal to the styloid [52]. At 50 to 85 mm proximal to the radial

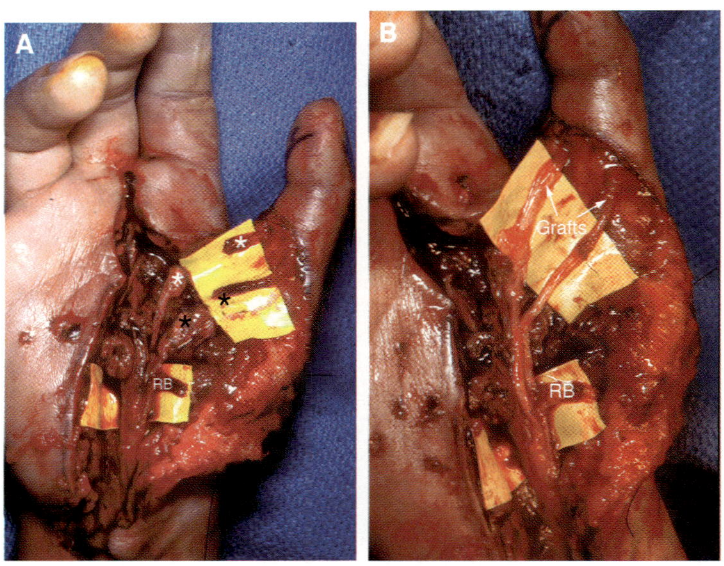

Fig. 11. Median nerve laceration. (*A*) Laceration of median nerve at junction of motor recurrent branch (RB) and digital sensory nerves to the thumb (*). (*B*) Repair of recurrent branch, LABCN grafts to digital nerves.

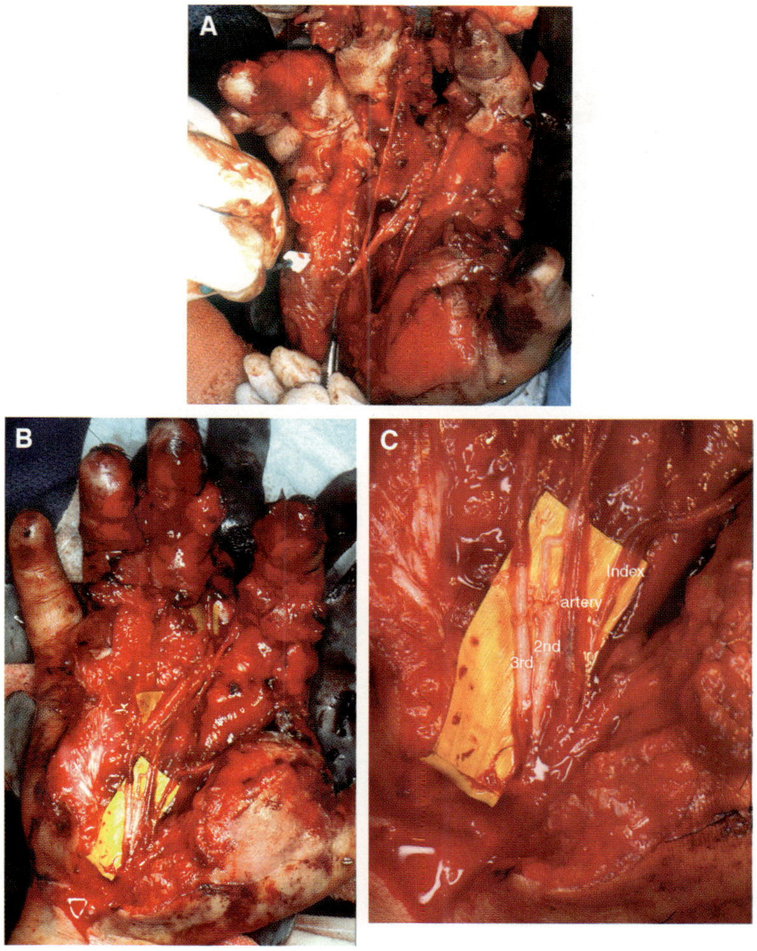

Fig. 12. Blast injury. (*A*) Disrupted common digital nerves and artery (forceps). (*B*) Repair of nerve to index, graft of second and third common digital nerves. (*C*) Close-up view.

styloid, the dorsal sensory branch joins the other groups. At the level of the midforearm, 50 mm from the ulnar styloid, the motor fascicles lie dorsal to the sensory fascicles [55]. A sural nerve graft should be placed in the dorsal quadrant of the proximal nerve end and the dorsoulnar quadrant of the distal nerve end to restore motor continuity.

Injury at the wrist

The ulnar nerve has 15 to 25 fascicles at the wrist. It can be divided into a volar sensory component and a dorsal motor component. The ulnar nerve is approached through an S-shaped incision over the volar ulnar forearm. The nerve is identified medial to the ulnar artery underneath the FCU muscle. If a muscle twitch is no longer present, the motor branch can be traced from the takeoff of the deep motor branch to the distal nerve end (see Fig. 7).

Hand

The nerve is approached through a volar ulnar incision in line with the ring finger. The deep motor and more superficial sensory fascicles are separated easily at this level and allow separate grafting (Fig. 14). The sural nerve, LABCN, or MABCN provides suitable sized grafts. The DCBUN usually is not grafted because neuromas of this nerve are uncommon.

Digits

Grafting in the digits is similar to grafting in the median nerve.

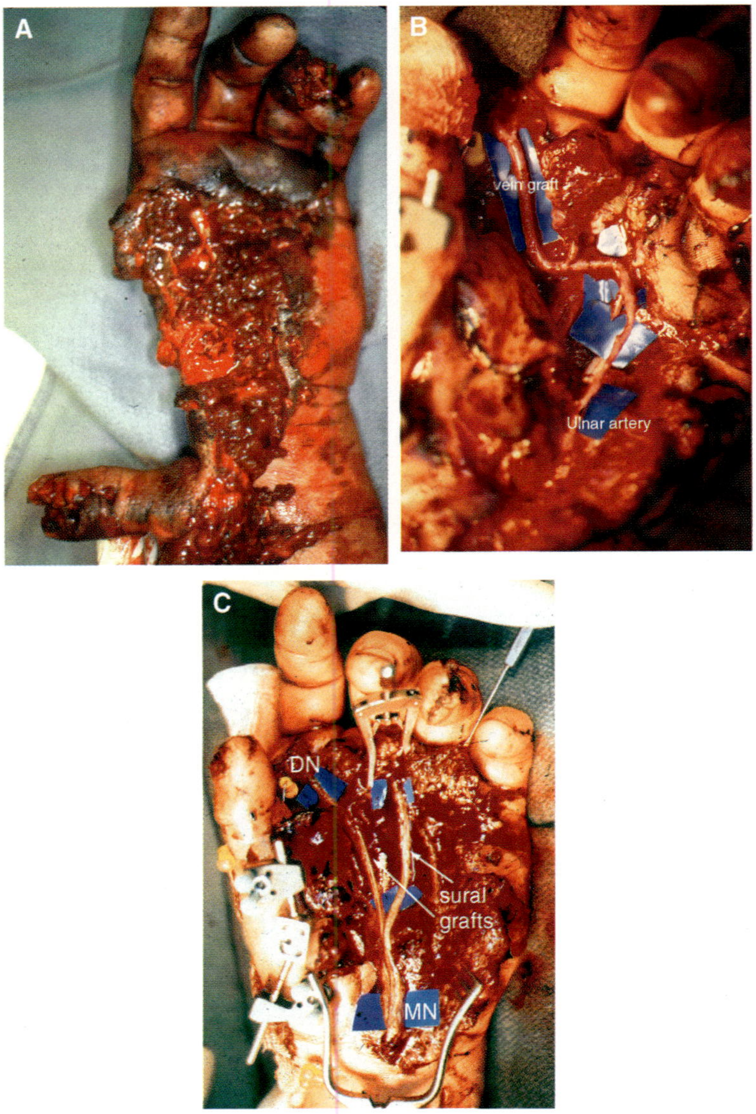

Fig. 13. Avulsion injury. (*A*) Thumb amputation associated with avulsion of the palmar arch and median nerve branches in the palm. (*B*) Thumb replant plus reconstruction of palmar arch with vein graft. (*C*) 12-cm sural nerve grafts from proximal median nerve to digital nerves (DN).

Guidelines for digital nerve graft selection

Higgins et al [68] investigated the fascicular cross-sectional area and number of fascicles of five nerve graft sites to specific digital nerve segments. In the fingertip distal to the DIP, the AIN, PIN, and MABCN all were appropriate choices for caliber-matched grafts. The LABCN was the only similar donor nerve, however, when number of fascicles was assessed. The LABCN also is the best match in caliber and fascicle number for digital nerve deficits from the metacarpophalangeal joint to the DIP joint and from the common digital nerve bifurcation to the metacarpophalangeal joint. The sural nerve was the most appropriate choice when grafting defects between the wrist and the common digital nerve bifurcation, even though there were considerably fewer fascicles and a smaller cross-sectional area than the common digital nerve.

Radial nerve

Anatomy

The radial nerve arises from the posterior cord of the brachial plexus. It receives contributions from C5-8 spinal roots. It runs medial to the axillary artery. At the level of the

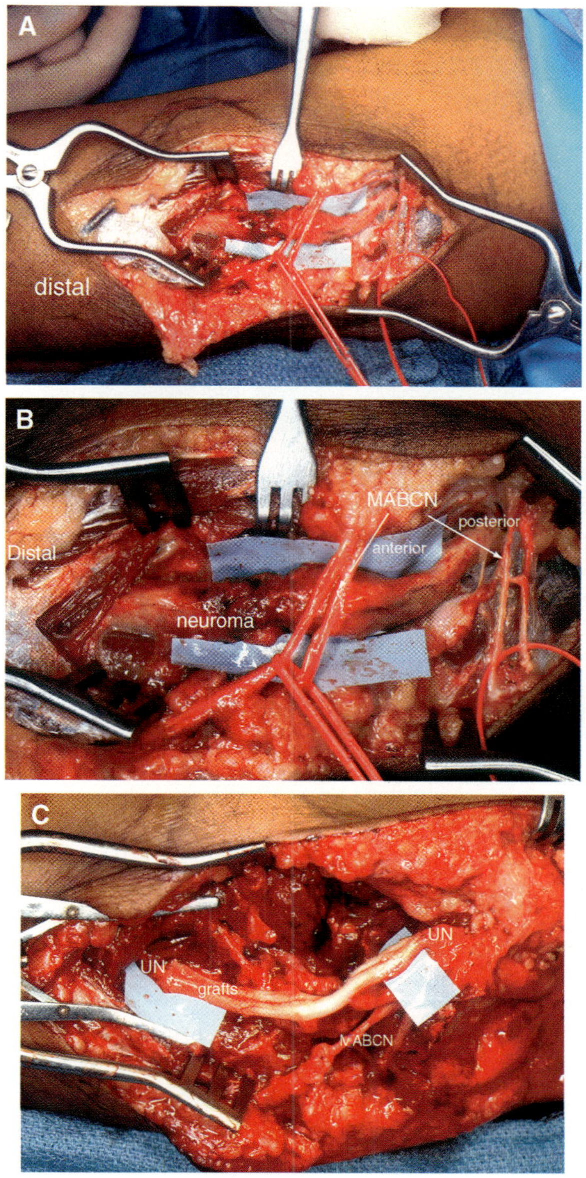

Fig. 14. Neuroma of ulnar nerve at elbow. (*A*) Medial aspect of the right elbow showing an ulnar nerve neuroma. (*B*) Close-up view of neuroma. Note the anterior and posterior branches of the MABCN. (*C*) Sural nerve grafts to ulnar nerve (UN).

coracobrachialis, it courses posteriorly to lie in the spiral groove of the humerus. In the lower arm, it pierces the lateral intermuscular septum to run between the brachialis and the brachioradialis. It divides 2 cm distal to the elbow into a superficial sensory branch and a deep motor branch, the PIN.

The radial nerve gives off branches to the extensor carpi radialis longus and brevis, brachioradialis, and anconeus before giving off the PIN branch. The PIN continues on between the superficial and deep head of the supinator muscle, to exit on the dorsal forearm. After it emerges from the distal border of the supinator, the PIN sends branches to the extensor digitorum communis, extensor carpi ulnaris, extensor digiti quinti, extensor pollicis longus and brevis, and extensor indicis proprius in descending order, although there may be considerable variation [69].

Injury at the elbow

The volar approach to the radial nerve is through an anterolateral incision, developing the intermuscular interval between the brachialis and the brachioradialis. Recurrent branches from

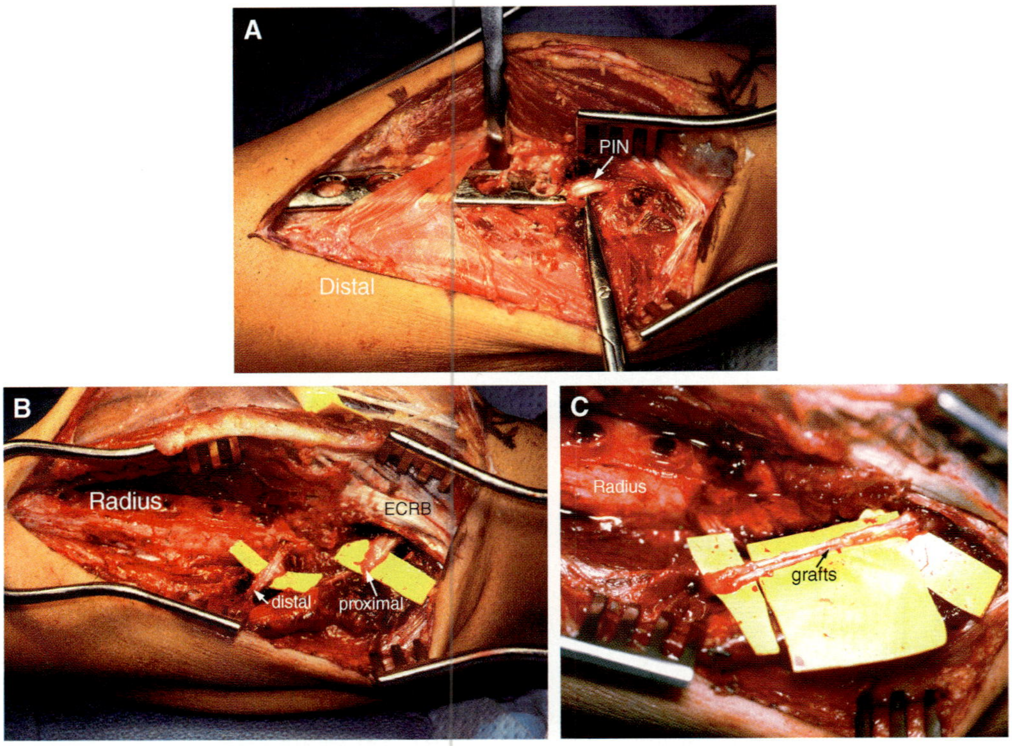

Fig. 15. Posterior Interosseous Nerve (PIN) injury. (*A*) Dorsal approach to left forearm showing a PIN injury after plating of a proximal radius fracture. (*B*) Proximal and distal nerve ends isolated. (*C*) Interposed nerve grafts. ECRL, extensor carpi radialis longus.

the radial artery must be divided to gain access to both nerve branches. Separate grafting of the superficial and deep branch are relatively straightforward (see Fig. 9).

Injury in the forearm and wrist

The PIN nerve is approached through a dorsolateral approach, developing the plane between the extensor carpi radialis brevis and the extensor digitorum communis. At this level, the PIN contains motor fibers only; separate fascicle identification is unnecessary (Fig. 15). The PIN also has a short distance to travel to reinnervate the motor end plates, which accounts for the generally favorable results [70]. Lacerations of the superficial branch in the forearm are not usually grafted, which allows harvest of the SRN for grafting adjacent nerve injuries. Some authors advocate grafting the SRN at the wrist, mostly to prevent symptomatic neuroma formation [71].

Summary

Nerve grafting is a century-old art [72] that is honed by experience and limited only by the imagination. Myriad factors may influence the type of graft and manner in which it is used. A sound knowledge of the intrafascicular topography combined with intraoperative aids for motor and sensory differentiation can lead to superior clinical results, especially with large nerve deficits. The basic tenets of managing the nerve gap will undoubtedly remain in vogue until the results of reinnervation through the use of synthetic conduits can reliably match the time-tested standards of the autogenous nerve graft.

References

[1] Lundborg G. Ischemic nerve injury: experimental studies on intraneural microvascular pathophysiology and nerve function in a limb subjected to temporary circulatory arrest. Scand J Plast Reconstr Surg Suppl 1970;6:3.

[2] Mellick RS, Cavanagh JB. Changes in blood vessel permeability during degeneration and regeneration in peripheral nerves. Brain 1968;91:141.

[3] Badalamente MA, Hurst LC, Stracher A. Calcium-induced degeneration of the cytoskeleton in monkey and human peripheral nerves. J Hand Surg 1986;11B:337.

[4] Haftek J, Thomas PK. Electron-microscope observations on the effects of localized crush injuries on the connective tissues of peripheral nerve. J Anat 1968;103:233.

[5] Thomas PK. Changes in the endoneurial sheaths of peripheral myelinated nerve fibres during wallerian degeneration. J Anat 1964;98:175.

[6] Lubinska L. Demyelination and remyelination in the proximal parts of regenerating nerve fibers. J Comp Neurol 1961;117:275.

[7] Yamada KM, Spooner BS, Wessells NK. Ultrastructure and function of growth cones and axons of cultured nerve cells. J Cell Biol 1971;49:614.

[8] Timpl R, Rohde H, Robey PG, et al. Laminin—a glycoprotein from basement membranes. J Biol Chem 1979;254:9933.

[9] Letourneau PC. Cell-to-substratum adhesion and guidance of axonal elongation. Dev Biol 1975;44:92.

[10] Mackinnon SE, Dellon AL, O'Brien JP. Changes in nerve fiber numbers distal to a nerve repair in the rat sciatic nerve model. Muscle Nerve 1991;14:1116.

[11] Buchthal F, Kuhl V. Nerve conduction, tactile sensibility, and the electromyogram after suture or compression of peripheral nerve: a longitudinal study in man. J Neurol Neurosurg Psychiatry 1979;42:436.

[12] Bevan S, Steinbach JH. Denervation increases the degradation rate of acetylcholine receptors at end-plates in vivo and in vitro. J Physiol 1983;336:159.

[13] Terzis JK, Michelow BJ. Sensory receptors. In: Gelberman R, editor. Operative nerve repair and reconstruction, vol. I. Philadelphia: JB Lippincott; 1991. p. 85.

[14] Levi-Montalcini R, Angeletti PU. Nerve growth factor. Physiol Rev 1968;48:534.

[15] Levi-Montalcini R, Hamburger V. Selective growth stimulating effects of mouse sarcoma on the sensory and sympathetic nervous system of the chick embryo. J Exp Zool 1951;116:321.

[16] Taniuchi M, Clark HB, Schweitzer JB, et al. Expression of nerve growth factor receptors by Schwann cells of axotomized peripheral nerves: ultrastructural location, suppression by axonal contact, and binding properties. J Neurosci 1988;8:664.

[17] Thanos PK, Okajima S, Terzis JK. Ultrastructure and cellular biology of nerve regeneration. J Reconstr Microsurg 1998;14:423.

[18] Nishiura Y, Brandt J, Nilsson A, et al. Addition of cultured Schwann cells to tendon autografts and freeze-thawed muscle grafts improves peripheral nerve regeneration. Tissue Eng 2004;10:157.

[19] Aguayo AJ, Kasarjian J, Skamene E, et al. Myelination of mouse axons by Schwann cells transplanted from normal and abnormal human nerves. Nature 1977;268:753.

[19a] Fansa H, Schneider W, Keilhoff G. Revascularization of tissue-engineered nerve grafts and invasion of macrophages. Tissue Eng 2001;7:519.

[20] Daly PJ, Wood MB. Endoneural and epineural blood flow evaluation with free vascularized and conventional nerve grafts in the canine. J Reconstr Microsurg 1985;2:45.

[21] Lind R, Wood MB. Comparison of the pattern of early revascularization of conventional versus vascularized nerve grafts in the canine. J Reconstr Microsurg 1986;2:229.

[22] Penkert G, Bini W, Samii M. Revascularization of nerve grafts: an experimental study. J Reconstr Microsurg 1988;4:319.

[23] Prpa B, Huddleston PM, An KN, et al. Revascularization of nerve grafts: a qualitative and quantitative study of the soft-tissue bed contributions to blood flow in canine nerve grafts. J Hand Surg 2002;27A:1041.

[24] Millesi H. Techniques for nerve grafting. Hand Clin 2000;16:73.

[25] Trumble TE, Parvin D. Physiology of peripheral nerve graft incorporation. J Hand Surg 1994;19A:420.

[26] Best TJ, Mackinnon SE, Evans PJ, et al. Peripheral nerve revascularization: histomorphometric study of small- and large-caliber grafts. J Reconstr Microsurg 1999;15:183.

[27] Kwan MK, Savio L- YW. Biomechanical properties of peripheral nerve. In: Gelberman R, editor. Operative nerve repair and reconstruction, vol. I. Philadelphia: JB Lippincott; 1991. p. 47.

[28] Beel JA, Groswald DE, Luttges MW. Alterations in the mechanical properties of peripheral nerve following crush injury. J Biomech 1984;17:185.

[29] Trumble TE, McCallister WV. Repair of peripheral nerve defects in the upper extremity. Hand Clin 2000;16:37.

[30] Lundborg G, Rydevik B. Effects of stretching the tibial nerve of the rabbit: a preliminary study of the intraneural circulation and the barrier function of the perineurium. J Bone Joint Surg Br 1973;55:390.

[31] Clark WL, Trumble TE, Swiontkowski MF, et al. Nerve tension and blood flow in a rat model of immediate and delayed repairs. J Hand Surg 1992;17A:677.

[32] Matsuzaki H, Shibata M, Jiang B, et al. Distal nerve elongation vs nerve grafting in repairing segmental nerve defects in rabbits. Microsurgery 2004;24:207.

[33] Ruch DS, Deal DN, Ma J, et al. Management of peripheral nerve defects: external fixator-assisted primary neurorrhaphy. J Bone Joint Surg Am 2004;86:1405.

[34] Terzis J, Faibisoff B, Williams B. The nerve gap: suture under tension vs. graft. Plast Reconstr Surg 1975;56:166.

[35] Millesi H. The current state of peripheral nerve surgery in the upper limb. Ann Chir Main 1984;3:18.

[36] Kalomiri DE, Soucacos PN, Beris AE. Nerve grafting in peripheral nerve microsurgery of the upper extremity. Microsurgery 1994;15:506.

[37] Millesi H. Healing of nerves. Clin Plast Surg 1977;4:459.

[38] Stevens WG, Hall JD, Young VL, et al. When should nerve gaps be grafted? An experimental study in rats Plast Reconstr Surg 1985;75:707.
[39] Frykman GK. Results of nerve grafting. In: Gelberman R, editor. Operative nerve repair and reconstruction, vol. I. Philadelphia: JB Lippincott; 1991. p. 545.
[40] Ross D, Mackinnon SE, Chang YL. Intraneural anatomy of the median nerve provides "third web space" donor nerve graft. J Reconstr Microsurg 1992;8:225.
[41] Vernadakis AJ, Humphreys DB, Mackinnon SE. Distal anterior interosseous nerve in the recurrent motor branch graft for reconstruction of a median nerve neuroma-in-continuity. J Reconstr Microsurg 2004;20:7.
[42] Masear VR, Meyer RD, Pichora DR. Surgical anatomy of the medial antebrachial cutaneous nerve. J Hand Surg 1989;14A:267.
[43] Nunley J. Donor nerves for grafting. In: Gelberman R, editor. Operative nerve repair and reconstruction, vol. I. Philadelphia: JB Lippincott; 1991. p. 545.
[44] Mackinnon SE, Dellon AL. The overlap pattern of the lateral antebrachial cutaneous nerve and the superficial branch of the radial nerve. J Hand Surg 1985;10A:522.
[45] Hall HC, MacKinnon SE, Gilbert RW. An approach to the posterior interosseous nerve. Plast Reconstr Surg 1984; 74:435.
[46] Greene TL, Steichen JB. Digital nerve grafting using the dorsal sensory branch of the ulnar nerve. J Hand Surg 1985;10B:37.
[47] Waters PM, Schwartz JT. Posterior interosseous nerve: an anatomic study of potential nerve grafts. J Hand Surg 1993;18A:743.
[48] Elgafy H, Ebraheim NA, Yeasting RA. The anatomy of the posterior interosseous nerve as a graft. J Hand Surg 2000;25A:930.
[49] Ustun ME, Ogun TC, Buyukmumcu M, et al. Selective restoration of motor function in the ulnar nerve by transfer of the anterior interosseous nerve: an anatomical feasibility study. J Bone Joint Surg Am 2001;83:549.
[50] Buntic RF, Buncke HJ, Kind GM, et al. The harvest and clinical application of the superficial peroneal sensory nerve for grafting motor and sensory nerve defects. Plast Reconstr Surg 2002;109:145.
[51] Millesi H. Indications and techniques of nerve grafting. In: Gelberman R, editor. Operative nerve repair and reconstruction, vol. I. Philadelphia: JB Lippincott; 1991. p. 525.
[52] Chow JA, Van Beek AL, Meyer DL, et al. Surgical significance of the motor fascicular group of the ulnar nerve in the forearm. J Hand Surg 1985;10A:867.
[53] Jabaley ME, Wallace WH, Heckler FR. Internal topography of major nerves of the forearm and hand: a current view. J Hand Surg 1980;5A:1.
[54] Watchmaker GP, Lee G, Mackinnon SE. Intraneural topography of the ulnar nerve in the cubital tunnel facilitates anterior transposition. J Hand Surg 1994;19A:915.
[55] Williams HB, Jabaley ME. The importance of internal anatomy of the peripheral nerves to nerve repair in the forearm and hand. Hand Clin 1986;2:689.
[56] Gaul JS Jr. Electrical fascicle identification as an adjunct to nerve repair. Hand Clin 1986;2:709.
[57] Deutinger M, Girsch W, Burggasser G, et al. Peripheral nerve repair in the hand with and without motor sensory differentiation. J Hand Surg 1993;18A:426.
[58] Hakstian RW. Funicular orientation by direct stimulation: an aid to peripheral nerve repair. J Bone Joint Surg Am 1968;50:1178.
[59] Landau WM. The duration of neuromuscular function after nerve section in man. J Neurosurg 1953;10:64.
[60] Chaudhry V, Cornblath DR. Wallerian degeneration in human nerves: serial electrophysiological studies. Muscle Nerve 1992;15:687.
[61] Happel LT, Kline DG. Nerve lesions in continuity. In: Gelberman R, editor. Operative nerve repair and reconstruction, vol. I. Philadelphia: JB Lippincott; 1991. p. 601.
[62] Tiel RL, Happel LT Jr, Kline DG. Nerve action potential recording method and equipment. Neurosurgery 1996;39: 103.
[63] Zhao X, Lao J, Hung LK, et al. Selective neurotization of the median nerve in the arm to treat brachial plexus palsy: an anatomic study and case report. J Bone Joint Surg Am 2004;86:736.
[64] Gunther SF, DiPasquale D, Martin R. The internal anatomy of the median nerve in the region of the elbow. J Hand Surg 1992;17A:648.
[65] Lanz U. Anatomical variations of the median nerve in the carpal tunnel. J Hand Surg 1977;2A:44.
[66] Tellioglu AT, Sensoz O. The dorsal branch of the digital nerve: an anatomic study and clinical applications. Ann Plast Surg 1998;40:145.
[67] Teboul F, Kakkar R, Ameur N, et al. Transfer of fascicles from the ulnar nerve to the nerve to the biceps in the treatment of upper brachial plexus palsy. J Bone Joint Surg Am 2004;86:1485.
[68] Higgins JP, Fisher S, Serletti JM, et al. Assessment of nerve graft donor sites used for reconstruction of traumatic digital nerve defects. J Hand Surg 2002;27A:286.
[69] Abrams RA, Ziets RJ, Lieber RL, et al. Anatomy of the radial nerve motor branches in the forearm. J Hand Surg 1997;22A:232.
[70] Young C, Hudson A, Richards R. Operative treatment of palsy of the posterior interosseous nerve of the forearm. J Bone Joint Surg Am 1990;72:1215.
[71] Wray RC Jr. Repair of sensory nerves distal to the wrist. Hand Clin 1986;2:767.
[72] Albert E. Einige Operationen an Nerven. Wiener Med Press 1885;26:1285.

ELSEVIER
SAUNDERS

Atlas Hand Clin 10 (2005) 93–99

Atlas of the
HAND
CLINICS

Functional Outcomes after Nerve Grafting

Christopher H. Allan, MD[a,*], Eric Vanderhooft, MD[b]

[a]*Department of Orthopaedics and Sports Medicine, Harborview Medical Center, University of Washington School of Medicine, 325 9th Avenue, 6th Floor, Seattle, WA 98104, USA*
[b]*Department of Orthopedic Surgery, Salt Lake Orthopedic Clinic, University of Utah Medical Center, 1160 East 3900 South, Suite 5000, Salt Lake City, UT 84124, USA*

Although most surgeons would choose primary repair of injured nerves when this is possible, nerve grafting still is necessary when gaps are too great to span. Attempting to approximate a nerve primarily under these conditions places the repair under undue tension. Dissection and mobilization of the nerve creates ischemia, which compromises the return of nerve function. This ischemia, and not suture pull-out, is believed to be the limiting factor in nerve elongation during acute repairs. If a 10% change in the original length of a nerve occurs during repair, nerve grafting is advocated [1].

Parameters thought to affect the recovery of a nerve repair—grafted or otherwise—include the nerve involved, the age of the patient, denervation time (the time from injury to repair), level of the injury (the distance of the injury from the receptor organ, proximal versus distal injury), gap (the length of the defect to be repaired), the vascularity of the soft tissue bed, the vascularity of the nerve, tension of the repair, and associated injuries. Of these parameters, only tension of the repair, vascularity, and potentially the timing of repair can be affected by the surgeon.

Sensibility testing

Numerous tests have been developed to assess sensibility. The most widely used means of reporting sensibility recovery is the British Medical Research Council scale, first proposed in 1953 in a government bulletin and later modified (Table 1) [2]. This scale is imperfect and has led other authors to attempt to improve on it. Moberg advocated that clinicians quantitate sensation in a way that correlates with hand function [3]. Although clinically useful, such functional testing does not always provide a mechanism for measuring and comparing specific clinical outcomes during research. In recent years, interest in and research on outcomes have been increasing.

When a nerve is recovering from an injury, the advancing edge of the regenerating nerve can be monitored with a Tinel test, percussing from distal to proximal until the growth cone of the regenerating axons is contacted. Loss of continuity of the sensory fiber with its end organ can be shown by failure of a denervated finger to wrinkle when placed in water. Neither of these tests provides quantitative, comparable, or functional data, however.

With the maturation of nerve fibers and receptor endings, a sensory threshold develops followed by improvements in perception and acuity of sensation. The first sensations to recover are pain and temperature, transmitted through the unmyelinated and small myelinated fibers. Such sensory recovery can be anticipated even with poor repairs, providing protective sensation to the patient. As regeneration progresses, perception from low-frequency vibrometry (30 Hz) receptors recovers, then moving touch stimuli, the perception of constant touch, and finally high-frequency vibration (256 Hz) [4].

* Corresponding author.
E-mail address: callan@u.washington.edu (C.H. Allan).

doi:10.1016/j.ahc.2004.10.001

handatlas.theclinics.com

Table 1
Sensibility grading*

Grade	Description
S0	No sensory recovery
S1	Recovery of deep cutaneous pain sensibility
S2	Recovery of superficial cutaneous pain sensibility
S2+	As in S2, but with overresponse
S3	Recovery of pain and touch sensibility with disappearance of overresponse 2-point discrimination >15 mm
S3+	As in S3, but localization of the stimulus is good 2-point discrimination 7–15 mm
S4	Complete recovery 2-point discrimination 2–6 mm

* British Medical Research Council classification with MacKinnon and Dellon's [2] modification delineating correlation with 2-point discrimination.

Data from MacKinnon SE, Dellon AL. Surgery of the peripheral nerve. New York: Thieme; 1988. p. 1–129.

The progression of sensory threshold can be monitored by vibrometry and later quantitated with monofilament testing. Semmes-Weinstein or Von Frey monofilament testing and vibrometry are tests of innervation threshold. Because the Semmes-Weinstein filaments measure the logarithm of force applied (Table 2) and not pressure, it is difficult to compare the results of monofilament testing with 2-point discrimination (2PD) testing or to determine which of the techniques is more accurate. The Semmes-Weinstein test has been reported to be more reproducible with repeated measurements and easier for examiners to monitor. Trumble et al [5] found no significant advantage for either of these techniques over the other.

Finally, as the population of nerve fibers and receptors increases, increasing innervation density is restored, which can be tested with 2PD. This testing reflects the number of nerve fiber receptors in an area. Moving 2PD (m2PD) differs from static 2PD (s2PD) in that it may be detected earlier and at narrower intervals (ie, 3 mm versus 6 mm). As with most of the other sensory tests, 2PD relies on patient cooperation and is subject to the ability or willingness of the patient to cooperate. Many authors consider an excellent functional result as an s2PD less than or equal to 6 mm or an m2PD less than or equal to 3 mm, and a good result as an s2PD between 7 and 15 mm or an m2PD between 4 and 7 mm [4]. The absence of 2PD (less than grade S3) is a poor result. Useful sensory recovery typically is defined as grade S3 (2PD $\leq$15 mm or monofilament testing $\leq$4.31).

Electrodiagnostic testing is perhaps the most objective test and should reflect the reinnervation of a nerve's end organs. Sensibility may be present (eg, the patient has perception), however, even when there is no electrical response; this has been shown in patients with peripheral nerve entrapment, such as carpal tunnel syndrome, in which electrodiagnostic findings may not correlate with the subjective severity of symptoms. MacKinnon and Dellon [2] showed that 20% of patients with mild carpal tunnel syndrome had normal electrodiagnostic testing, but that 20% of patients with clinically severe carpal tunnel syndrome also had normal electrodiagnostic testing. Electrodiagnostic testing may be of limited value in quantitating nerve recovery.

Table 2
Monofilament testing

Logarithm of force to bend, in milligrams	Description
1.65–2.83	Normal sensation
3.22–3.63	Diminished light touch and intact texture discrimination
3.84–4.31	Absent light touch and diminished texture discrimination; temperature discrimination and stereognosis remain
4.56	Loss of some protective sensation with absent texture discrimination and diminished stereognosis and temperature sensation
6.65	Absent texture and stereognosis discrimination with sparing of deep cutaneous pain sensibility with maintenance of some protective sensation
>6.65	No protective sensation

Motor testing

Muscle power grading provides a semiquantitative measure of strength with similar interobserver biases as sensory grading. The most commonly used means for reporting motor function was devised by the British Medical Research Council (Table 3), and attempts to improve on this are ongoing. Muscle bulk (or atrophy) and electromyography studies can provide information regarding the innervation of muscles, but are not quantifiable indicators of functional nerve recovery. Grip and pinch dynamometers can provide quantitative measures of strength. Trumble et al [5–7] have expanded this concept, devising force plates that can measure quantitatively isolated motor functions, such as metacarpophalangeal joint extension (ie, radial nerve), thumb abduction (ie, median nerve), and plantar flexion of the foot (ie, peroneal nerve) to assess motor nerve recovery.

Functional recovery after nerve grafting of the upper extremity

Because most surgeons and centers treat too few patients to allow a meaningful assessment of outcomes, data often are pooled from multiple sites. This pooling requires that treatment, patient assessment, and reporting be consistent across surgeons and centers, but such consistency and uniformity are often absent. Frykman and Gramyk [8] analyzed the literature before 1990 on nerve grafting and found that few of the series they reviewed had greater than 20 cases. For inclusion in their review, they required that appropriate grading be noted, assessment parameters be reported (ie, age, graft length, denervation time), and a minimum of 1-year follow-up be provided.

Digital nerves

Frykman and Gramyk's [8] review of six series of digital nerve grafting identified 151 cases. S3 sensory recovery was achieved in 88% of cases reported. The two series of repairs performed before 1955 (32 patients) achieved less than 50% S3 recovery. Although delayed repair often is cited as a factor negatively affecting outcome, delays of 6 months were associated with useful recovery in 90% of patients; this may be due in part to the shorter distance necessary for regeneration from the nerve graft to the end organ in a digital nerve as opposed to a forearm or arm injury. Other important factors affecting outcome included patient age and graft length. All patients younger than age 20 achieved some degree of 2PD, and useful innervation was achieved in all patients age 40 or younger. Graft lengths less than 50 mm achieved at least grade S3 sensibility in 80% of cases.

Table 3
Muscle strength grading*

Grade	Description
M0	None: No evidence of contractility
M1	Trace: Evidence of slight contractility; no joint motion; return of perceptible contraction of the proximal muscles
M1+	Proximal muscles contract against gravity, but intrinsics paralyzed
M2	Poor: Complete range of motion with gravity eliminated Same as M1+ with perceptible intrinsic contraction
M2+	Proximal and distal muscles are all active against gravity
M3	Fair: Complete range of motion against gravity; return of function in proximal and distal muscles to such a degree that all important muscles are sufficiently powerful against gravity
M4	Good: Complete range of motion against gravity with some resistance; all muscles act against strong resistance, and some independent movements are possible; some intrinsic weakness
M5	Normal: Complete range of motion against gravity with full resistance; full recovery in all muscles

* British Medical Research Council motor grades with Highet and Sanders modification.

Data from Woodhall B. Peripheral nerve regeneration: a follow-up study of 3656 World War II injuries. Washington, DC: VA Medical Monograph; 1957. US Government Printing Office.

Kallio [9] found that only 4 of 26 patients with gaps exceeding 5 cm who underwent grafting of digital nerves had a useful result. Grade S3 or better was obtained in 8 cases with gaps less than 2 cm and in 9 of 12 cases in which gaps measured 4 to 5 cm.

Wang et al [10] reported a series of digital nerve injuries in 1996 and correlated outcome with age, the degree of innervation overlap, and the recovery of nerve repairs versus nerve grafts. Only 14 of the 90 injured digits they analyzed underwent nerve grafting. These investigators pointed out that care must be taken when comparing repair versus grafting because most sharp, clean injuries (grade I) were repaired primarily, whereas more severe injuries required grafting. Overall, injuries of lesser severity had better recovery, as did the primary repairs or grafts compared with the secondary repairs or grafts. In attempting to account for the various degrees of injury, Wang et al [10] reported that nerve grafts seemed to perform better than primary nerve repairs for mild crush injuries (grade 2, blunt, saw-type injuries with limited soft tissue injury). The five nerve grafts achieved a median m2PD of 4 mm and s2PD of 3 mm compared with an m2PD of 6 mm and s2PD of 8 mm in the 37 primary repairs. Although this improved result might be attributed to increased tension and ischemia occurring when primarily repairing these injuries, the investigators recognized that there were too few patients to allow any definitive conclusions to be drawn.

MacKinnon and Dellon [11] evaluated 15 patients with digital nerve injuries with gaps ranging from 0.5 to 3 cm. They eliminated patients with underlying diseases (ie, alcoholism, diabetes, vasculitis), which might adversely influence neural regeneration. Additionally, they substituted polyglycolic tubes for autogenous grafts. Even with this artificial conduit, most patients (86%) achieved grade S3 or better (33% achieved S4). Four patients complained of pain at the surgical site postoperatively, but of eight patients who had preoperative pain attributed to the nerve injury, only one patient did not obtain relief by grafting.

An alternative strategy to nerve grafting or synthetic guidance tubes is the use of autogenous vein as a conduit for digital nerve regeneration. Multiple studies suggest functional outcomes approximately equivalent to outcomes seen with standard nerve grafting [12–16]. Although the authors have limited experience with this technique, it may have value in cases in which donor graft material is limited.

Median nerve

Frykman and Gramyk's [8] review of median nerve grafting included eight studies (four of which were part of the above-discussed digital nerve group). Of 167 patients reviewed, 81% achieved grade M3. Patients younger than age 20 fared better with 88% useful motor return, although even patients older than 40 were reported to obtain a 64% success rate. Gap length seemed to have a more profound effect in injuries of the median nerve with a 95% success rate with gaps less than 5 cm compared with 66% for gaps greater than 10 cm. A time delay of greater than 6 months and a more proximal nerve injury (ie, cubital fossa versus forearm or wrist) also adversely affected the outcome.

With respect to sensory recovery, 79% achieved S3. Age again correlated with recovery, with 98% of patients younger than 20 obtaining S3 versus only 58% of patients older than 40. Delays of more than 6 months, gaps greater than 10 cm, and location (ie, high median nerve injuries) compromised the final outcome.

Of concern in evaluating motor recovery in median nerve injuries is the crossover of ulnar innervation allowing functional opposition of the thumb. Frykman and Gramyk [8] estimated that 50% of the evaluated patients would have had satisfactory thumb opposition even if no median reinnervation occurred. Of their 73 median nerve injuries, 93% achieved grade M3 (55% grade M4). They believed that age and denervation interval correlated with improved function but did not provide data to support this contention. These investigators also implied sensory grade and motor grade are correlated (ie, a grade S3+ or S4 is anticipated with grade M4 recovery).

Similarly, Walton and Finseth [17] showed a correlation between sensory and motor recovery in their limited series of patients with median nerve injuries. Although their description and analysis are limited, they showed remarkable recovery in motor grade and sensory recovery despite large gaps (5–13 cm) and prolonged delays from injury to treatment (4 months to

7 years). Four of their seven patients were reported to have grade M4, and only two had less than grade S3+.

Daoutis et al [18] published a brief report on 47 of 100 patients who underwent grafting for median nerve injuries; 68% of their patients achieved grade M3 or greater (51% grade M4). All of the patients achieved at least grade S3, with 51% obtaining grade S3+ or greater. Although no analysis of their data was provided, review of their data shows that shorter denervation times and gaps typically improved outcomes.

In 2001, Kim et al [19] reported on a large series of median nerve injuries that included 50 patients treated with nerve grafting. Sensory and motor recovery of grade 3 or better was seen in 36 (72%) of 50 who patients received graft repair.

Ulnar nerve

Ulnar nerve injuries often are depicted as the least favorable injury to the upper extremity. Frykman and Gramyk [8] found the results better than they expected. Reviewing six series (all included in the median nerve series) for a total of 104 patients, they reported that 63% obtained grade M3 or better, and 75% obtained grade S3 or better. In contrast to the median nerve results, neither a delay of 6 months nor level of injury affected the results. A gap of more than 10 cm significantly diminished the sensory and higher motor grades, however. Improved useful sensory recovery occurred in 87% of patients younger than 20 compared with 70% of patients older than 20.

Kalomiri et al [20] evaluated 85 ulnar nerve injuries. Useful motor recovery was achieved in 94% of injuries (61% grade M4). Daoutis et al [18] obtained 85% useful motor recovery (71% grade M4) and 88% useful sensory recovery in 41 of 96 patients with ulnar nerve injuries. Vastamaki et al [21] grafted 76 patients and secondarily repaired 34. These patient populations were not delineated in the evaluation, but the investigators concluded that the level of injury, gap, delay to surgery, and age (for sensory outcomes) all affected the end results.

In 2003, Kim et al [22] reported another large series of patients with ulnar nerve injuries, including 36 cases treated with nerve grafting. Sensory and motor recovery to grade 3 was seen in 24 (67%) of the 36. These investigators noted that fewer patients exceeded grade 3 after ulnar nerve grafting than was true for patients treated with median or radial nerve grafting.

Radial nerve

Radial nerve injuries have been reported less commonly, with only three of the series Frykman and Gramyk [8] reviewed including radial nerve injuries, for a total of 60 patients. Although 78% of the patients obtained useful motor recovery, 16% obtained none at all. Worse results were seen with patients older than 40, gaps exceeding 10 cm, and more proximal level of injury. Sensory recovery closely paralleled motor recovery.

Kalomiri et al [20] reported only 35 radial nerve injuries with 97% achieving useful motor recovery (60% grade M5). Daoutis et al [18] reported only five patients, with all achieving grade M3 or better. Kallio's [9] series of 21 patients obtained only 38% useful motor recovery. Kallio [9] believed that a gap greater than 5 cm, a delay greater than 3 months, and associated injuries significantly diminished useful outcomes. Tendon transfers for this injury were readily available to achieve subsequent functional results.

Nunley et al [23] reviewed 20 patients with radial nerve grafting. They reported a 72% useful motor recovery with 44% of patients obtaining a motor grade of M4. Nunley et al [23] did not find a correlation between recovery and patient age or length of graft, but did find that for nerve grafting within 6 months, a motor grade of M3 was achieved in 85% of patients. Injuries to the posterior interosseous nerve did better than high radial nerve injuries.

In 2001, Kim et al [24] reported their large series of radial nerve injuries, which included 54 treated with nerve grafting. At a minimum 18-month follow-up, motor function of M3 or better was seen in 43 (80%) of the 54 patients so treated.

Discussion

Despite differences in means by which outcomes are reported, some summary statements can be derived from the series presented here. In their review of nerve grafting results, Frykman and Gramyk [8] reported that the four most important factors affecting outcome were age of the patient, length of gap to be spanned, time (delay) from injury to nerve grafting, and level of injury (proximal versus distal). This conclusion is supported by more recent investigations [5,7,18,20,21,25,26]. It has been found that gaps greater than 5 cm, delays of 3 months, age older than 20 years, and nature of the injury (blunt versus sharp) adversely affect the desired outcome. These factors should not be construed as restrictions to grafting patients, however. Even the limited results seen in lower extremity injuries provide a useful level of function.

Surgeons must strive to recognize and modify the factors that affect patient outcomes. Series such as the ones reported here help surgeons to understand better how they can intervene to improve outcomes for patients with these challenging injuries. Nerve grafting provides a tool to restore some meaningful level of function in situations in which primary repair is not feasible. As newer conduits and bioactive materials become available, standardized and rigorous outcomes measures must be applied to help clarify their potential value in surgical practice. Future techniques making use of the ability of the peripheral nerve to regenerate after injury will offer opportunities that can only be imagined today. Until that time, careful reporting of results and application of those data will best allow surgeons to meet the needs of patients.

References

[1] Trumble T. Overcoming defects in peripheral nerves. In: Gelberman RH, editor. Operative nerve repair and reconstruction. Philadelphia: JB Lippincott; 1991. p. 507–24.

[2] Mackinnon SE, Dellon AL. Surgery of the peripheral nerve. New York: Thieme; 1988.

[3] Dellon A. The sensational contributions of Erik Moberg. J Hand Surg Br 1990;15(1):14–29.

[4] Dellon A. Sensibility testing. In: Gelberman RH, editor. Operative nerve repair and reconstruction. Philadelphia: JB Lippincott; 1991. p. 135–58.

[5] Trumble TE, Vanderhooft E, Khan U. Sural nerve grafting for lower extremity nerve injuries. J Orthop Trauma 1995;9:158–63.

[6] Trumble TE, Kahn U, Vanderhooft E, Bach AW. A technique to quantitate motor recovery following nerve grafting. J Hand Surg [Am] 1995;20:367–72.

[7] Trumble T, Vanderhooft E. Nerve grafting for lower-extremity injuries. J Pediatr Orthop 1994;14:161–5.

[8] Frykman G, Gramyk K. Results of nerve grafting. In: Gelberman RH, editor. Operative nerve repair and reconstruction. Philadelphia: JB Lippincott; 1991. p. 553–67.

[9] Kallio PK. The results of secondary repair of 254 digital nerves. J Hand Surg [Br] 1993;18:327–30.

[10] Wang WZ, Crain GM, Baylis W, Tsai TM. Outcome of digital nerve injuries in adults. J Hand Surg [Am] 1996;21:138–43.

[11] Mackinnon SE, Dellon AL. Clinical nerve reconstruction with a bioabsorbable polyglycolic acid tube. Plast Reconstr Surg 1990;85:419–24.

[12] Walton RL, Brown RE, Matory WE Jr, Borah GL, Dolph JL. Autogenous vein graft repair of digital nerve defects in the finger: a retrospective clinical study. Plast Reconstr Surg 1989;84:944–52.

[13] Tang JB, Gu YQ, Song YS. Repair of digital nerve defect with autogenous vein graft during flexor tendon surgery in zone 2. J Hand Surg [Br] 1993;18:449–53.

[14] Malizos KN, Dailiana ZH, Anastasiou EA, Sarmas I, Soucacos PN. Neuromas and gaps of sensory nerves of the hand: management using vein conduits. Am J Orthop 1997;26:481–5.

[15] Stahl S, Rosenberg N. Digital nerve repair by autogenous vein graft in high-velocity gunshot wounds. Milit Med 1999;164:603–4.

[16] Risitano G, Cavallaro G, Merrino T, Coppolino S, Ruggeri F. Clinical results and thoughts on sensory nerve repair by autologous vein graft in emergency hand reconstruction. Chir Main 2002;21:194–7.

[17] Walton R, Finseth F. Nerve grafting in the repair of complicated peripheral nerve trauma. J Trauma 1977;17:793–6.

[18] Daoutis NK, Gerostathopoulos NE, Efstathopoulos DG, Misitizis DP, Bouchlis GN, Anagnostou SK. Microsurgical reconstruction of large nerve defects using autologous nerve grafts. Microsurgery 1994;15:502–5.

[19] Kim DH, Kam AC, Chandika P, Tiel RL, Kline DG. Surgical management and outcomes in patients with median nerve lesions. J Neurosurg 2001;95:584–94.

[20] Kalomiri DE, Soucacos PN, Beris AE. Nerve grafting in peripheral nerve microsurgery of the upper extremity. Microsurgery 1994;15:506–11.

[21] Vastamaki M, Kallio PK, Solonen KA. The results of secondary microsurgical repair of ulnar nerve injury. J Hand Surg [Br] 1993;18:323–6.

[22] Kim DH, Han K, Tiel RL, Murovic JA, Kline DG. Surgical outcomes of 654 ulnar nerve lesions. J Neurosurg 2003; 98:993–1004.

[23] Nunley JA, Saies AD, Sandow MJ, Urbaniak JR. Results of interfascicular nerve grafting for radial nerve lesions. Microsurgery 1996;17:431–7.

[24] Kim DH, Kam AC, Chandika P, Tiel RL, Kline DG. Surgical management and outcome in patients with radial nerve lesions. J Neurosurg 2001;95:573–83.

[25] Demuynck M, Zuker RM. The peroneal nerve: is repair worthwhile? J Reconstr Microsurg 1987;3:193–9.

[26] Kallio PK, Vastamaki M, Solonen KA. The results of secondary microsurgical repair of radial nerve in 33 patients. J Hand Surg [Br] 1993;18:320–2.

ELSEVIER
SAUNDERS

Atlas Hand Clin 10 (2005) 101–124

Atlas of the
HAND
CLINICS

Vascularized Nerve Grafts: A Review

Julia K. Terzis, MD, PhD, FACS, FRCS(C)[a,*],
Vasileios K. Kostopoulos, MD[a,b]

[a] *Eastern Virginia Medical School, Division of Plastic and Reconstructive Surgery, Microsurgery Program, Microsurgical Research Center, 700 Olney Road, Lewis Hall, #2055, Norfolk, VA 23507, USA*
[b] *Athens Naval Hospital, 70 Denokratous Street, Athens, Greece*

For the last few decades, surgeons have tried to improve the outcome of reconstruction in patients with peripheral nerve injuries. The advent of microsurgery, the knowledge of the nature of these injuries, and the experience gained over the years has produced improved results in the last two decades. The vascularization of the nerve grafts contributes to this progress. Vascularized nerve grafts were introduced in 1976 [1]. Since then experimental and clinical studies have suggested the superiority of vascularized nerve grafts [2–15]. The senior author (JKT) has used vascularized ulnar, sural, saphenous, superficial radial, superficial, and deep peroneal nerves for 181 reconstructions in cases of brachial plexus injuries and in peripheral nerve injuries of upper and lower extremity.

History

The first nerve graft was done by Phillipeaux and Vulpian in 1870 [16]. In 1878, Albert described the first nerve graft in a human [17]. A defect in the median nerve created after resection of a tumor was bridged by an allograft removed from the amputated foot of another patient. In 1939 Bunnell and Boys introduced the concept of cable grafting for reconstruction of large peripheral nerves [18]. They used multiple strands of a sensory cutaneous nerve bound into a cable of equal diameter to the nerve to be reconstructed. In 1942 Tarlov and Epstein described the process of revascularization in conventional nerve grafts [19]. In 1945 St. Clair Strange reported on the first vascularized nerve pedicle for reconstruction of large nerve grafts; the ulnar nerve was transferred in two stages to reconstruct the median nerve [20].

In 1976 Taylor and Ham reported the first free vascularized nerve graft: 24 cm of the superficial branch of the radial nerve based on the radial artery were used to reconstruct a median nerve damaged by Volkmann ischemic contracture [1]. In 1981 Terzis and Breindenbach performed an extensive anatomic dissection study on fresh specimens using injection techniques in which they evaluated the blood supply of all possible peripheral nerves that could be used as vascularized nerve grafts and introduced a classification of the blood supply of nerves based on the number of dominant vascular pedicles [21]. Also in 1981 Fachinelli et al reported on the use of free vascularized sural nerve graft and introduced a technique of folding the nerve without destroying the blood supply of each segment [22]. The same year Terzis, for the bridging of large defects in brachial plexus injuries with lower root avulsions, introduced the use of the ulnar nerve as a free vascularized graft based on the superior ulnar collateral artery [21,23], and in 1984 Bonney et al presented 12 cases of vascularized ulnar graft based on the ulnar artery [3]. The first step in vascularization of the nerve graft had been accomplished.

* Corresponding author.
E-mail address: jktmd1@aol.com (J.K. Terzis).

doi:10.1016/j.ahc.2004.08.004

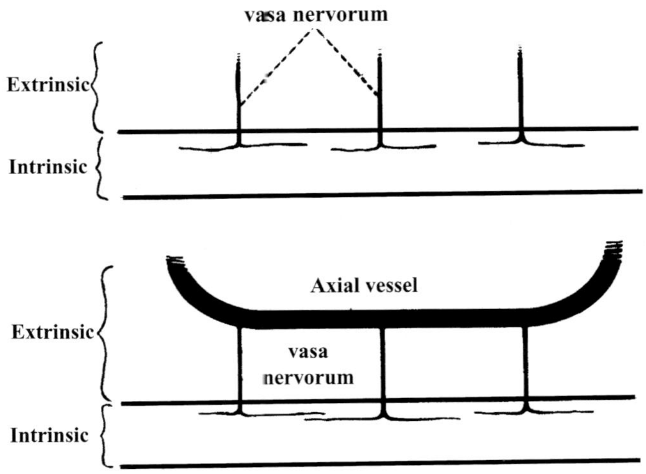

Fig. 1. Diagram showing the blood supply to nerves, extrinsic vessels, vasa nervosum, and intrinsic vessels. *Used with permission from* Breindenbach WC, Terzis JK. The blood supply of vascularized nerve grafts. J Reconstr Microsurg 1986;3:43.

Blood supply to nerves

The blood supply of nerves is divided into two systems: an extrinsic and an intrinsic blood supply [24]. All vessels outside the epineurium are extrinsic, whereas those within the epineurium are intrinsic. The extrinsic system serves as a nutrient system, providing flow to the intrinsic system. The intrinsic system is responsible for the cellular metabolism of the nerve and functions as an exchange system. Vasa nervosum are vessels that originate external to the nerve and terminate intraneurally [25]. These are the nutrient vessels of the nerve and were classified as part extrinsic and part intrinsic by Terzis [21] (Fig. 1).

Dominant pedicle is a pedicle of vessels that have sufficient size for microsurgical transfer ($\geq$0.8 mm) and run for a significant distance alongside the nerve [21,23]. The remaining portion of the nerve is referred as free segment (Fig. 2).

Terzis and Breindenbach performed an extensive anatomic dissection and they classified the nerves according to the number of the dominant vascular pedicles [21,23]. In the type I pattern there are no dominant pedicles [21,23]. The nerve receives its blood supply through the intrinsic system or through those extrinsic vessels that originate from musculocutaneous perforators or fascia and directly enter the nerve, not running along its length. These vessels are of small caliber and not suitable for microsurgical transfer. The medial brachial cutaneous, the medial antebrachial cutaneous, the lateral cutaneous of the thigh, and the femoral cutaneous nerves have no dominant vessels.

In the type II pattern there is one dominant vessel that runs with the nerve for a significant distance of its length and in type III pattern there are multiple dominant pedicles (Fig. 3). The superficial radial nerve (radial artery), the deep peroneal nerve (anterior tibial artery), the superficial peroneal nerve (superficial peroneal artery), the posterior cutaneous nerve of

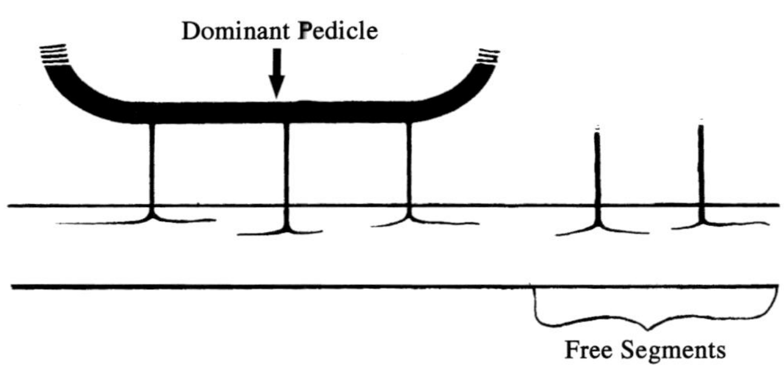

Fig. 2. Diagram showing that the dominant pedicle is an axial vessel supplying a nerve. These vessels are of sufficient size for microsurgical transfer. In contrast, the vessels arising from fascia, musculocutaneous perforators, and periosteal vessels are normally of small caliber. The segment of these smaller vessels is called free segment.

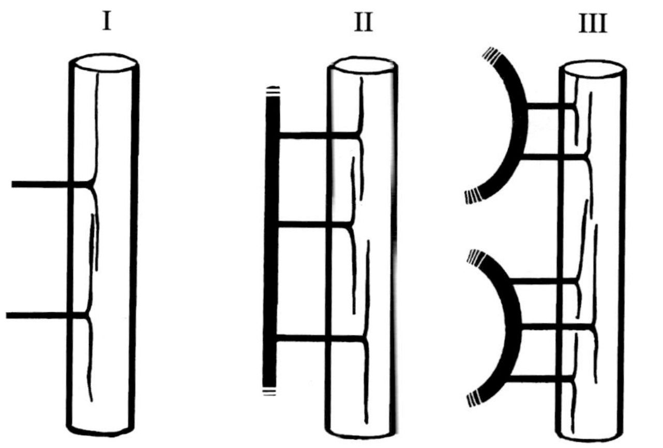

Fig. 3. Classification of blood supply to nerves. *Used with permission from* Breindenbach WC, Terzis JK. The blood supply of vascularized nerve grafts. J Reconstr Microsurg 1986;3:43.

the thigh (branch from inferior gluteal vessels), the sural (superficial sural artery), and the intercostal nerves have one dominant pedicle, so they adhere to type II pattern. The ulnar nerve (ulnar artery and ulnar superior collateral artery) and saphenous nerve (femoral and saphenous vessels) have two dominant vessels, so they have type III pattern of blood supply.

The ideal nerve graft would have one dominant vessel (type II) that runs for most of its length. Nerves with multiple dominant pedicles (type III) may be used as vascularized nerve grafts after their conversion to one dominant system (type II).

Terminology

If a nerve graft is used as a graft without its blood supply, it is referred to as a non-vascularized nerve graft or as a conventional nerve graft. If it is transferred with its blood supply it is called vascularized nerve graft. Vascularized nerve grafts may be pedicled or free vascularized nerve grafts.

Pedicled vascularized

The ulnar nerve has been used on occasion as a pedicled vascularized nerve graft when there are confirmed preganglionic avulsion lesions of C8 [21] and T1 roots in an adult patient and the sural nerve for lower extremity nerve injuries. The first successful vascularized pedicled nerve graft was reported by St. Clair Strange in 1947. He transferred in two stages a pedicled ulnar nerve graft into a 12-cm median nerve gap [20].

Free vascularized

A nerve graft is transferred with its accompanying artery and vein. The anastomoses with the recipient vessels are usually end to side, but they may be end to end. Blood flows from the recipient artery to the artery of the graft and then from the capillaries to the vein of the graft and finally to the recipient vein. Taylor and Ham reported the first free vascularized nerve graft [1]. They transferred the superficial radial nerve based on the radial artery for repair of a median nerve injury. Faschinelli et al (1981) and Gilbert (1984) used the sural nerve based on the superficial sural artery [22,26]. Bonney reported on a free ulnar nerve transfer based, however, on the ulnar artery, which is a major artery necessary for adequate vascularization of the injured upper limb [3]. Terzis introduced in 1981 the free vascularized ulnar nerve transfer based on the superior ulnar collateral vessels without the need of sacrifice of a major extremity vessel [21,27,28].

Arterialized nerve graft

A free vascularized nerve graft may be transferred only with the associated artery. The blood flows from the recipient artery into the graft dominant artery and then into the distal recipient vein. Rose and Kowalski [12] used the deep peroneal nerve with the dorsalis pedis artery to repair digital nerves in scarred digits.

Alternative perfusion methods may be used to carry out a vascularized nerve graft based on the assumption that they facilitate nerve survival.

Arterialized venous fistula nerve graft

A nerve graft may be transferred with an associated vein. Blood flows from the recipient artery into the graft-associated vein and then out into the recipient bed vein. Rose and Kowalski et al [13] used the deep peroneal nerve graft based on the dorsalis pedis venae. The sural nerve has been used in the authors' center with the lesser saphenous vein for upper and lower extremity injuries, especially when the superficial sural artery is not of adequate size.

Arterialized venous nerve graft

The nerve graft is transferred with the vein. The blood flows from the recipient artery into the vein associated with the graft and then into the recipient artery. Townsend and Taylor [29] and Gu et al [30] reported on successful results with the use of the sural nerve based on reverse lesser saphenous vein.

Arakaki et al [31] used a type of vascularized venous nerve graft: the blood flows from the recipient vein into the graft-associated vein and then back into the recipient vein. There is no arterial blood supply.

Factors affecting the selection of a vascularized donor nerve graft

The vascular supply is not the only criterion for the selection of a vascularized nerve graft. Obviously a nerve with no dominant system is not a good candidate as a free vascularized graft. One can use alternative methods of vascularization, however. Sural nerve can be used as a vascularized graft without harvesting the superficial sural artery (associated artery). It can be used as an arterialized venous nerve graft based on the short saphenous vein or it can be harvested with its nutrient perforators in association with the vascularized posterior calf fascia. According to Terzis et al [28], factors that influence the selection of a vascularized donor nerve graft are the following:

1. Type of vascular supply: the ideal vascularized nerve graft would have one dominant system that runs most of its length.
2. Neural tissue area: the cross-section of the neural tissue transferred by the donor graft ideally should approximate the cross-section of the neural tissue to be reconstructed.
3. Length of the nerve graft: the donor nerve must be sufficiently long.
4. Accessibility: the donor nerve should be easily accessible.
5. Expendability: the nerve should be expendable without loss of function.

The superficial radial and the deep peroneal nerves require sacrifice of a major vessel of the upper and lower extremity, respectively. The deep peroneal nerve can be used not only with the associated artery [12] but also with the associated vein [13].

Revascularization of the nerve grafts

The blood flow is increased after manipulation of the nerve [32], which represents a response to help protect the nerve from ischemia [33]. The blood flow was found higher in divided and folded vascularized grafts [34]. Vascularized nerve grafts displayed increased blood flow from the first postoperative day. At the same period in nonvascularized nerve grafts blood flow is not detectable and it exceeds normal values after the fourth postoperative day [35,36]. At 4–6 days it was observed in conventional grafts greater flow than the flow in vascularized grafts [35,37]. When a vascularized nerve graft is used, the initial period of ischemia is avoided because the nerve is transferred with its own blood supply.

When a conventional nerve graft is placed on the recipient area a revascularization procedure takes place. Revascularization of a nerve graft is performed in two ways: vessels from the surrounding tissue bed grow into the graft tissue (centripetal revascularization) and vessels from the end of the graft sprout (hook up) into the existing vascular tree (inosculation). Wongtrakul, Bishop, and Friedrich in 2002 found that on the third postoperative day only 42% of the grafts had partial longitudinal neovascularization [38]. Vascular sprouting from the surrounding tissues is superior to that of longitudinal revascularization [39,40] and for this reason the status of the recipient bed is important: Conventional nerve grafts, if of small diameter, can be used on a well vascularized recipient bed, whereas vascularized nerve grafts are at an advantage when they are used on a compromised recipient bed Some investigators [41] believe in the predominance of inosculation over the centripetal revascularization. In this case vascularized nerve grafts may be advantageous because of impaired conditions of the graft as it awaits revascularization [41]. Revascularization depends on the cross-section of the neural tissue. In an experimental study [42] small-diameter nerve grafts revascularized spontaneously 4 days after graft placement. In contrast larger caliber nerves did not revascularize well (were not perfused at 7 days and were poorly perfused at 40 days).

Indications

Experimental studies have shown that nonvascularized nerve grafts undergo an initial period of ischemia even in a normal recipient bed. As the recipient bed gets increasingly scarred, the nerve graft becomes more vulnerable to ischemic damage. The same effect is operable, because the diameter of the nerve graft or the deficit in the recipient nerve increases in size. Several factors can determine whenever a nerve graft should be used as a vascularized or as a conventional graft.

The vascular supply of the recipient bed

Successful transfer of a conventional nerve graft requires a well vascularized bed. The clinical indication for a vascularized nerve graft is a scarred recipient bed that will not support a nonvascularized nerve graft. The use of vascularized nerve graft seems to be the best choice when there is inadequate vascularization (such as in Volkmann contracture or as a result of irradiation injury) or when the conventional nerve graft has failed already.

The thickness of nerve graft

When a trunk graft is used as an interposition nerve graft it should be transferred as a vascularized graft. If it is used as a nonvascularized graft, central necrosis follows. This was the most common cause of failure in the past when attempts were made to transplant entire nerve trunks.

The length of the missing neural tissue

There is no definite indication what the exact length of the nerve gap has to be for one to use vascularized grafts. The more the nerve deficit increases in size (especially in scarred beds), the greater the need for the use of a vascularized nerve graft. Some investigators determine this length is 6 cm or greater when the recipient bed is not well vascularized [5].

The necessity of rapid axonal regeneration

A relative indication is when the patient presents for reconstruction late, after prolonged denervation time. Vascularized grafts may allow more rapid axonal growth and could be used for the same reason in the repair of proximal lesions.

Vascularized versus nonvascularized nerve graft experimental and clinical results

Several experimental and clinical studies have addressed the question regarding the superiority of vascularized nerve grafts compared with conventional nerve grafts.

Experimental results

Most investigators provided experimental evidence of superiority of the vascularized nerve graft [43]. Koshima and Harii in 1985 used 1.5-cm rat sciatic nerve transferred into silicone tubes [8]. They found that the diameters of myelinated axons were larger in the vascularized group and that there was a significant increase in the number of large myelinated axons. The same investigators reported on faster motor nerve conduction velocity, earlier regeneration of axons, and greater density of large regenerated axons when the nerves were transferred into an acute burn wound [7].

Restrepo et al in 1985, in an experimental study in the rabbit sciatic nerve, found that the myelin thickness and the fiber number were greater in vascularized nerve grafts 15 weeks after the graft placement in a 4.5-cm gap [11].

Shibata et al in 1988 used pedicled vascularized nerve grafts to bridge a 3.0-cm median nerve gap in the rabbit. They found differences in muscle contraction and axon number (better results for vascularized group) at 24 weeks. No differences were found in conduction velocity, compound action potential, muscle weight, and axon diameter [15].

Kanaya et al in 1992 used pedicled vascularized nerve grafts to bridge a 2.5-cm gap in the sciatic nerve of the rat [9]. They found better recovery of nerve conduction velocity, peak amplitude, compound action potential area, contraction force, and sciatic function index in the vascularized group as compared with the conventional group. They did not find a significant difference in muscle weight or axon counts.

Gu and Chen in 1994, in an experimental study of contralateral C7 transfer with vascularized and nonvascularized ulnar grafts to treat brachial plexus root avulsion, found that vascularized grafts were superior to conventional grafts in the recovery of motor nerve latency, axonal count and area, muscle weight, and muscle fiber area and muscle power in the rat [6].

Schutles et al in 2001 found a lower degree of intraneural fibrosis and vesicular degeneration of the myelin sheath in vascularized nerve transfers as compared with the conventional grafts [14].

Mani et al in 1993 found a delay in revascularization of more than 14 days in 30-mm nonvascularized nerve grafts in completely avascular graft beds [44]. Over a period of 44 weeks, however, this prolonged ischemia did not affect nerve regeneration and vascularized nerve grafts did not differ significantly with respect to the rate of regeneration, motor conduction velocity, fiber diameter, and thickness of myelin sheath.

There are only a few experimental studies in which investigators did not find differences between vascularized and conventional nerve grafts. McCullough et al in 1984 reported on no difference in the rate of axonal regeneration in a 2.5-cm rat sciatic nerve graft [45]. They believed that nerves of small cross-sectional area such as used in that study (3 mm in diameter) are likely to be vascularized even in adverse conditions.

Pho et al in 1985 [46] did not find any difference in the degree of vascularization, rate and extent of axonal regeneration, and remyelination between vascularized and conventional grafts when they used pedicled grafts in a 2-cm gap in the rat femoral nerve. Seckel et al in 1986 [47] used 1-cm peroneal nerve in rats placed in a well vascularized bed, and they noted no increase in axon number, in axon diameter, and in myelin thickness.

Clinical results

Bonney, Birch, et al in 1984 [3] analyzed the use of ulnar nerve based on the ulnar artery in 12 brachial plexus reconstructions and they found superior results with vascularized grafts.

Birch, Bonney, et al in 1988 [2] reported 42 cases of supraclavicular brachial plexus injuries treated with vascularized ulnar nerve grafts. Thirty months later the functional recovery for the proximal limb was superior to that of patients who were treated with nonvascularized ulnar grafts.

In the previous reports there was no control. In place of conventional grafts the investigators used their clinical experience. They concluded that vascularized ulnar nerve grafts produced a superior result compared with their clinical experience with nonvascularized conventional ulnar nerve grafts.

Several investigators have reported superior results when they placed vascularized nerve grafts where previous conventional nerve grafts had failed already.

Rose, Kowalski, et al restored the sensibility of anesthetic scarred digits with the use of vascularized deep peroneal nerve graft based on the dorsalis pedis artery [12] or on reverse dorsalis pedis venae [13].

There are only a few clinical well controlled comparative studies, because it is difficult to design a study to evaluate the clinical effect of the vascularized procedure in nerve grafting. Doi et al [5] used 27 vascularized and 22 conventional sural nerve grafts to multiple upper extremity recipients. Their conclusion was that vascularized sural nerve grafting is indicated when a nerve gap of more than 6 cm in length is associated with a large skin defect or amputation. They also demonstrated superior results in normal recipient bed, however, and in cases with small nerve defects.

In contrast Okinaga and Nagano [48] found that vascularization had little clinical benefit in intercostals nerve transfer when the recipient bed had normal vascularity. They transferred vascularized and nonvascularized intercostal nerves in patients with brachial plexus injury. The nerves were dissected for 11–12 cm and directly coapted to the musculocutaneous nerve. No obvious difference between the two groups were found in any of the five evaluated values (time interval between surgery and the appearance of the Tinel sign, rate of advancement of Tinel sign, time interval between surgery, and the electrical appearance of reinnervation potentials in needle electromyography (EMG) of the biceps muscle, isometric elbow flexion strength, and elbow flexor strength).

There are two case reports that allowed a comparison between vascularized and conventional nerve grafts. Boorman and Sykes [4] published a case report in which two lengths of 5 cm of the lateral antebrachial cutaneous nerve were used, one vascularized and one nonvascularized, to reconstruct both digital nerves of the thumb. At 9 months the side with the vascularized graft was found to have better sensory recovery. Mackinnon et al [10] used one superficial vascularized radial nerve graft and one conventional sural nerve graft to reconstruct the defect of a median nerve in two stages. Histologic examination (biopsies were taken in the second stage, 7 months after the initial proximal coaptation) and sensory function were superior in the side that a vascularized nerve graft was used.

Ulnar nerve

Terzis in 1984 [21,23] first introduced the free vascularized ulnar nerve graft based on the superior ulnar collateral artery for cases with lower brachial plexus avulsions. Since 1981 the ulnar nerve has been routinely transferred based on the superior ulnar collateral artery to bridge long gaps during brachial plexus reconstruction and especially in global plexopathies with C8, T1 avulsions. Bonney et al in 1984 [3] used the ulnar nerve as a vascularized nerve graft but transferred it on the ulnar artery, thus sacrificing the dominant artery in the injured upper extremity. They later adopted the superior ulnar collateral vascular pedicle and used it in more recent experience.

Surgical anatomy

The ulnar nerve has a multiple dominant blood supply pattern (type III). In the axilla it is supplied by a branch of the lateral thoracic artery or directly by the axillary artery. In the arm the ulnar nerve is supplied by the superior ulnar collateral artery. The superior ulnar collateral artery arises from the brachial artery 14–22 cm above the medial epicondyle (average, 16.6 cm), runs with the nerve for 10.5 cm (from 4–15 cm) [21,23], is separated from the nerve 1 cm above the medial epicondyle, and finally is anastomosed to the posterior recurrent ulnar artery. Similar anatomic findings were reported 20 years later by Xu et al in 2001 [49]. Below the elbow the ulnar nerve is supplied by the ulnar artery

The vascular supply of the vascularized ulnar nerve graft is based on the superior ulnar collateral artery. This transforms the blood supply of this trunk nerve from a multiple dominant system (type III) to one dominant system (type II) that runs with the nerve for several centimeters (4–15 cm). Proximal and distal to this part, the nerve is transferred without extrinsic blood supply and for this reason protection of the epineurial vasculature during harvesting is of high priority. An average of 55.6 cm of this nerve is harvested routinely starting from its exit from the infraclavicular plexus to distal to the wrist [21,23].

The average diameter of the superior ulnar collateral artery at its origin is 1.8 mm (0.2–2.5 mm) and can be used easily for a free vascularized transfer of the nerve.

Indications

Under normal circumstances the ulnar nerve is not available for nerve grafting. In severe adult plexopathies, however, in which roots C8 and T1 have been avulsed, the ulnar nerve is available for harvesting as a vascularized trunk graft.

A second indication is whenever there is compromise of the vascular supply of the upper extremity. Terzis and Vekris [50] found that 28% of the patients with brachial plexus injury presented with an associated vascular injury and most of these lesions involved the subclavian or axillary vessels (69%). The authors usually perform a preoperative angiography and laser Doppler studies to investigate vascularization of the extremity and to identify any vascular compromise. If there is any vascular insufficiency, the authors usually reconstruct the previous injured vessel (usually subclavian) to improve vascularization of the extremity before the use of the vascularized ulnar graft.

Harvesting technique

The ulnar nerve is explored proximal to the elbow and the superior ulnar collateral artery and vein are identified several centimeters proximal to the cubital tunnel. The ulnar nerve is elevated distally by transecting the branches holding it to the ulnar recurrent vessels. Dissection then is carried proximally, maintaining the superior collateral vessels on the nerve with a cuff of epineural tissue around the whole neurovascular complex and is continued proximally until the ulnar nerve joins the infraclavicular brachial plexus. The nerve should be transected there.

Dissection then begins from the level of the cubital tunnel distally. The flexor carpi ulnaris fascia and muscle is split and the nerve is harvested from the elbow to the wrist. Attention is given to preserve the ulnar artery and venae comitante while maintaining a rich adventitia layer around the nerve. The dorsal ulnar cutaneous branch is identified and must be harvested distally with the remainder of the ulnar nerve. The ulnar nerve is traced distally and is transected distal to the Guyon tunnel (Fig. 4).

Pedicled or free

The ulnar nerve can be used as a free vascularized or as a pedicle vascularized nerve graft. The decision is determined from

1. the position of the dominant vascular leash (superior ulnar collateral artery)
2. the amount of nerve graft tissue needed to reconstruct the defect

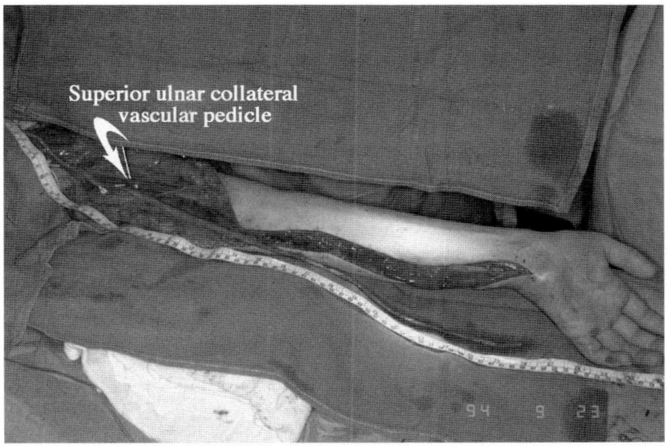

Fig. 4. Intraoperative image of vascularized ulnar nerve graft harvesting.

Use of the vascularized ulnar nerve for cross-chest neurotization

The authors use the vascularized ulnar nerve as a single long graft whenever we want to bridge long gaps, especially when we need extraplexus donors from the contralateral side (contralateral C7). When the vascular pedicle is high near the axilla and the length of the graft is long enough, the nerve can be used as a pedicled graft. The high pedicle is identified and marked. The nerve subsequently is elevated and harvested as described previously. Subsequently the distal nerve is flipped over and tunneled across the chest with special tunnelers so that the distal part of the ulnar nerve faces the anterior or posterior divisions of the contralateral C7. The proximal end is coapted to the desired target (Fig. 5).

When the pedicle is situated more distally, the authors use the nerve graft as a free vascularized graft. Recipient vessels in the normal side are identified; often the transverse cervical artery is used as the recipient artery. The external jugular vein may serve as the recipient vein. End to side or end to end anastomoses are performed.

When several proximal nerve roots are available for reconstruction or there is more than one distal target the nerve is divided into segments corresponding to each of the defects to be bridged.

Terzis' technique for the use of free vascularized ulnar nerve for intraplexus reconstruction

Cases of global plexopathy with avulsion of the lower roots and rupture of the upper roots provide the best indication for using the ipsilateral ulnar as a vascularized graft for intraplexus reconstruction.

The ulnar nerve is harvested as described previously (see Fig. 4). The ipsilateral brachial plexus has been explored, the neuroma excised, and the proximal stumps of the upper donor roots have been prepared for coaptation. More distally the recipient nerves (usually these include musculocutaneous, median, axillary, and so on) also have been readied under the operating microscope. The recipient vessels have been identified (usually these consist of the transverse cervical vascular leash) and adequately mobilized. The superior ulnar collateral pedicle is prepared for microvascular anastomosis. Usually end-to-side or end-to-end anastomoses of artery and vein are accomplished in the supraclavicular area. The most proximal part of the ulnar nerve (which is optimally vascularized) is dedicated for reconstruction of the musculocutaneous nerve. Using high magnification, the epineurium of the ulnar nerve is split longitudinally with great care being taken not to injure the longitudinally running epineurial vessels. The epineurium is pushed gently aside to express the intraneural contents. Great attention is given to transect the fascicles sharply without injury to the epineural vessels, which are preserved meticulously. Following transaction of the neural bundles, microcoaptation with proximal donors and distal targets takes place while the blood supply to the entire nerve is preserved (Fig. 6).

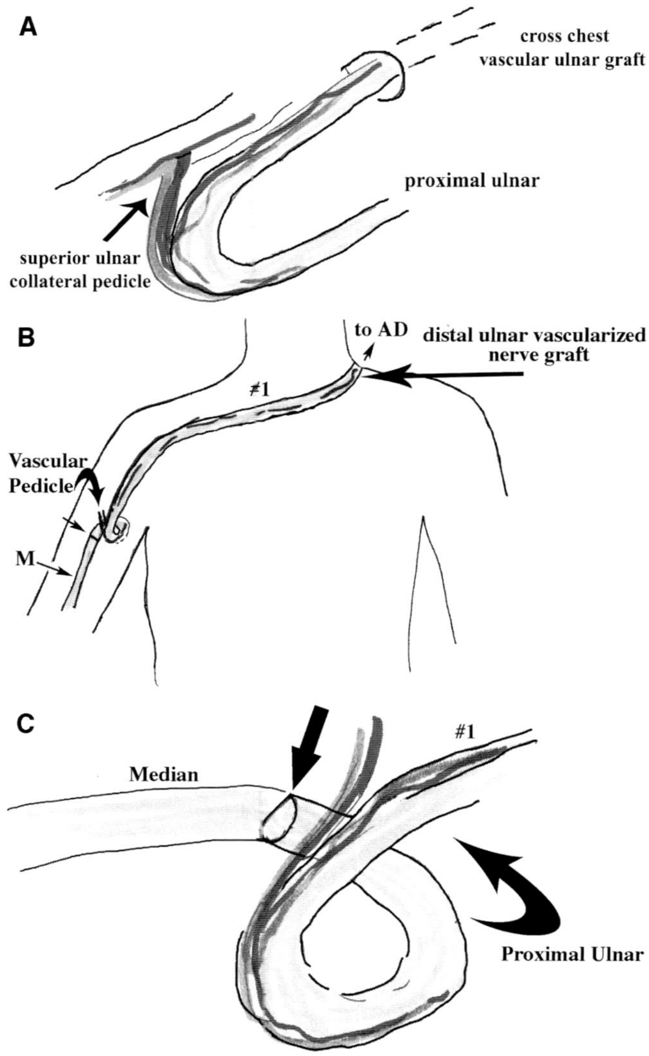

Fig. 5. Ulnar nerve has been used as pedicled, vascularized nerve graft for neurotization of median nerve from contralateral C7 (anterior division). (*A*) The ulnar nerve is dissected and the nerve is rotated based on the superior ulnar collateral artery. (*B*) The distal portion of the nerve is transferred across the chest in such a way that the distal end is approximated for coaptation with the donor root of the contralateral side. (*C*) The proximal end is approximated to the recipient nerve (median nerve).

Clinical experience

The vascularized ulnar nerve graft was used in 63 patients for 143 nerve reconstructions. More than 90% of the patients treated with vascularized ulnar nerve grafting had a global plexopathy usually with sparing of the upper roots (Fig. 7). In 44 patients the ulnar nerve was used to accomplish neurotization of distal targets from intraplexus donors (22 free and 22 pedicled). Mostly C5 or C6 roots were used as donors for distal target neurotizations. Four patients did not have an avulsion of the C8, T1 roots, but the denervation time was long enough and the authors did not expect any recovery from ulnar nerve-innervated intrinsic muscles. In 18 patients the vascularized ulnar nerve was used for neurotizations on the contralateral side, using the contralateral C7 root as the donor.

Ulnar nerve is long enough to be used as a pedicled, vascularized graft to reach the contralateral C7 root, and in 16 patients it was used as a long, single, pedicled graft to accomplish neurotization from the contralateral C7 root (Terzis' selective contralateral C7 technique, which refers to selective use of the entire anterior or posterior division of the root or partial use of each division). In 40 patients the ulnar nerve was used as a pedicled graft based on

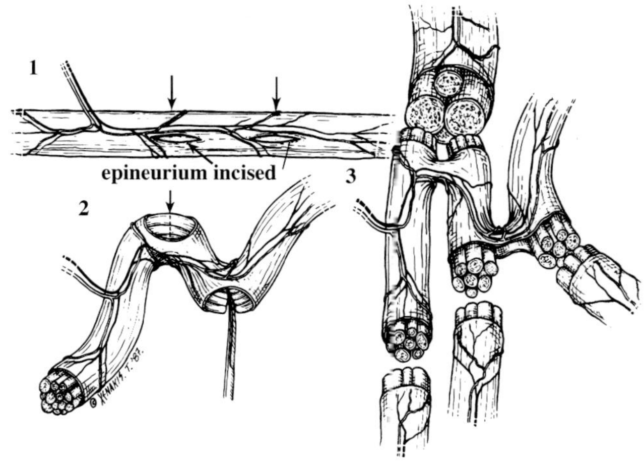

Fig. 6. Terzis' method for the use of the free vascularized ulnar nerve for ipsilateral intraplexus reconstruction. The epineurium is transected longitudinally without compromising the longitudinal epineurial blood supply and the fascicles are transected transversely. Blood supply is maintained through the folded epineurium. *Used with permission from* Terzis JK, Skoulis TG, Soucacos PN. Vascularized nerve grafts. Int Angiol 1995;14:264–77.

the superior ulnar collateral vessels (Fig. 8). In 23 patients it was transferred as a free vascularized nerve graft and the superior ulnar collateral artery was anastomosed to the transverse cervical artery (Fig. 9).

Vascularization always enhances the speed of regeneration of the nerve grafts. The mean rate of Tinel sign advancement was found to be 6.8 cm/month (range, 5–12 cm/month). In contrast, conventional nerve grafts have a regeneration rate of 2–4 cm/month. The authors strongly disagree with Okinaga and Nagano [48], who reported on rates of Tinel sign advancement equal to those of conventional nerve grafts. The authors found that the rate of the Tinel sign advancement gets lower with time (Fig. 10). After a period of 22 months it is difficult to discern any difference between vascularized and conventional nerve grafts.

The vascularized ulnar nerve was used for neurotization of median nerve, musculocutaneous, radial, triceps, and axillary nerves (Fig. 11).

The authors' strategy of reconstruction is as follows.

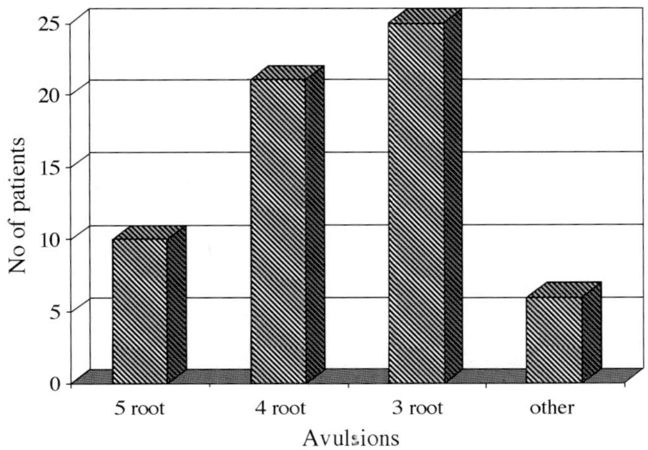

Fig. 7. Intraoperative findings in 63 patients who were treated with vascularized ulnar nerve graft. When all five roots were avulsed (first column) the ulnar nerve was used for neurotizations from the contralateral C7. Ipsilateral intraplexus neurotizations with sparing of the upper roots are depicted in the remaining columns.

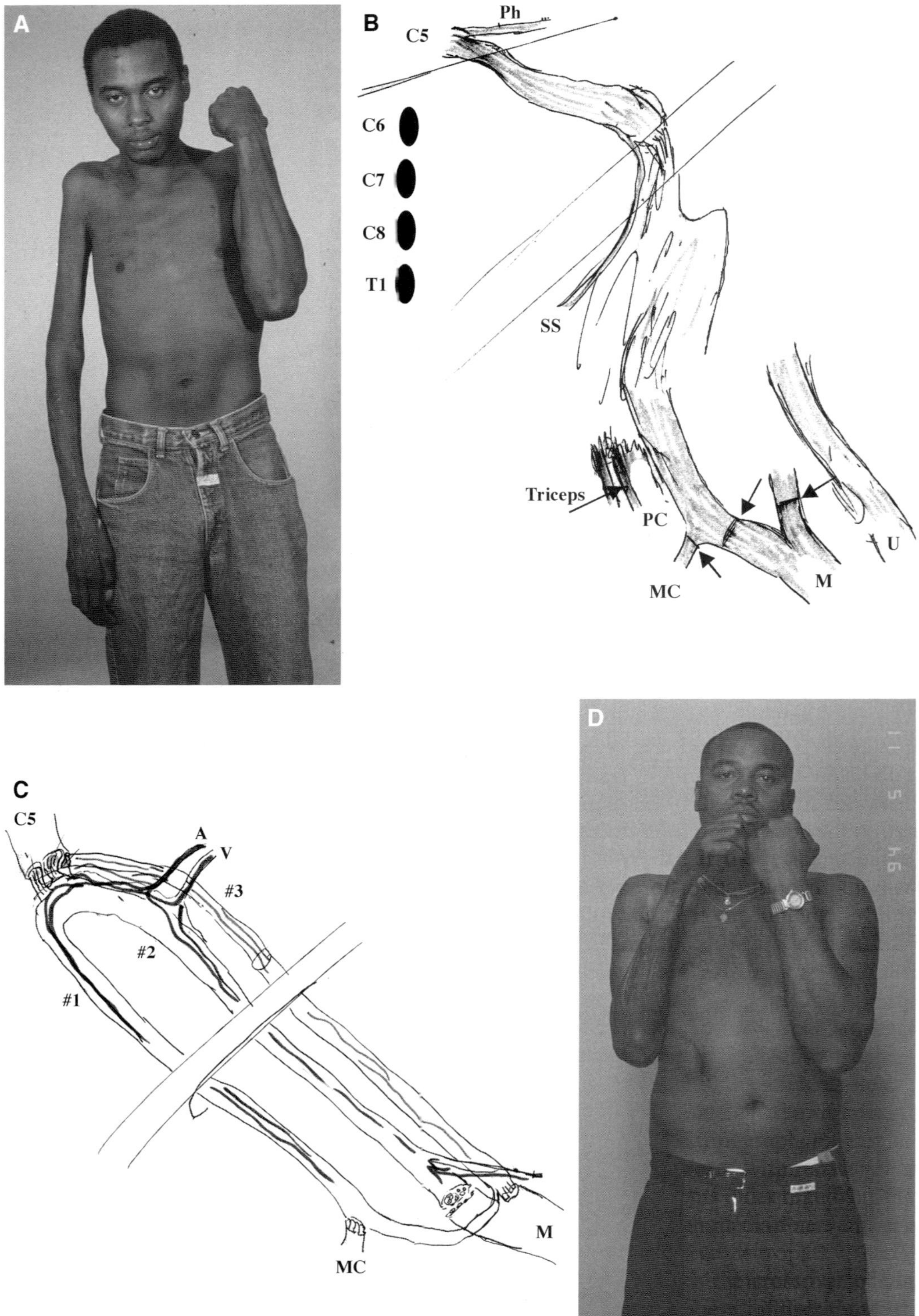

Fig. 8. A 23-year-old black man sustained a right brachial plexus injury in April 1986. He was unloading sandblasting material when his arm was caught between a conveyor belt roller and the belt itself. He sustained fractures of radius, ulna, triquetral, and capitate bones. He underwent emergency fasciotomy and external fixation in his forearm. (*A*) Preoperatively the patient presented with a flail anesthetic arm. (*B*) On August 28, 1986 an exploration of the right brachial plexus revealed C5 rupture and C6–T1 avulsion. (*C*) The ulnar nerve was transferred as a free vascularized graft. It was folded three times to neurotize the right median and right musculocutaneous nerves from C5 root. (*D* and *E*) Patient seen 8 years after brachial plexus repair demonstrating strong elbow flexion.

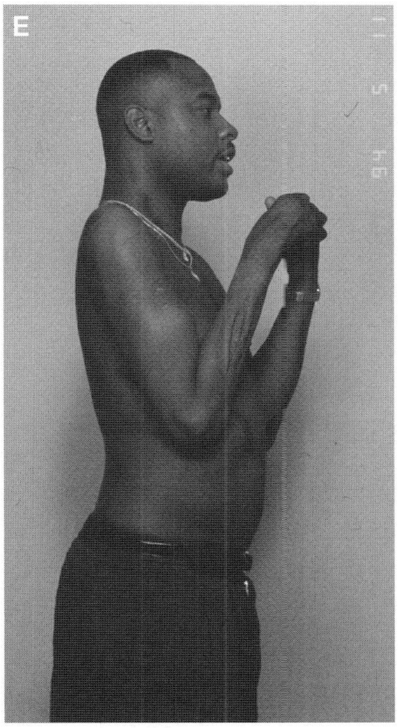

Fig. 8 (*continued*)

To improve sensation of the upper extremity, especially of the hand

The authors used vascularized ulnar nerve to carry out median nerve neurotizations in 59 cases (39% of the patients). All the patients but one (87.5%) achieved at least protective sensation. On the contrary only 65% of the patients, treated with vascularized or conventional grafts in an extensive study with 204 brachial plexus reconstructions, achieved protective sensation in the hand [50].

To eliminate the problem of long graft failure

Whenever a contralateral donor is used, the length of the cross-chest nerve grafts imposes a necessary delay before target connectivity. The authors used vascularized ulnar nerve, even for non compromised beds, to eliminate this delay. In one case the authors used vascularized ulnar and conventional saphenous nerve grafts to neurotize from the contralateral C7 root (anterior and posterior divisions), the median and radial nerves, respectively. After 12 months the Tinel sign was found across the course of median nerve at a distance of 85 cm from the contralateral C7 root (regeneration rate of 7 cm/month for the vascularized ulnar nerve). At the same time the distance across the course of the radial nerve (nonvascularized saphenous) was only 50 cm (4 cm/month). In another case vascularized and conventional nerve grafts also have been used simultaneously to neurotize median and radial nerve from intraplexus donors. In that case (the authors did not use long nerve grafts), we found differences between the rates of Tinel sign advancement (6.4 and 4 cm/month, respectively).

The problem of long graft failure has been minimized with the use of vascularized nerve grafts. The intraneural environment is optimally preserved and axonal carry-through is not compromised.

To improve muscle function

Biceps was the first priority (25% of the patients with vascularized ulnar had a neurotization of the musculocutaneous nerve).

Preliminary unpublished data from the biggest series of vascularized ulnar nerve grafts show that:

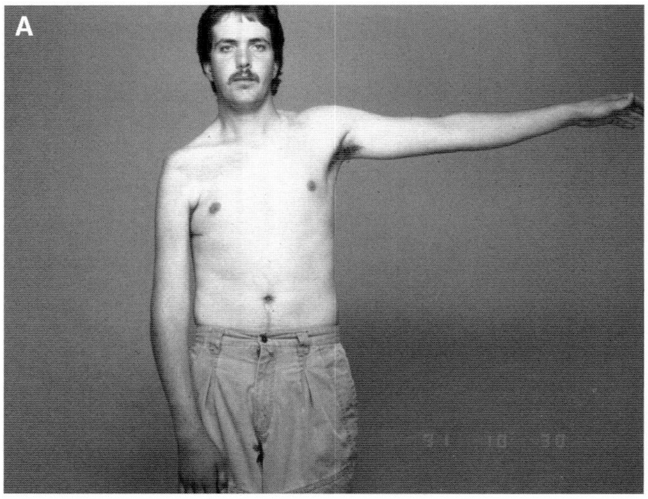

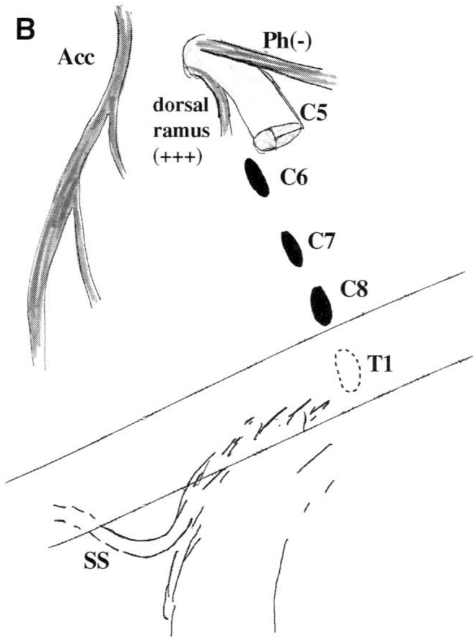

Fig. 9. On June 13, 1991 a 24-year-old man sustained right brachial plexus injury. He was driving a small pickup at a speed of 45 mph when he fell asleep and the pickup hit a tree. A right subclavian artery injury was diagnosed and repair of the artery was performed with a Gore-Tex patch. (*A*) Preoperative patient presented with a total flail anesthetic right arm. (*B*) On November 14, 1991 an exploration of the right brachial plexus revealed C5 root rupture and C6–T1 root avulsion. (*C*) Reconstruction of right brachial plexus was performed with interposition free vascularized ulnar nerve graft from C5 to musculocutaneous, axillary, and median nerves. The superior ulnar collateral artery was anastomosed with the transverse cervical artery (end-to-side) and the associated vein with the external jugular vein (end-to-side). (Reconstruction also included accessory to suprascapular direct neurotization and reconstruction of the thoracodorsal and triceps nerves from C5 with interposition sural nerve grafts.) Seven years postoperatively the patient had excellent (*D*) abduction and (*E*) elbow flexion.

1. Even after long denervation time, the degree of muscle strength recovered was adequate. Excellent elbow flexion and shoulder abduction was achieved even after 24 and 48 months postinjury.
2. The degree of advancement of the Tinel sign at 12 months may have predictability value for the final strength recovery by the neurotized muscle. Rates of advancement of more than 6 cm/month correlated well with muscle grade of more than 4°. There was no correlation, however, between the Tinel sign advancement at 4 or 6 months (even for rates of 10 cm/month) and muscle function.
3. Vascularized ulnar also was used (as a free and as a pedicle nerve transfer) to accomplish neurotization of free muscle (gracilis for finger flexion) from intraplexus donors. Free muscles achieved useful function (mean muscle grading more than three plus), although it is

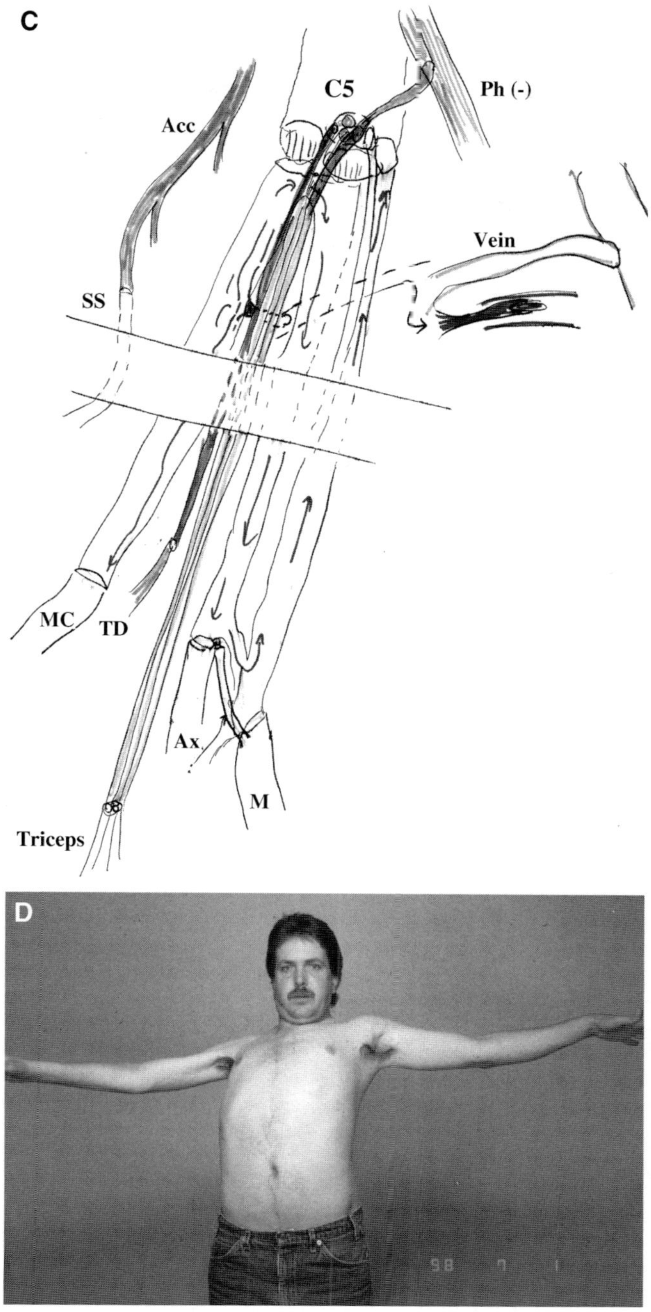

Fig. 9 (*continued*)

always a difficult decision which part of the ulnar nerve to coapt to obturator nerve because of the large cross-sectional discrepancy between graft and recipient nerve.

Sural

The medial sural nerve has been used as a vascularized nerve graft based on the superficial sural artery [22] or based on the perforator vessels that supply the fascia [51] or as an arterialized venous nerve graft when it is transferred with the associated lesser saphenous vein [29].

Usually it is folded into cables. When the nerve is harvested and it has one dominant pedicle that runs the entire length of the nerve it can be divided easily into cables [22].

The senior author (JKT) used vascularized sural nerves to reconstruct peripheral nerve defects in the upper and lower extremity. For the lower extremity the sural nerve was used as a pedicled vascularized nerve graft, and for upper extremity it was used as a free vascularized

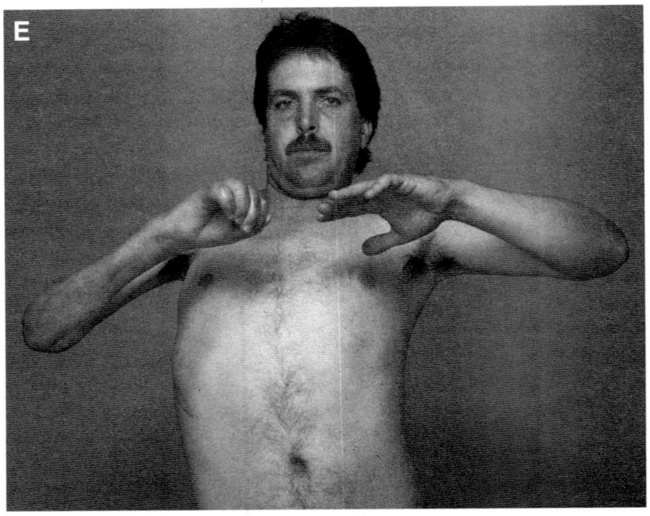

Fig. 9 (*continued*)

nerve graft, based on the lesser saphenous vein. The superficial sural artery was used in the upper extremity for vascularization of the transferred deep calf fascia and it was anastomosed with muscular branches of the radial or ulnar artery. In the lower extremity the superficial sural artery was used as a pedicle vessel to provide more vascular support for fascia and sural nerve graft.

Surgical anatomy

The sural nerve is nourished by the superficial sural artery proximally, but distally it receives multiple contributions from musculocutaneous and fasciocutaneous perforators of the posterior tibial and peroneal arteries. The superficial sural artery arises directly from the popliteal artery or from the sural arteries. The superficial sural artery is present in 30% [23] to 91% [52] of the dissections. It gives off several cutaneous branches and follows the sural nerve along almost its entire length. At the origin the mean diameter of the artery is 1.5 mm and can be used for free transfer of the nerve [23]. After the nerve penetrates the deep fascia, several segmental vessels enter the nerve. In the middle third of the calf, the muscular perforating branch of the posterior tibial artery joins the segmental vessels. In the distal third of the calf, cutaneous branches of the peroneal artery join the segmental vessels. There are vascular anastomoses between them and the sural nerve is vascularized through either pedicle [51].

Doi et al harvest the vascularized sural nerve with posterior calf fascia and perforator vessels that supply the fascia. These vessels usually are identified within the intermuscular septum or

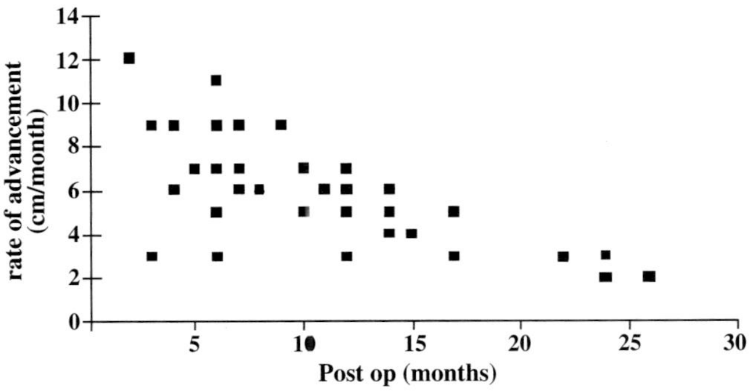

Fig. 10. The rate of Tinel sign advancement for vascularized nerve grafts was found (mean rate, 6.8 cm/month) to be more than the rate of Tinel sign advancement for nonvascularized nerve grafts (3–4 cm/month). The figure shows the rates for vascularized nerve grafts in relation to the postoperative time of the examination. The rate of Tinel sign advancement gets slower with time.

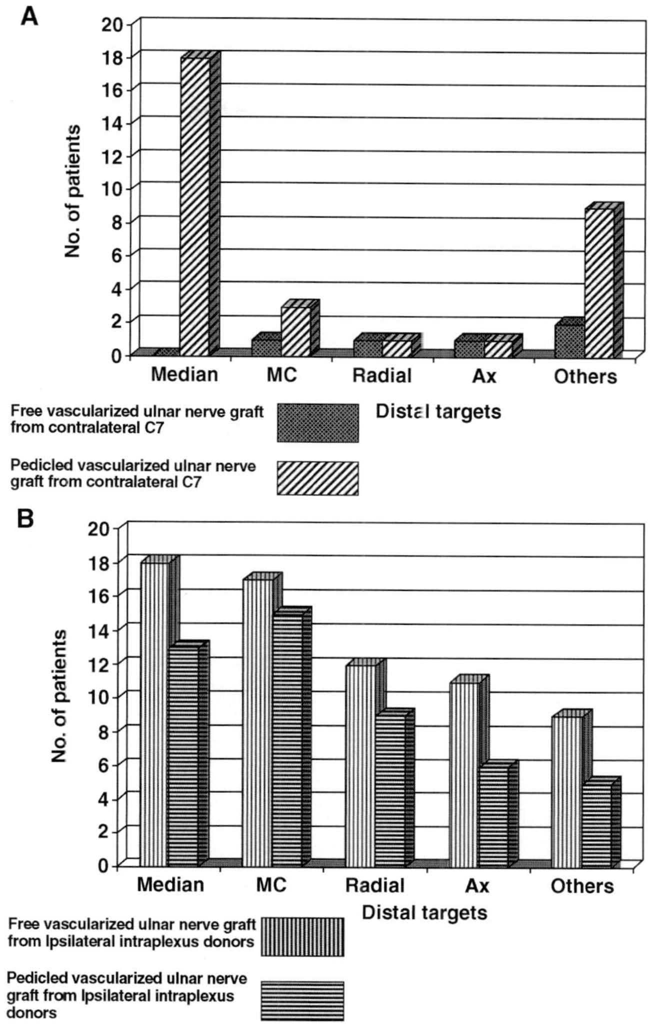

Fig. 11. Ulnar nerve was used as an interposition nerve graft from ipsilateral and contralateral donors. (*A*) From the contralateral C7 donor root the ulnar nerve was used mostly as a pedicled, vascularized nerve graft (columns with oblique lines) especially for median nerve neurotization. (*B*) From ipsilateral intraplexus donors (mostly C5 or C6 roots) ulnar nerve graft was used to median, musculocutaneous, radial, and axillary nerves. It was transferred as a pedicled (columns with vertical lines) or as free (columns with horizontal lines) vascularized nerve graft.

they course directly through the muscle. If the recipient artery is large they use a section of the peroneal vessel as the main pedicle.

They reported good results in multiple upper extremity reconstructions [5,51]. Townsend and Taylor [29] and Gu et al [30] also reported good results with the sural nerve–saphenous vein complex transferred as an arterialized venous nerve graft.

In the authors' center, since 1984 11 vascularized nerve grafts have been used to reconstruct upper extremity nerve injuries. In five cases the authors used the vascularized sural nerve graft. The authors also used the superficial radial nerve as a pedicled vascularized graft, the free vascularized saphenous nerve in four cases, and the sensory component of the deep and superficial peroneal nerves as a free vascularized nerve graft for upper extremity reconstruction.

Four patients suffered from median nerve injury and one patient from ulnar nerve injury. Whenever the injury was in the elbow region the authors did an end-to-side anastomosis of the lesser saphenous vein with the brachial artery proximally and with the basilic vein distally (arterialized venous nerve graft). Whenever the injury was in the wrist the authors used the radial artery as the donor vessel and anastomosed the lesser saphenous vein in an end-to-side manner. Distally the lesser saphenous vein was anastomosed to a dorsal forearm vein (arterialized venous nerve graft).

The appropriate length of the nerve grafts was determined by measuring the nerve defect after the resection of the neuroma. The nerve grafts were folded into segments maintaining their vascular connections. The appropriate number of nerve grafts for median and ulnar nerve reconstruction in the mid-forearm was usually four or five grafts. In case the nerve gap was too long, vascularized nerve graft was placed in association with conventional nerve grafts to cover the cross-sectional area of the injured nerve.

Most nerve gaps were more than 12 cm. At the wrist on occasion the vascularized sural nerve graft was used in conjunction with vascularized fascia to improve the vascularization of the area and the gliding of the adjacent tendons in the area of the carpal tunnel. Most injuries involved their dominant hand (four right, one left). There were four male and one female patients ranging in age from 7–48 years. Denervation time ranged from 23 months to 15 years.

Most of the patients had a work-related injury (eg, power saw, jet engine injury), one patient had a fall from a high altitude, and one fell in a glass door.

The indications were prolonged denervation time, failure of the previously used conventional nerve grafts, and inappropriate vascularization of the area with excessive scar formation.

The Tinel sign was noted to be progressing rapidly at a rate of 2.8–6.5 cm per month. Usually the rate of axon progression along the nerve transplant was greater than the expected in conventional nerve grafts but less than vascularized nerve grafts used for brachial plexus reconstruction.

Taylor reported similar results in the upper extremity [53].

Two-point discrimination tests (static and moving) were improved to near equal rates compared with the contralateral, normal hand (Fig. 12).

Lower extremity

Whenever the authors used a vascularized nerve graft to reconstruct lower extremity nerve injuries we used sural nerve. The authors harvested it as a pedicled nerve graft based on the superficial sural artery. In three cases the sural nerve was used as an arterialized venous nerve graft. Proximally the lesser saphenous vein was anastomosed end-to-side with superior genicular artery or the femoral artery and distally with the distal part of remaining saphenous vein. Two grafts received double vascular supply from arterialized saphenous vein and pedicled superficial sural artery.

In six patients the authors harvested vascularized sural nerve and vascularized posterior calf fascia to improve the vascularization of the recipient bed and to eliminate the postoperative scar formation.

Eleven patients were men and one was a woman ranging in age from 20–53 years. Mean denervation time was 9.5 months (range, 3–23 months) and average nerve graft length was 18.5 cm (range, 6–35 cm). Postoperative follow-up ranged from 27 months to 7 years.

In four patients the nerve was found in continuity because of neuroma or huge scar formation. Most patients suffered from a dislocation or valgus injury during sport participation. There were also motor vehicle accidents, fall from height, farm injur, and gunshot wound injury.

Six patients had a common peroneal nerve injury, three patients had posterior tibial and peroneal nerve injuries, and two patients had a sciatic nerve injury.

Tinel sign advancement for the lower extremity was found at a rate of 3.875–7.300 cm per month (more than 2 or 4 cm/month in conventional grafts).

Sensation of the extremity also improved postoperatively. Most patients regained improved sensibility.

Muscle strength was estimated with the British Medical Research Council Grading expanded further with intermediate grades of + and −. Regression analysis for the preoperative and the postoperative differences in muscle grading was correlated with denervation time. All patients with denervation time between 3 and 6 months regained muscle strength to near a preinjury level (muscle grade more than 4) even when long grafts were used for gaps of 20 cm or more (Fig. 13). Hasagawa et al in 2004 reported on successful repair of large nerve gaps (20–30 cm) after severe extremity trauma with vascularized sural nerve grafts. Late cases with denervation time more than 20 months uniformly yielded inadequate muscle function even with the use of vascularized grafts.

A patient with 23 months denervation time received vascularized and nonvascularized nerve grafts for repair of lesions of the deep and superficial peroneal nerves subsequent to high velocity sport injury. The deep peroneal nerve was grafted with vascularized sural and his sensation to the first webspace returned to near normal levels. In contrast he had no sensation in the distribution of superficial peroneal nerve. The latter was grafted with nonvascularized nerve graft.

The authors' choice to use vascularized grafts in elderly patients was justified. Vascularization seems to improve the results even in the group of elder patients. The authors used 6-cm vascularized sural nerve graft to bridge the gap in a common peroneal nerve lesion in a 53-year-old woman with damage of the common peroneal nerve after the excision of schwannoma

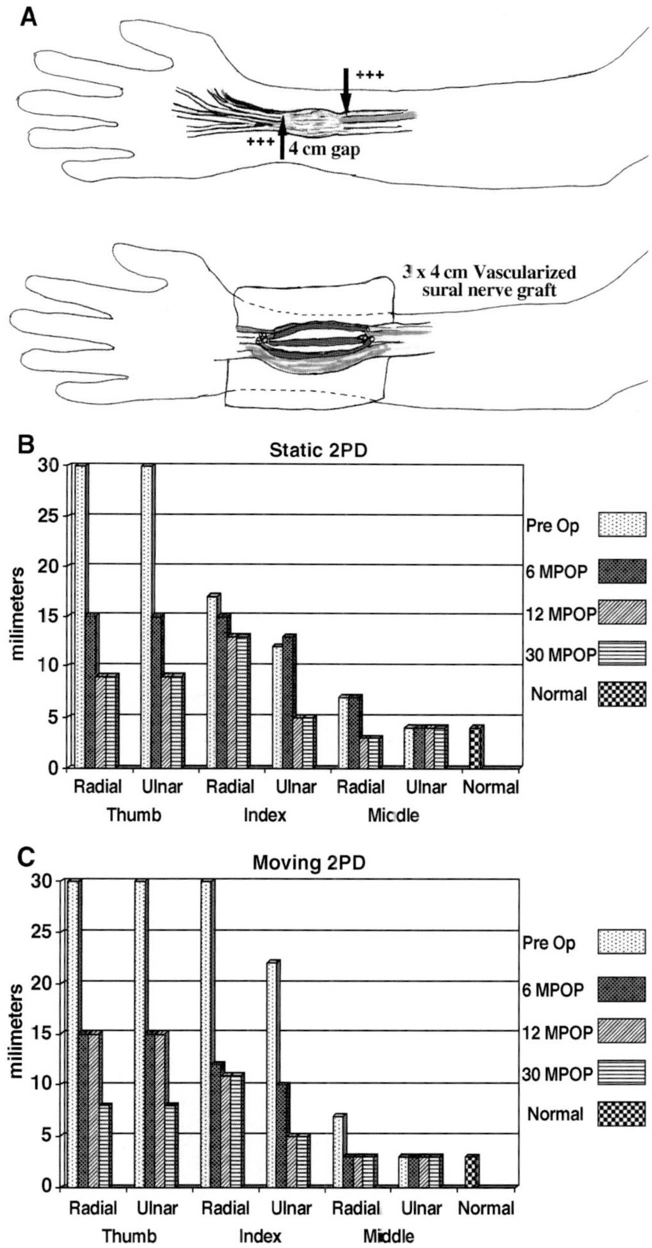

Fig. 12. A 23-year-old patient underwent multiple resections and revisions of traumatic neuroma of his right median nerve at the wrist at another facility. Vascularized sural nerve graft based on reverse lesser saphenous vein was transferred with vascularized posterior calf fascia. The lesser saphenous vein was anastomosed proximally (end-to-side) with the anterior interosseous artery and distally (end-to-end) with the distal ulnar artery. (*A*) Intraoperative findings and surgical reconstruction. Functional return over time depicted in (*B*) and (*C*). MPOP = months postoperatively. Note improvement with time.

(denervation time, 4 months). The patient has been able to walk without external support (muscle grade 4) and she recovered a rewarding degree of sensation.

Vascularized saphenous nerve

The saphenous nerve has excellent length, is expendable, and is situated anteriorly [27], but the dissection is extensive, requiring exposure of the Hunter canal. Saphenous nerve has a multiple dominant blood supply. Proximally it is supplied by the femoral vessels. In the region of the lower thigh and knee it is supplied by the saphenous vessels. Below the knee there is no dominant blood supply [23]. The saphenous nerve can be used as a vascularized graft based on the saphenous artery and vein.

Surgical anatomy and harvesting technique

The patient must be in supine position, the thigh must be abducted, and the knee must be flexed slightly over a sterile blanket.

With a long curvilinear skin incision on the medial aspect of the thigh from the femoral triangle to the region of the medial epicondyle of the knee the muscular interval between the sartorius and the adductor longus is identified proximally. The saphenous nerve is the medial component of the femoral nerve and comes to lie directly to the lateral side of the femoral artery. The nerve and artery proceed in close proximity down the leg into the Hunter canal. The nerves to the vastus medialis and branches to sartorius are adjacent to it and must be identified and preserved. Stimulation of this nerve should not yield muscle contraction. With the use of a disposable nerve stimulator one should ensure that motor branches are not contained in the harvested saphenous nerve. The sartorius muscle is identified and reflected laterally to expose beneath the adductor's canal. In the adductor's canal the nerve crosses medially over the femoral artery.

Usually in this region the saphenous artery and vein leave the femoral vessels and run 2–6 cm to join the saphenous nerve. These vessels join the nerve 17–42 cm from its origin in the groin. The vessels accompany the nerve for 17–23 cm [27]. The main pedicle must be identified, isolated, and preserved while the remaining nerve is being dissected.

The saphenous nerve courses posterior to the sartorius muscle, then pierces the fascia between the tendons of the sartorius and gracilis muscles and becomes subcutaneous on the

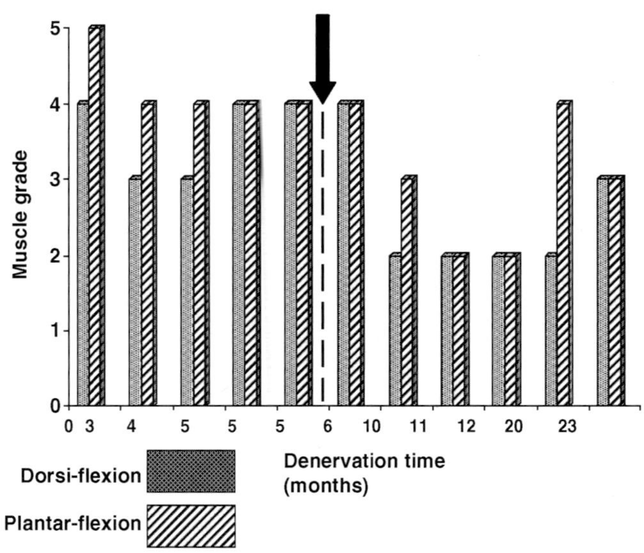

Fig. 13. Eleven patients with lower extremity nerve injury were treated with pedicled, vascularized sural nerve, and in six of these patients a concomitant vascularized posterior calf fascia was used. Postoperative results (muscle strength) versus denervation time show that patients with denervation time less than 6 months regained excellent muscle strength.

medial aspect of the knee where it gives off a large infrapatellar branch. The length of the nerve graft can range from 31–49 cm (sometimes 63 cm in patients with long legs).

Clinical experience

Since 1981 nine saphenous vascularized nerve grafts has been harvested in the authors' center. In all cases a pedicle was present, but in one case the pedicle came off in the popliteal fossa. Eight nerves were transferred successfully, all for upper extremity reconstruction. Depending on where the lesion was, the pedicle was anastomosed end-to-side with the transverse cervical, subclavian, thoracoacromial, brachial, or radial artery.

The authors used vascularized saphenous for brachial plexus and upper extremity peripheral nerve injuries.

For the peripheral nerve injuries the mean length of the recipient nerve gap was 23.5 cm (range, 14–40 cm). The authors used the vascularized saphenous nerve as an ultimate solution after multiple failures of conventional nerve grafts for reconstruction of bilateral upper extremity nerve injury and in a case of multiple level injuries. For brachial plexus injuries, vascularized saphenous nerve has the same indications for use as the vascularized ulna, except it is used primarily in patients with intact C8 and T1 roots.

Other vascularized nerve grafts

Superficial radial nerve

In 1976 Taylor and Ham established the applicability of the procedure of grafting with a free vascularized nerve graft; 24 cm of the superficial branch of the radial nerve with the radial artery was used to reconstruct a median nerve damaged by Volkmann ischemic contracture.

The senior author (JKT) successfully used the superficial radial nerve as a vascularized nerve graft for upper extremity reconstruction (twice for brachial plexus injury and once for distal nerve injury). Because the authors didn't want to sacrifice a major vessel, the senior author (JKT) simultaneously reconstructed the radial artery with interposition vein graft. As a vascularized nerve graft, the superficial radial nerve has many advantages. There now are alternate nerves one can use, however, whenever one needs a vascularized nerve graft, without the sacrifice of a major vessel in the upper extremity.

Superficial peroneal nerve

In August 1984 the senior author (JKT) used the superficial peroneal nerve as a free vascularized graft. This was the first time this nerve was used clinically. The graft may be taken proximally from the last motor branch (1–12 cm from the origin from common peroneal nerve) to the bifurcation distally at the level of the ankle. The length of the graft ranges from 14–30 cm [27]. The senior author (JKT) transferred deep and superficial peroneal nerves on their common pedicle to reconstruct the median nerve in a case of double level injury of median and ulnar nerve from a boat propeller injury. The ulnar nerve was reconstructed with a vascularized saphenous nerve.

Vascularization allows a nerve graft to avoid the initial period of ischemia and ensures continuous nutrition of the nerve graft. Intraneural fibrosis is avoided and axonal regeneration and target connectivity is enhanced. Vascularized nerve graft was developed not to replace conventional grafting techniques but to provide a potential solution to specific problems (large defects, scarred beds, proximal lesions, trunk grafts)

To compare a vascularized with a nonvascularized graft the following questions should be addressed [23]: Is there any difference between a vascularized and a nonvascularized nerve graft in a normal bed or a scarred bed? Will a vascularized nerve graft improve results over nonvascularized nerve grafts if the nerve defect is large? With a proximal lesion should one use a vascularized nerve graft because it will produce more rapid axonal regeneration?

Vascularized nerve grafts already have been used for almost three decades and these questions have been answered with clinical and experimental studies.

Most clinical studies referred to scarred beds and some of them to long nerve defects. Rose and Kowalski displayed the superiority of vascularized nerve grafts over the nonvascularized nerve grafts. In their clinical study they found fair to excellent sensory return in severely scarred digits in patients with previously failed nonvascularized nerve grafts [12].

Doi et al successfully used free vascularized sural nerve graft to reconstruct peripheral nerve defects in the upper extremity. The mean nerve defect was not long (7 cm), but all the repairs were done in severely scarred beds [51]. Compared with the nonvascularized grafts, results were found to be superior [5].

Taylor presented four cases with very good functional results after long-term follow-up (greater than 20 years). The nerve gap was more than 20 cm and the recipient bed was heavily scarred [53].

The authors successfully used vascularized saphenous nerve graft after multiple failures of conventional nerve grafts to reconstruct long nerve gaps (mean length, 23.5 cm) in the upper extremity. The authors' experience in the lower extremity was the same. Patient regained muscle strength to near a preinjury level even when long grafts were used for gaps of 20 cm or more.

Most experimental studies also showed better results for vascularized nerve grafts in scarred beds. Koshima and Harii found that vascularized grafts produced better results in scarred and acute burn wound beds [7,8]. Mani et al, however, did not find any significant difference between vascularized and nonvascularized nerve grafts in avascular graft beds even after the prolonged initial period of revascularization for nonvascularized nerve grafts [44].

Normal recipient bed experimental studies are conflicted as to which produces the best results. Restrepo et al [11], Shibata et al [15], Kanaya et al [9], and Schultes et al [14] reported better results with vascularized nerve grafts, whereas McCullough et al [45], Pho et al [46], and Seckel at al [47] did not find any difference.

In an experimental study for brachial plexus injuries Chen and Gu in a rat model of contralateral C7 transfer with vascularized and nonvascularized ulnar grafts found that vascularized grafts were superior to conventional nerve grafts [6].

Brachial plexus injuries fulfill the second and third criteria (proximal lesions, large defects) and occasionally fulfill the first (whenever there is a compromise of the vascularization) and can be used as a clinical model to investigate this hypothesis.

Birch et al have used successfully vascularized ulnar nerve graft to bridge gaps of up to 16 cm for supraclavicular brachial plexus injuries (proximal lesions) [2].

On the contrary Okinaga and Nagano, who used intercostal nerves transfer into normal recipient beds for brachial plexus injuries, did not find any obvious difference between vascularized and nonvascularized nerve grafts [48].

The authors' belief is that vascularized ulnar nerve graft should be used in global plexopathies and in global root avulsions. In these cases one is always short of graft material and the quality of the vascularized ulnar nerve as an interposition graft far surpasses that of the sural nerve [21]. The injury is proximal and usually long grafts are needed.

Multiple factors play a role in determining the end results of a nerve grafting procedure: the type of injury, the age of the patient, the level of the injury, the length of the graft, the particular nerve involved, the denervation time, and the technique of repairs are some of the variables that influence the results. Case reports that allow the comparison between vascularized and nonvascularized nerve grafts are the best way to control these factors. Each one of the two case report studies of Boorman and Sykes [4] and Mackinnon et al [10] confirm the superiority of the vascularized grafts.

In the authors' studies there are control cases in brachial plexus reconstruction in which there are used vascularized and nonvascularized nerve grafts in the same patient. In these cases, rates of Tinel sign advancement were higher in vascularized nerve graft.

In a lower extremity case that was repaired with vascularized and nonvascularized nerve grafts the authors also found better restoration of sensation in the area that was reinnervated with a vascularized graft.

Experimental and clinical evidence indicates that in proximal lesions as brachial plexus injuries and in long nerve gaps especially when the recipient bed is heavily scarred, microsurgical nerve transfer of a free or pedicled vascularized nerve graft should be used.

Vascularized nerve grafts are not widely accepted, not only because of increased technical difficulty and because it is a time-consuming procedure, but also because the exact indications for their use are not understood clearly and the literature sometimes is controversial. This review study, however, emphasizes that in the authors' center, 25 years of experience with vascularized nerve grafts did not change significantly the criteria and indications for their use. The authors still recommend vascularized ulnar nerve graft for global plexopathies and vascularized sural nerve grafts for lower and distal upper extremity lesions. For brachial plexus injuries only a few changes have been made over time: (1) the authors do not use vascularized nerve graft for multiple targets, (2) if there is a high pedicle, the vascularized ulnar nerve is used as a pedicle rather than as a free vascularized nerve graft and (3) the authors do not use the contralateral C7 with vascularized ulnar nerve for neurotizations of motor nerves. The authors' strategy regarding the use of vascularized ulnar nerve graft at present is as follows: (1) In global plexopathy, if the C5 or C6 roots are ruptured (but the proximal stumps are in continuity with the spinal cord) with simultaneous lower root avulsions, then during the initial reconstruction the ipsilateral ulnar nerve is used as a vascularized graft to reconstruct the musculocutaneous, median, and, on occasion, the axillary or radial nerves. (2) If there is global avulsion, then ipsilateral extraplexus donors are used. Subsequently the authors use the vascularized ulnar nerve graft during the second stage of brachial plexus reconstruction as an interposition long nerve graft to neurotize the median nerve from the anterior division of the contralateral C7 root.

References

[1] Taylor GI, Ham FJ. The free vascularized nerve graft. Plast Reconstr Surg 1975;56:166.

[2] Birch R, Dunkerton M, Bonney G, et al. Experience with the free vascularized ulnar nerve graft in repair of supraclavicular lesions of the brachial plexus. Clin Orthop 1988;237:96–104.

[3] Bonney G, Birch R, Jamieson AM, et al. Experience with vascularized nerve grafts. Clin Plast Surg 1984;1:137–42.

[4] Boorman JG, Sykes PJ. Vascularised versus conventional nerve grafting: a case report. J Hand Surg [Br] 1987;2: 218–20.

[5] Doi K, Tamaru K, Sakai K, et al. A comparison of vascularized and conventional sural nerve grafts. J Hand Surg [Am] 1992;4:670–6.

[6] Chen L, Gu YD. An experimental study of contralateral C7 root transfer with vascularized nerve grafting to treat brachial plexus root avulsion. J Hand Surg [Br] 1994;1:60–6.

[7] Koshima I, Harii K. Experimental study of vascularized nerve grafts: multifactorial analyses of axonal regeneration of nerves transplanted into an acute burn wound. J Hand Surg [Am] 1985;1:64–72.

[8] Koshima I, Harii K. Experimental study of vascularized nerve grafts: morphometric study of axonal regeneration of nerves transplanted into silicone tubes. Ann Plast Surg 1985;3:235–43.

[9] Kanaya F, Firrell J, Tsai TM, et al. Functional results of vascularized versus nonvascularized nerve grafting. Plast Reconstr Surg 1992;5:924–30.

[10] Mackinnon SE, Kelly L, Hunter DA. Comparison of regeneration across a vascularized versus conventional nerve graft: case report. Microsurgery 1988;4:226–34.

[11] Restrepo Y, Merle M, Michon J, et al. Free vascularized nerve grafts: an experimental study in the rabbit. Microsurgery 1985;2:78–84.

[12] Rose EH, Kowalski TA. Restoration of sensibility to anesthetic scarred digits with free vascularized nerve grafts from the dorsum of the foot. J Hand Surg [Am] 1985;4:514–21.

[13] Rose EH, Kowalski TA, Norris MS. The reversed venous arterialized nerve graft in digital nerve reconstruction across scarred beds. Plast Reconstr Surg 1989;4:593–604.

[14] Schultes G, Gaggl A, Kleinert R. Vascularized versus non-vascularized nerve transfers: histologic study in rats. J Reconstr Microsurg 2001;8:637–42.

[15] Shibata M, Tsai TM, Firrell J, et al. Experimental comparison of vascularized and nonvascularized nerve grafting. J Hand Surg [Am] 1988;3:358–65.

[16] Phillipeaux JM, Vulpian A. Note sur.es Essais de greffe d'un troncon de nerf lingual entre les deux bouts de l'hypoglose. Archs Physiol Norm Path 1870;3:618.

[17] Albert E. Einige Operationen an Nerven. Wien Med Presse 1885;26:1285.

[18] Bunnel S, Boys JH. Nerve grafts. Am J Surg 1939;44:64.

[19] Tarlov IM, Epstein JA. Nerve grafts: the importance of an adequate blood supply. J Neurosurg 1945;2:49.

[20] Strange SC. An operation for nerve pedicle grafting. Preliminary communications. Br J Surg 1947;34:423.

[21] Terzis JK, Breidenbach WC. The anatomy of free vascularized nerve grafts. In: Terzis JK, editor. Microreconstruction of nerve injuries. Philadelphia: WB Saunders; 1987. p. 101–16.

[22] Faschinelli A, Masquelet AC, Restrepo J, et al. The vascularized sural nerve. Int J Microsurg 1981;3:57.

[23] Breidenbach W, Terzis JK. The anatomy of free vascularized nerve grafts. Clin Plast Surg 1984;1:65–71.

[24] Lundborg G. Intraneural microvascular pathophysiology as related to ischemia and nerve injury. In: Daniel RK, Terzis JK, editors. Reconstructive microsurgery. Boston: Little Brown & Co.; 1977. p. 334–41.

[25] Sunderland S. Blood supply of the peripheral nerves. Practical considerations. Arch Neurol. Psychiatr 1945;54:280.
[26] Gilbert A. Vascularized sural nerve graft. Clin Plast Surg 1984;1:73–7.
[27] Breidenbach WC, Terzis JK. The blood supply of vascularized nerve grafts. J Reconstr Microsurg 1986;1:43–58.
[28] Terzis JK, Skoulis TG, Soucacos PN. Vascularized nerve grafts. Int Angiol 1995;14:264–77.
[29] Townsend PL, Taylor GI. Vascularised nerve grafts using composite arterialised neuro-venous systems. Br J Plast Surg 1984;1:1–17.
[30] Gu YD, Wu MM, Zheng YL, et al. Arterialized venous free sural nerve grafting. Ann Plast Surg 1985;4:332–9.
[31] Arakaki A, Tsai TM, Firrell JC, et al. Vascular filling and protein extravasation in three varieties of vascularized venous nerve grafts. J Reconstr Microsurg 1994;3:165–70.
[32] Lundborg G. Structure and function of the intraneural microvessels as related to trauma, edema formation, and nerve function. J Bone Joint Surg [Am] 1975;7:938–48.
[33] Lundborg G. Ischemic nerve injury. Experimental studies on intraneural microvascular pathophysiology and nerve function in a limb subjected to temporary circulatory arrest. Scand J Plast Reconstr Surg Suppl 1970;6:3–113.
[34] Kanaya F, Firrell J, Breidenbach WC. Blood flow of segmentally divided and folded nerve. J Reconstr Microsurg 1993;6:429–33.
[35] Settergren CR, Wood MB. Comparison of blood flow in free vascularized versus nonvascularized nerve grafts. J Reconstr Microsurg 1984;2:95–101.
[36] Daly PJ, Wood MB. Endoneural and epineural blood flow evaluation with free vascularized and conventional nerve grafts in the canine. J Reconstr Microsurg 1985;1:45–9.
[37] Lux P, Breidenbach W, Firrell J. Determination of temporal changes in blood flow in vascularized and nonvascularized nerve grafts in the dog. Plast Reconstr Surg 1988;1:133–44.
[38] Wongtrakul S, Bishop AT, Friedrich PF. Vascular endothelial growth factor promotion of neoangiogenesis in conventional nerve grafts. J Hand Surg [Am] 2002;2:277–85.
[39] Lind R, Wood MB. Comparison of the pattern of early revascularization of conventional versus vascularized nerve grafts in the canine. J Reconstr Microsurg 1986;4:229–34.
[40] Penkert G, Bini W, Samii M. Revascularization of nerve grafts: an experimental study. J Reconstr Microsurg 1988; 4:319–25.
[41] Best TJ, Mackinnon SE. Peripheral nerve revascularization: a current literature review. J Reconstr Microsurg 1994; 3:193–204.
[42] Best TJ, Mackinnon SE, Evans PJ, et al. Peripheral nerve revascularization: histomorphometric study of small- and large-caliber grafts. J Reconstr Microsurg 1999;3:183–90.
[43] Terzis JK, Dupree J, D'Antonio M, et al. Vascularized versus nonvascularized nerve grafts: the controversy persists. Presented at the Plastic Surgery Research Council Meeting. San Francisco, May 19–21, 1988.
[44] Mani GV, Shurey C, Green CJ. Is early vascularization of nerve grafts necessary? J Hand Surg [Br] 1992;5:536–43.
[45] McCullough CJ, Gagey O, Higginson DW, et al. Axon regeneration and vascularisation of nerve grafts: an experimental study. J Hand Surg [Br] 1984;3:323–7.
[46] Pho RW, Lee YS, Rujiwetpongstorn V, et al. Histological studies of vascularised nerve graft and conventional nerve graft. J Hand Surg [Br] 1985;1:45–8.
[47] Seckel BR, Ryan SE, Simons JE, et al. Vascularized versus nonvascularized nerve grafts: an experimental structural comparison. Plast Reconstr Surg 1986;2:211–20.
[48] Okinaga S, Nagano A. Can vascularization improve the surgical outcome of the intercostal nerve transfer for traumatic brachial plexus palsy? A clinical comparison of vascularized and non-vascularized methods. Microsurgery 1999;4:176–80.
[49] Xu J, Gu Y, Lao J. Anatomic basis of vascularized ulnar nerve graft by the pedicle of the superior collateral ulnar artery. Clin J Traumatol 2001;4:195–8.
[50] Terzis JK, Vekris MD, Soucacos PN. Outcomes of brachial plexus reconstruction in 204 patients with devastating paralysis. Plast Reconstr Surg 1999;5:1221–40.
[51] Doi K, Kuwata N, Kawakami F, et al. The free vascularized sural nerve graft. Microsurgery 1984;5:175.
[52] Riordan CL, Nanney LB, Upton J III, Wolfort SF. Vascularized medial sural cutaneous nerve based on the superficial sural artery: a reliable nerve graft. J Reconstr Microsurg 2002;3:147–52.
[53] Taylor GI. Free vascularized nerve transfer in the upper extremity. Hand Clin 1999;4:673–95.

ELSEVIER
SAUNDERS

Atlas Hand Clin 10 (2005) 125–133

Atlas of the HAND CLINICS

Nerve Conduits in Peripheral Nerve Repair

Charles K. Herman, MD, John F. Diaz, MD, Berish Strauch, MD*

Department of Plastic and Reconstructive Surgery, Albert Einstein College of Medicine and Montefiore Medical Center, 1625 Poplar Street, Suite 200, Bronx, NY 10461, USA

Motor and sensory deficits resulting from injury to the peripheral nervous system can be devastating. Reconstruction of peripheral nerve injuries remains one of the greatest challenges in plastic surgery. In recent years significant progress has been made in repairing tendon and vessel damage and soft tissue defects that accompany trauma to the extremities. Unless satisfactory restoration of sensory and motor innervation is accomplished, however, the extremity may be rendered functionally impaired or useless.

The treatment of choice for transected peripheral nerves today is still primary tensionless end-to-end repair. In cases involving significant loss of nerve substance, delay in treatment, and other associated injuries, primary repair may not be possible. Excessive tension at the site of coaptation has been demonstrated to result in increased scar formation between nerve ends and decreased nerve conduction velocities and amplitudes [1,2].

Several techniques have been developed to bridge nerve gaps. Autologous nerve grafting has proven to be an effective modality but is associated with donor-site morbidity. Nerve conduits have been used with success in bridging nerve gaps up to 3 cm. These conduits can be of biologic or nonbiologic origin. Biologic conduits include autologous venous conduits, arterial conduits, and muscular conduits. Some research also has investigated the usefulness of conduits derived from bone, fascia, and intestinal wall. Nonbiologic conduits are derived from a variety of prosthetic materials that are either absorbable or nonabsorbable.

Biologic conduits

Autologous venous nerve conduits (Fig. 1)

Buengner reported the first use of a vascular conduit in 1891, bridging a canine sciatic nerve gap using a segment of human brachial artery [3]. As a consequence of the morbidities associated with donor artery harvest, attention subsequently has focused on autologous venous nerve conduits. Wrede in 1909 used a vein graft to regain some motor and sensory function in a patient with a median nerve defect [4].

In 1982, Chiu presented histologic and electrophysiologic evidence of nerve regeneration using a vein graft in his landmark animal study [5]. Numerous histologic and electrophysiologic studies have been performed since then. Independent studies by Chiu and by Suematsu showed that nerves repaired with vein grafts demonstrated comparable electrophysiologic behavior to nerves repaired with conventional nerve grafts [6,7]. These studies showed that nerve conduction velocities were similar. Action potentials generated in a nerve repair using a vein graft, however, were of lesser magnitude in relation to those in nerves repaired with nerve grafts. Janecka demonstrated that the density of axons that regenerate through a venous conduit is similar to that in an unoperated nerve [8].

* Corresponding author.
E-mail address: bstrauch@montefiore.org (B. Strauch).

1082-3131/05/$ - see front matter
doi:10.1016/j.ahc.2004.08.002

handatlas.theclinics.com

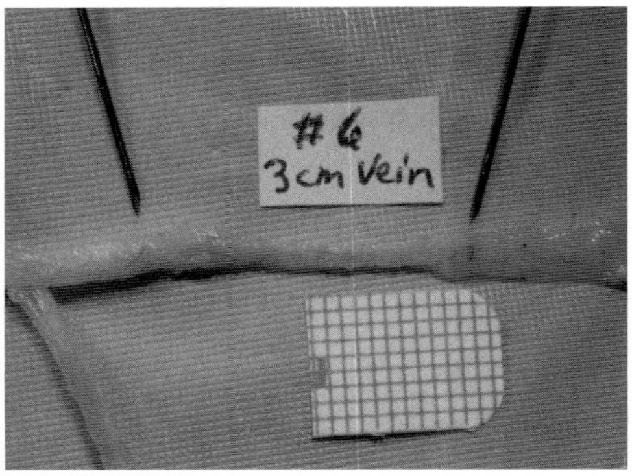

Fig. 1. Photograph of a 3-cm autologous vein conduit repair.

In the late 1980s and early 1990s several investigators demonstrated axonal regrowth through venous conduits for nerve gaps up to 3 cm [7,9–13]. Chiu and Strauch in 1990 established the clinical effectiveness of vein grafts for sensory nerve defects up to 3 cm in length [14]. Return of good sensibility was achieved, measured by two-point discrimination and the ten test [15]. Initial studies questioned the applicability of venous conduits in delayed repair [16]. Chiu and Strauch, on the other hand, demonstrated that autologous venous nerve conduits were effective in immediate and delayed repairs. Tang has presented evidence that vein grafts can be used for sensory nerve defects up to 4.5 cm [17].

Some investigators have hypothesized that the limiting factor in nerve repair seems not to be the technique of coaptation but the mechanism of regeneration itself [12,18,19]. For this reason considerable research has been dedicated to the investigation of ways to improve the ability of nerve conduits to enable nerve regeneration. These efforts have focused largely on the addition of neurotrophic factors to the conduits. Other strategies have included the addition of Schwann cells and other autologous tissues into nerve conduits. Recently Strauch et al were able to drive axonal regeneration through 6-cm gaps by inserting a Schwann cell matrix into autologous venous conduits [20]. Other investigators have coupled a variety of growth factors with vein grafts, including basic fibroblast growth factor [21].

Arterial conduits

The morbidity associated with obtaining donor arterial material has deterred investigation into arterial conduits despite the promising early historical findings by Buengner. As a result few experimental and clinical studies have been conducted.

Muscle conduits

Studies demonstrating axonal growth through muscle basal laminae provided the impetus for research into muscle conduits for nerve regeneration [22,23]. In addition, the type IV collagen and laminin contained in muscle tissue have been shown to promote nerve fiber growth [24,25]. Glasby et al used freeze-thawed muscle grafts to bridge sciatic nerve gaps in rats [26]. This information has been applied to several human investigations. Norris et al used muscle grafts to repair digital nerve injuries [27]. Pereira et al reported the use of muscle conduits in digital nerve reconstructions for defects up to 28 mm [28] and in posterior tibial and median nerve defects up to 60 mm [29].

Muscle conduits have some recognized disadvantages. Nerve fibers can grow out of a freeze-thawed denatured muscle tissue conduit, prompting investigators to place muscle tissue within nerve guides [30]. Studies have suggested that Schwann cells may be limited in their ability to migrate into muscle grafts [31]. Stirrat et al noted some sensory but no motor recovery in seven patients with mixed nerve injuries repaired with muscle grafts [32]. The clinical usefulness of muscle conduits has not been elucidated yet.

Nonautologous biologic conduits

Small intestinal submucosa

The use of porcine small intestinal submucosa (SIS) has been examined recently in the laboratories of Strauch (B. Strauch, unpublished data, 2003). SIS conduits used to bridge nerve gaps of 1 and 3 cm in a rabbit model have demonstrated excellent potential for nerve growth and myelination (Figs. 2 and 3). These results were demonstrated using optical and electron microscopy. In the same study the SIS conduits showed comparable results to those obtained from conventional gluteal vein conduits for nerve gaps of 3 cm. Good nerve growth and excellent myelination were seen in the 1-cm grafts. Good nerve growth and inconsistent myelination were seen in the SIS and vein grafts when used for 3-cm defects. SIS conduits therefore may possess efficacy similar to vein conduits without the need for vein harvest and its associated morbidities.

Collagen

Nerve conduits from collagen can be semipermeable and biodegradable. For these reasons collagen has been investigated as a potential material for nerve repair. In 1991 Archibald et al studied collagen conduits for the repair of nerve transections in rat and primate models [33]. Muscle evoked action potentials were measured to compare direct microneurosurgical repair, nerve autografts, and collagen conduits to bridge 4-mm gaps in transected rat sciatic nerves. Results were comparable among all three groups at 12 weeks post-repair. Similarly no statistically significant differences were found between nerve autograft and collagen conduit repairs of distal median nerve gaps of 4 mm in the primate model. Additional studies by Archibald et al comparing nerve autografts and collagen conduits for median and ulnar nerve gaps of 5 mm yielded similar results [34].

In summary, collagen possesses many characteristics that make it attractive for use as a nerve conduit. Further studies investigating its use in humans and for longer defects are needed before its clinical usefulness is elucidated.

Nonbiologic conduits

Using autologous tissue for nerve repair has many advantages. The use of autologous tissues, however, will always be associated with additional operative time and labor to harvest the material and with some donor site morbidity, no matter how theoretically minor that morbidity may be. It is for these reasons that substantial effort has been dedicated to the research and design of synthetic materials that can be used for nerve repair.

Reports of the experimental use of nonautologous conduits date from 1901 [35]. Early materials included gelatin tubes, agar, and parchment. Poor results discouraged further studies. Treatment of injuries during World War II renewed interest in the development of synthetic materials for nerve conduits.

Attempts to create synthetic nerve conduits have used a vast array of materials. A major distinguishing feature of these different synthetic conduits is their susceptibility to

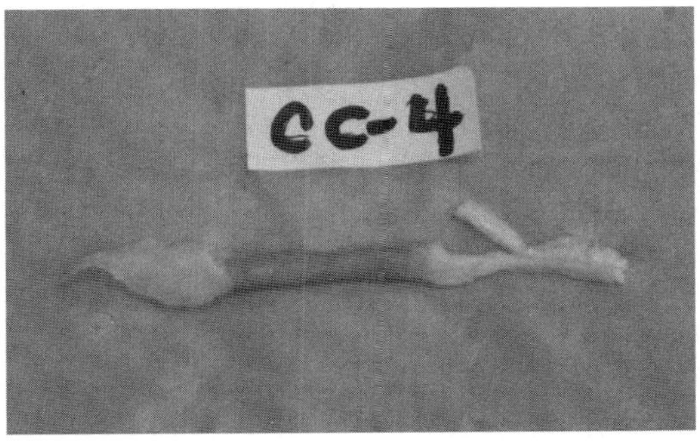

Fig. 2. Photograph of a 3-cm porcine small intestinal submucosal conduit repair.

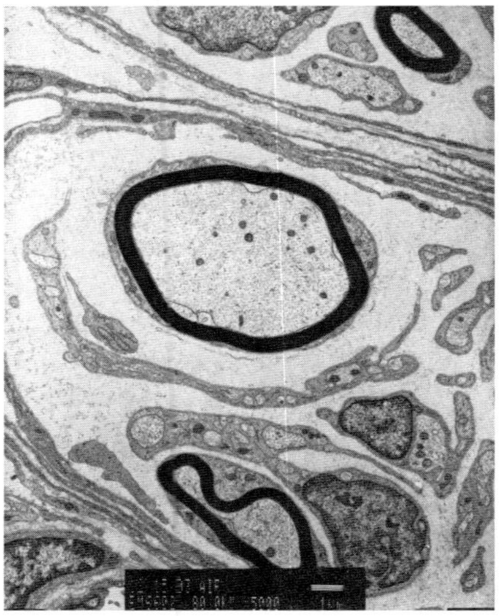

Fig. 3. Electron micrograph demonstrating nerve growth and myelination within a 1-cm porcine small intestinal submucosal conduit.

biodegradation. It is thus useful to categorize synthetic nerve conduits into those that are bioabsorbable and those that are not.

Nonabsorbable conduits

The basic goal of any nerve conduit is to provide regenerating axons with a passage to the distal nerve stump while protecting it from the surrounding environment. Nonbiodegradable conduits can provide this protective environment. Non-bioabsorbable conduits, however, have been associated with several disadvantages. Because they remain as foreign bodies in the tissue, they can cause foreign body reactions. This can lead to scar formation and inflammation. Excessive scar formation may result in compression of the conduit. Inflammation may cause irritation and discomfort at the site of implantation. Many of the patients who have received non-bioabsorbable conduits thus have required a second procedure to remove the conduit. Nevertheless these materials constantly are researched and improved. Further studies are needed to explore fully the potential clinical usefulness of these materials.

Silicone

Silicone has been used in a multiplicity of clinical applications. Merle et al were the first to use this material clinically as a nerve guide in 1989 [36]. Successful regeneration of peripheral nerves was demonstrated in three patients. Significant complications with the procedure were reported, however. After 2 years the patients began complaining about nerve impairment and irritation at the surgical site, subsequently requiring a second procedure to remove the silicone tubes.

Lundborg et al have written extensively about their experience with silicone nerve guides. In a case report from 1991 they described the use of a silicone chamber to repair an ulnar nerve injury at the level of the wrist in a 21-year-old man [37]. Although motor and sensory functions were excellent, the patient ultimately required removal of the silicone chamber because of local irritation. In another study from 1997 they randomized 18 patients with median or ulnar nerve injuries into two groups. One group was repaired using conventional microsurgical repair. The other group was repaired using a silicone tube. After 1 year there were no significant differences between the two groups with respect to motor or sensory recovery except for the perception of touch, which was significantly better in the group repaired with the silicone tube [38]. Recently Lundborg et al reported their 5-year follow-up results in this study group. After 5 years they found there was no significant difference in outcome between the two techniques except that cold intolerance was significantly less severe with the tubular technique [39]. Dahlin and Lundborg reviewed the use of silicone tubes as a nerve conduit and suggested that it can be a useful technique for the repair of a maximum of 5-mm gaps in human median and ulnar nerves [40].

In summary, silicone nerve conduits may be used for small defects of 5 mm or less. Their usefulness in longer nerve gaps has not been validated. The material can be associated with significant foreign body reaction, excessive scar formation, and subsequent nerve compression. It may cause local irritation requiring later removal. Clinical experience is limited with this material.

Polytetrafluoroethylene (PTFE)

PTFE (Gore-Tex) has widespread and successful use in vascular surgery. Investigators have theorized that it can also, therefore, serve as a potentially useful nerve conduit. Stanec and Stanec have presented two studies using PTFE as a nerve conduit. The first was a report on the use of PTFE to bridge a 29-mm defect of the ulnar nerve in the forearm [41]. Although there was excellent motor and sensory recovery, the graft required removal because of complaints of irritation at the repair site. In a second article they reported their experience using PTFE to repair nerve defects in 43 patients [42]. Their experience consisted of secondary reconstructions of 21 injuries to the median nerve and 22 injuries to the ulnar nerve at various levels. The investigators concluded that PTFE can be used as a nerve guide for reconstruction of nerve gaps up to 4 cm.

In another study of seven patients, PTFE tubes were used to repair nerve defects of the lingual and inferior alveolar nerves [43]. The nerve defects were smaller than 3 mm. Two patients had return of sensation (one lingual and one inferior alveolar); the remaining five patients did not have any return of function. The investigators concluded that PTFE tubes may not be effective for nerve regeneration. They pointed out, however, that only one patient was operated on within the conventionally accepted time for optimum repair of 3–6 months postinjury. The patients, therefore, might not have had functional recovery with any type of repair used.

In general, nonabsorbable conduits seem to have had some experimental and clinical success. They have not had widespread clinical acceptance, however. Prospective randomized clinical trials are needed to determine the efficacy of nonabsorbable conduits.

Absorbable conduits

Nerve conduits function as a passage for regenerating axons to bridge a nerve defect. Once the nerve fibers have bridged the gap between the proximal and distal nerve stumps, the conduits theoretically are no longer needed. As stated previously, synthetic nonabsorbable conduits have the potential disadvantages of causing foreign body reactions, excessive scar formation, and nerve compression. These results would negate the very reason for their use [44].

Ideally, synthetic bioabsorbable nerve conduits should be noncytotoxic, noncarcinogenic, and nonimmunogenic. Their absorption rate should be matched with the growth rate of the regenerating axons such that they are degraded at the time regeneration is completed or shortly thereafter. Numerous bioabsorbable materials have been investigated in clinical and animal studies.

Polyglycolic acid (PGA)

Several studies have been performed investigating the potential use of this bioabsorbable material. Mackinnon and Dellon described the use of PGA conduits for digital nerve repair [45]. In their study, 15 patients underwent secondary reconstruction of digital nerve injuries. Results showed excellent functional sensibility in 33% and good functional sensibility in 53%. In addition, they found that for defects up to 30 mm the PGA tubes produced comparable results to classic nerve graft repair.

Weber et al performed a prospective, randomized, multicenter study to compare PGA tubes with standard end-to-end nerve repair [46]. All patients received postoperative sensory re-education and were followed for 12 months. Excellent results were obtained in 91% of the PGA tube-treated patients, compared with 40% in the patients treated with end-to-end repair. The average length of the defects was 7 mm.

In summary, multiple studies have supported the use of PGA tubes for nerve reconstruction. Successful regeneration has been shown in nerve defects of less than 3 cm.

Microbraided poly (L-lactide-coglycolide)

The proposed advantages of this material include its biocompatibility, permeability to nutrients, and flexibility for use in different areas and defects. Bini et al have reported their study of this material in rat sciatic nerve defects up to 12 mm [47]. The investigators noted that there was no inflammatory reaction to the material. After 1 month, 9 of 10 rats showed evidence of regeneration across the gap.

Poly(DLLA-epsilon-CL)

Varejao et al have studied the use of this material. The conduits were filled with skeletal muscle grafts before repair. They showed successful nerve regeneration across a 1-cm gap in the rat sciatic nerve [48]. Histomorphometric analysis showed good regeneration across this conduit [49].

Poly 3-hydroxybutyrate (PHB)

Mohanna et al studied the use of PHB in a rabbit model [50]. In this study, PHB conduits were used to bridge gaps of 2–4 cm in the rabbit common peroneal nerve. They found successful axonal regeneration across a 2-cm nerve gap. Young et al compared PHB conduits with nerve autografts to bridge nerve gaps of up to 4 cm in the rabbit common peroneal nerve. They found that by 42 days, regenerating axons had bridged nerve gaps of all lengths in groups with nerve autografts and in those with PHB conduits. The investigators concluded that PHB can be used to support nerve regeneration up to 4 cm [51].

These animal studies suggest that PHB may be useful to repair nerve defects of up to 4 cm. Human clinical studies are needed to assess its ultimate usefulness.

Poly(L-lactic acid) (PLLA)

Evans et al have investigated the use of this bioabsorbable material. In one study they used conduits made of PLLA to bridge nerve defects of up to 10 mm in the rat sciatic nerve [52]. Nerve isografts were used as controls. Walking track analysis, gastrocnemius muscle evaluation, and nerve fiber analysis revealed evidence of regeneration across these conduits. The use of isografts demonstrated superior regrowth, however.

In another study they showed evidence of successful regeneration across a 12-mm defect of the rat sciatic nerve [53]. Analysis after 8 months revealed that the PLLA conduit remained structurally intact and demonstrated tissue incorporation and vascularization. There was no evidence of conduit collapse or breakage with limb ambulation.

Poly(phosphoester) (PPE)

The proposed advantages of PPE are its biocompatibility and its adjustable biodegradability. Wang et al investigated the feasibility of using this material as a nerve conduit [54]. Using a rat sciatic nerve model, 10-mm nerve gaps were repaired using PPE tubes. Successful regeneration was demonstrated in their study.

Poly-L-lactide-epsilon-caprolactone (PLC)

Valero-Cabre et al performed a study comparing the use of PLC conduits with silicone tubes and nerve grafts [55]. Nerve gaps measuring 8 mm were repaired using the various tubes in a rat sciatic nerve model. Nerve regeneration was assessed by measuring compound muscle action potential (CMAP) amplitudes. In addition, histologic analysis was used to evaluate the branching pattern of regenerating axons. The CMAP amplitudes were similar in nerve autograft and PLC tube implantation groups but lower in the silicone tube group. Furthermore, the percentage of neurons with multiple projections was lower in the autograft and PLC tube groups than in the silicone tube group. The investigators suggest that PLC tubes may be a suitable conduit for nerve repair.

Gelatin

Mligiliche, Tabata, and Ide looked at the feasibility of using gelatin tubes as nerve guides [56]. In this study, 7-mm nerve gaps were created in mice sciatic nerves. The defects were repaired using a gelatin conduit. The investigators reported successful regeneration with the use of this material in this model.

Polyphosphazene (poly-[bis-(ethylalanate)-phosphazene])

Polyphosphazenes are biodegradable and biocompatible. Two studies have demonstrated the potential applicability of this material for nerve repair. In both, 10-mm nerve gaps in the rat sciatic nerve were repaired. Histologic examination and electron microscopy revealed nerve regeneration across the conduit [57,58].

Maxon (glycolide trimethylene carbonate)

In one study using a primate model, 2- and 5-cm nerve defects were repaired using either Maxon or collagen conduits [59]. At 14 months excellent regeneration was noted across the 2-cm nerve gap through the collagen and Maxon conduits. At 5 cm, regeneration as determined by morphometric analysis was significantly better across the Maxon conduit, although there was no difference by electrophysiologic assessment.

Since the introduction of vein conduits into the clinical realm by Chiu and Strauch in 1990, the race to find the most suitable and clinically useful conduit has produced advocates for many different types. Autologous material, although clinically successful, probably will not satisfy the need because of the requirement to harvest the graft, creating additional scarring and associated donor-site morbidities. Other biologic or nonbiologic conduits probably will prove to be the most clinically useful. The ability to serve as a guide and subsequently to develop an intrinsic circulation or to disintegrate are most attractive concepts.

Nerve conduits may play a future role in one of two ways: as replacements for long defects or for short defects with small gaps or no gap at all. In long segment replacements, they will need to be modified with nerve growth factors or cultured Schwann cell contents to overcome defects of 3 cm or greater on a consistent basis. Use of nerve conduits for short gaps of a few millimeters or for no gap at all may be a valid technique, theoretically allowing nerves to find their own distal tubules without epineurial sutures. This was advocated recently by Taras in his report on digital nerve repairs [60]. Lundborg in his latest evaluation of silicone tubes in distal ulnar and median nerve repairs in fresh lacerations found similar results between standard micro-neurosurgical repairs and repairs performed with silicone conduits that left a 5-mm gap [39].

Summary

The use of nerve conduits is still in its infancy. The promise of being able to provide a substitute for longer nerve defects or even to allow for improved healing of primary disruptions is close at hand.

References

[1] Millesi H, Meissl G, Berger A. The interfascicular nerve grafting of the median and ulnar nerves. J Bone Joint Surg 1972;54A:727.

[2] Terzis JK, Faibisoff B, Williams B. The nerve gap: suture under tension vs. graft. Plast Reconstr Surg 1975;56:169.

[3] Buengner OV. Ueber die degenerations-und regenerationsvorgaenge am nerven nach verletzungen. Beitr Pathol Anat 1891;10:321.

[4] Wrede L. Ueberbruckung eines nervendefektes mittles seidennaht and lebenden venenstuckes. Deutsches Medezin Wochenschrift 1909;35:1125.

[5] Chiu DTW, Janecka I, Krizek TJ, Wolff M, Lovelace RE. Autologous vein graft as a conduit for nerve regeneration. Surgery 1982;91:226.

[6] Chiu DTW, Lovelace RE, Yu LT, Wolff M, Stengel S, Middleton L, et al. Comparative electrophysiologic evaluation of nerve grafts and autologous vein grafts as nerve conduits: an experimental study. J Reconstr Microsurg 1988;4(4):303.

[7] Suematsu N, Atusuta Y, Hirayama T. Vein graft for repair of peripheral nerve gap. J Reconstr Microsurg 1984;4(4): 313.

[8] Janecka IP. Peripheral nerve regeneration: an experimental study. Laryngoscope 1987;97:942.

[9] Benito-Ruiz J, Navarro-Monzonis A, Piqueras A, Baena-Montilla P. Invaginated vein graft as nerve conduit: an experimental study. Microsurgery 1994;15:105.

[10] Berger A, Lassner F, Schaller E. The Dellon tube in injuries of peripheral nerves. Handchir Mikrochir Plast Chir 1994;26:44.

[11] Keeley R, Atagi T, Sabelman E, Padilla J, Kadlcik S, Keeley A, et al. Peripheral nerve regeneration across 14-mm gaps: a comparison of autograft and entubulation repair methods in the rat. J Reconstr Microsurg 1993;9:349.

[12] Strauch B, Ferder M, Lovelle-Allen S, Moore K, Kim DJ, Llena J. Determining the maximal length of a vein conduit used as an interposition graft for nerve regeneration. J Reconstr Microsurg 1996;12:521.

[13] Wang KK, Costas PD, Jones DS, Miller RA, Seckel BR. Sleeve insertion and collagen coating improve nerve regeneration through vein conduits. J Reconstr Microsurg 1993;9:39.

[14] Chiu DTW, Strauch B. A prospective clinical evaluation of autologous vein grafts used as a nerve conduit for distal sensory nerve defects of 3 cm or less. Plast Reconstr Surg 1990;82:928.

[15] Strauch B, Lang A, Ferder M, Keyes-Ford M, Freeman K, Newstein D. The 10 test: use of an analog scale for sensibility testing. Plast Reconstr Surg 1997;99:924.

[16] Walton RL, Brown RE, Matory WE, Boral GL, Dolph JL. Autologous vein graft repair of digital nerve defects in the finger: a retrospective clinical study. Plast Reconstr Surg 1989;84:944–9.

[17] Tang JB. Vein conduits with interposition of nerve tissue for peripheral nerve defects. J Reconstr Microsurg 1995; 11:21.

[18] Jabaley ME. Peripheral nerve repair. In: McCarthy JG, editor. Plastic surgery. Philadelphia, PA: WB Saunders Co.; 1990.

[19] Strauch B. Use of nerve conduits in peripheral nerve repair. Hand Clin 2000;16(1):123–30.

[20] Strauch B, Rodriguez DM, Diaz J, Yu HL, Kaplan G, Weinstein DE. Autologous Schwann cells drive regeneration through a 6-cm autologous venous nerve conduit. J Reconstr Microsurg 2001;17(8):589–95.

[21] Li CY, Cao DC. Experimental study on repair of peripheral nerve defect by basic fibroblast growth factor combined with autologous vein graft conduit. Zhongguo Xiu Fu Chong Jian Wai Ke Za Zhi 2000;14(1):14–6.

[22] Ide C. Nerve regeneration through the basal lamina scaffold of the skeletal muscle. Neurosci Res 1984;1:379.

[23] Keynes RJ, Hopkins WB, Huang CLH. Regeneration of mouse peripheral nerves in degenerating skeletal muscle: guidance by residual muscle fiber basement membrane. Brain Res 1984;295:275.

[24] Lundborg G, Dahlin L, Danielsen N, Zhao Q. Trophism, tropism and specificity in nerve regeneration. J Reconstr Microsurg 1994;10:345–54.

[25] Satou T, Nishida S, Hiruma S, Tanji K, Takahashi M, Fujita S, et al. A morphological study of the effects of collagen gel matrix on regeneration of severed rat sciatic nerve in silicone tubes. Acta Path Jpn 1986;36:199–208.

[26] Glasby MA, Gschmeissner SG, Hitchcock RJI, Huang CL-H. Regeneration of the sciatic nerve in rats. J Bone Joint Surg 1986;68B:829–33.

[27] Norris RW, Glasby MA, Gattuso JM, Bowden REM. Peripheral nerve repair in humans using muscle autografts: a new technique. J Bone Joint Surg 1988;70:530.

[28] Pereira JH, Palande DD, Subramanian A, Narayanakumar TS, Curtis J, Turk JL. Denatured autologous muscle graft in leprosy. Lancet 1991;16:1239–40.

[29] Pereira JH, Bowden RE, Gattuso JM, Norris RW. Comparison of results of repair of digital nerves by denatured muscle grafts and end-to-end sutures. J Hand Surg 1991;16B:519–23.

[30] Meek MF, Robinson PH, Stokroos I, Blaauw EH, Kors G, den Dunnen WF. Electronmicroscopical evaluation of short term nerve regeneration using a thin-walled biodegradable poly (DL-lactide-epsilon-caprolactone) nerve guide filled with modified denatured muscle tissue. Biomaterials 2001;22:1177–85.

[31] De Franzo AJ, Morykwas MJ, La Rosse JR, Jennings DA, Challa V, Argenta LC. Autologous denatured muscle as a nerve graft. J Reconstr Microsurg 1994;10(3):145–9.

[32] Sirrat AN, Birch R, Glasby MA. Applications of muscle autograft in peripheral nerve injury. Brighton, UK: Abstracts of the British Orthopedic Association; 1991. p. 8.

[33] Archibald SJ, Krarup C, Shefner J, Li ST, Madison RD. A collagen-based nerve guide conduit for peripheral nerve repair: an electrophysiological study of nerve regeneration in rodents and nonhuman primates. J Comp Neurol 1991;306(4):685–96.

[34] Archibald SJ, Shefner J, Krarup C, Madison RD. Monkey median nerve repaired by nerve graft or collagen nerve guide tube. J Neurosci 1995;15(5 Pt 2):4109–23.

[35] Weiss P. The technology of nerve regeneration: a review. Tubulation and related methods of nerve repair. J Neurosurg 1944;1:400.

[36] Merle M, Dellon AL, Campbell JN, Chang PS. Complications from silicone polymer entubulation of nerves. Microsurgery 1989;10:130–3.

[37] Lundborg G, Dahlin LB, Danielsen N. Ulnar nerve repair by the silicone chamber technique: case report. Scand J Plast Reconstr Hand Surg 1991;25:79–82.

[38] Lundborg G, Rosen B, Dahlin L, Danielsen N, Holmberg J. Tubular versus conventional repair of median and ulnar nerves in the human forearm: early results from a prospective, randomized, clinical study. J Hand Surg 1997; 22A:99–106.

[39] Lundborg G, Rosen B, Dahlin L, Holmberg J, Rosen I. Tubular repair of the median or ulnar nerve in the human forearm: a 5-year follow-up. J Hand Surg [Br] 2004;29(2):100–7.

[40] Dahlin LB, Lundborg G. Use of tubes in peripheral nerve repair. Neurosurg Clin N Am 2001;12(2):341–52.

[41] Stanec S, Stanec Z. Reconstruction of upper extremity peripheral nerve injuries with ePTFE conduits. J Reconstr Microsurg 1998;14:227–32.

[42] Stanec S, Stanec Z. Ulnar nerve reconstruction with an expanded polytetrafluoroethylene conduit. Br J Plast Surg 1998;51:637–9.

[43] Pogrel MA, McDonald AR, Kaban LB. Gore-Tex tubing as a conduit for repair of lingual and inferior alveolar nerve continuity defects: a preliminary report. J Oral Maxillofac Surg 1998;56:319–21.

[44] Meek MF, Coert JH. Clinical use of nerve conduits in peripheral nerve repair: review of the literature. J Reconstr Microsurg 2002;18(2):97–109.

[45] Mackinnon SE, Dellon AL. Clinical nerve reconstruction with a bioabsorbable polyglycolic acid tube. Plast Reconstr Surg 1990;85:419–24.

[46] Weber RA, Breidenbach WC, Brown RE, Jabaley ME, Mass DP. A randomized prospective study of polyglycolic acid conduits for digital nerve reconstruction in humans. Plast Reconstr Surg 2000;106:1036–45.

[47] Bini TB, Gao S, Xu X, Wang S, Ramakrishna S, Leong KW. Peripheral nerve regeneration by microbraided poly(L-lactide-co-glycolide) biodegradable polymer fibers. J Biomed Mater Res 2004;68A(2):286–95.

[48] Varejao AS, Cabrita AM, Meek MF, Fornaro M, Geuna S. Nerve regeneration inside fresh skeletal muscle-enriched synthetic tubes: a laser confocal microscope study in the rat sciatic nerve model. Ital J Anat Embryol 2003;108(2): 77–82.

[49] Varejao AS, Cabrita AM, Meek MF, Fornaro M, Geuna S, Giacobini-Robecchi MG. Morphology of nerve fiber regeneration along a biodegradable poly (DLLA-epsilon-CL) nerve guide filled with fresh skeletal muscle. Microsurgery 2003;23(4):338–45.

[50] Mohanna PN, Young RC, Wiberg M, Terenghi G. A composite poly-hydroxybutyrate-glial growth factor conduit for long nerve gap repairs. J Anat 2003;203(6):553–65.

[51] Young RC, Wiberg M, Terenghi G. Poly-3-hydroxybutyrate (PHB): a resorbable conduit for long-gap repair in peripheral nerves. Br J Plast Surg 2002;55(3):235–40.

[52] Evans GR, Brandt K, Widmer MS, Lu L, Meszlenyi RK, Gupta PK, Mikos AG, Hodges J, Williams J, Gurlek A, Nabawi A, Lohman R, Patrick CW Jr. In vivo evaluation of poly(L-lactic acid) porous conduits for peripheral nerve regeneration. Biomaterials 1999;20(12):1109–15.

[53] Evans GR, Brandt K, Niederbichler AD, Chauvin P, Herrman S, Bogle M, et al. Clinical long-term in vivo evaluation of poly(L-lactic acid) porous conduits for peripheral nerve regeneration. J. Biomater Sci Polym Ed 2000; 11(8):869–78.

[54] Wang S, Wan AC, Xu X, Gao S, Mao HQ, Leong KW, Yu H. A new nerve guide conduit material composed of a biodegradable poly(phosphoester). Biomaterials 2001;22(10):1157–69.

[55] Valero-Cabre A, Tsironis K, Skouras E, Perego G, Navarro X, Neiss WF. Superior muscle reinnervation after autologous nerve graft or poly-L-lactide-epsilon-caprolactone (PLC) tube implantation in comparison to silicone tube repair. J Neurosci Res 2001;63(2):214–23.

[56] Mligiliche NL, Tabata Y, Ide C. Nerve regeneration through biodegradable gelatin conduits in mice. East Afr Med J 1999;76(7):400–6.

[57] Nicoli Aldini N, Caliceti P, Lora S, Maltarello MC, Fini M, Rocca M, Martini L, Giavaresi G, Veronese FM, Giardino R. Polymer biomaterials (polyphosphazenes) in the repair of peripheral nervous system. Ann Ital Chir 1996;67(6):843–8.

[58] Nicoli Aldini N, Fini M, Rocca M, Giavaresi G, Giardino R. Guided regeneration with resorbable conduits in experimental peripheral nerve injuries. Int Orthop 2000;24(3):121–5.

[59] Mackinnon SE, Dellon AL. A study of nerve regeneration across synthetic (Maxon) and biologic (collagen) nerve conduits for nerve gaps up to 5 cm in the primate. J Reconstr Microsurg 1990;6(2):117–21.

[60] Taras J. Use of nerve conduits for acute digital nerve repairs. Presented at the combined meeting of the American Society for Reconstructive Microsurgery and the American Society for Peripheral Nerve, Palm Springs, CA, January 14–17, 2004.

ELSEVIER
SAUNDERS

Atlas Hand Clin 10 (2005) 135–140

Atlas of the
HAND
CLINICS

Application of Autogenous Venous Nerve Conduits for Digital Nerve Reconstruction

David T.W. Chiu, MD, FACS*, James M. Savundra, MBBS, FRACS

Institute of Reconstructive Plastic Surgery, New York University Medical Center, 560 First Avenue, TH-169, New York, NY 10016, USA

The use of an autogenous tube to reconstruct a gap in a nerve has been described by many authors in the last 150 years. Various structures have been used to provide a tube, including decalcified bone (Gluck [1]), brachial artery (Bungnar [2]), and vein (Foramitti [3] and Nageotte [4]), but little success was obtained, and these procedures were abandoned. There were many more unsuccessful reports of biologic tubes used for nerve reconstruction during the first half of the twentieth century. Chiu et al [5–7] revisited this previous work in the animal model and subsequently in humans. Their work showed good histologic and clinical evidence of nerve regeneration across a gap in a nerve bridged by an autogenous vein. The autogenous venous nerve conduit (AVNC) works in conjunction with the influence of various nerve factors to allow the preferential growth of a nerve down a hollow biologic conduit [8].

Anatomy

Digital nerves

The digital nerves are branches from the median and ulnar nerves. They branch off the main nerves as either individual or common digital nerves at the level of the distal end of the transverse carpal ligament, just proximal to the superficial palmar arterial arch. These nerves pass deep to this arch and remain deep to the common digital arteries until the superficial transverse metacarpal ligament, where they change their position in relation to the digital arteries to lie superficial to them. The common digital nerves branch into their individual digital nerves at this superficial transverse metacarpal ligament, which is proximal to where the common digital arteries branch into their individual digital arteries. In the palm, the digital nerves and arteries lie under the palmar fascia and its specialized transverse fibers of Skoog. They lie in the space to the side of the long flexor tendons. In the digits, there is a digital nerve on each side. They lie superficial to the digital arteries, and this neurovascular bundle lies between specialized digital fascial sheets called *Grayson's ligaments* palmarly and *Cleland's ligaments* dorsally. Along the length of the nerve, there is a degree of glide as the fingers and wrist flex and extend, so this region, which contains the neurovascular bundles, contains loose connective tissue and fat so that glide may occur.

Veins

The venous anatomy of the upper limb has far more variability. The major venous drainage can be categorized into superficial and deep systems. The superficial system lies in the

* Corresponding author. Center for Restorative Surgery, 900 Park Avenue, New York, NY 10021, USA.
E-mail address: dtwc@davidchiumd.com (D.T.W. Chiu).

doi:10.1016/j.ahc.2004.11.001

subcutaneous plane along with the cutaneous nerves. The veins on the dorsum of the hand tend to be fairly large, and these drain into main venous systems—preaxial (cephalic) and postaxial (basilic). On the distal volar forearm, the veins are finer and more proximally in the volar forearm drain into the median cubital vein. The deep system lies with the major arteries, and the veins are usually paired (one on each side of the artery) and referred to as the *venae comitantes*. The veins of the upper limb contain valves that assist venous return to the heart along with the activation of muscles within the limb, which tend to send blood in the same direction. The donor veins used in AVNCs usually are from the same limb as the nerve defect, and they usually are harvested from the superficial system. For digital nerve defect reconstruction, the veins on the dorsum of the hand are of appropriate caliber. There is a fairly constant vein running longitudinally on the dorsum of the hand in the line of the fourth web space, and this lies adjacent to the dorsal branch of the ulnar nerve.

Other treatment options

Direct repair of nerves is the preferred choice of treatment, and several authors have shown that this provides better recovery than any other form of treatment for a complete division of a nerve [6]. Several options for reconstruction of nerve defects exist when direct repair is not possible. For defects in digital nerves of up to 3 cm, the authors' preference is AVNCs. For larger nerves and nerve trunks, other techniques may be appropriate. There are advantages and disadvantages to all forms of reconstruction, and these should be understood before undertaking such surgery.

Nerve graft

Nerve graft remains the gold standard for treatment of defects in nerves where direct repair is not possible. The donor nerves include the sural nerve, the distal posterior interosseous nerve of the upper limb, and the lateral antebrachial nerve. Only the posterior interosseous nerve has no cutaneous sensory deficit after sacrifice, but its size varies, and sometimes it is too small to be of use. The sural nerve graft for facial nerve defects is commonly used because the nerve gap tends to be large. The nerve graft has the advantage of containing the various cytokines of nerve origin, which have been shown to be beneficial in experimental nerve reconstruction. The disadvantage of a nerve graft is the morbidity associated with the harvest of a sensory nerve and sensory loss in the distribution of that nerve.

Denatured muscle

Freeze-thawed muscle has been used as a conduit to reconstruct nerve defects. The advantage has been a low donor site morbidity and an almost unlimited supply of conduit material. The basal lamina is thought to act in a similar manner to other biologic conduits encouraging nerve growth in a certain direction. The results of this technique have been variable [9].

End-to-side nerve repair

Several authors have found end-to-side nerve repair to be successful, especially in sensory nerves. This technique relies on the distal stump of the divided digital nerve being transferred onto an adjacent intact digital nerve, with or without an epineural window. There is apparently no loss of function in the intact nerve with recovery in the distribution of the injured nerve [10].

Synthetic conduits

Various materials have been used to create hollow conduits to allow nerve regeneration across gaps. Polyglycolic acid is a resorbable substance that has been used in the past. Synthetic

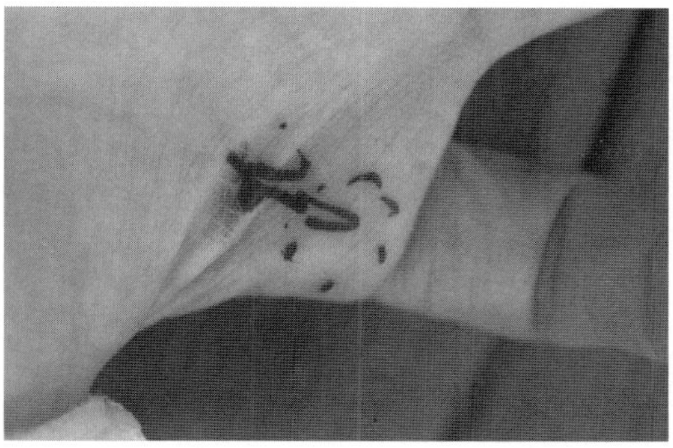

Fig. 1. Preoperative marking of digital nerve.

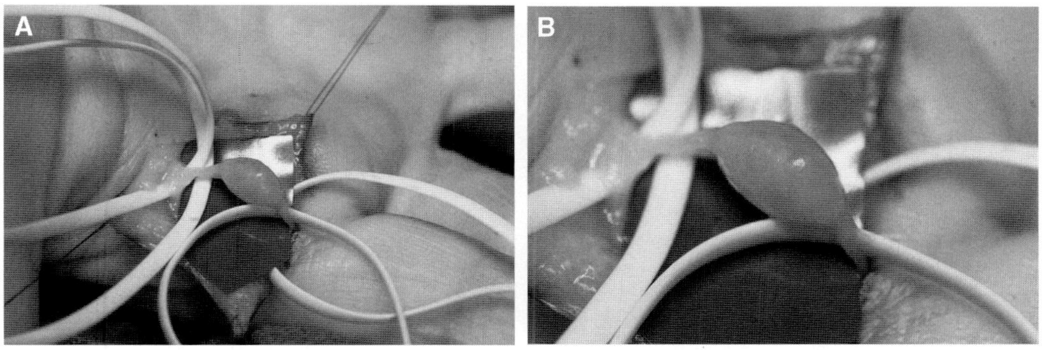

Fig. 2. (*A* and *B*) Pathology of digital nerve.

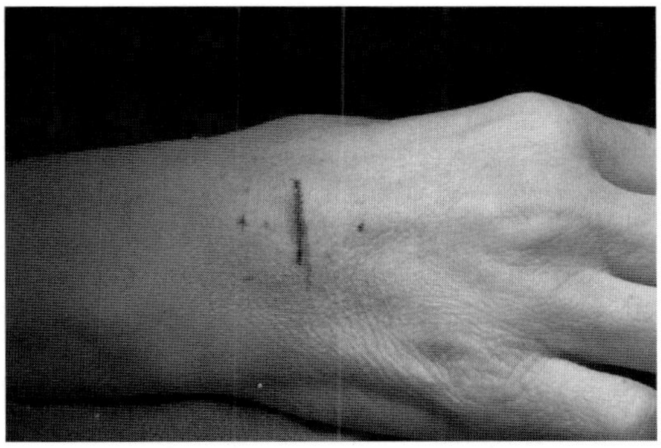

Fig. 3. Preoperative marking for vein donor site.

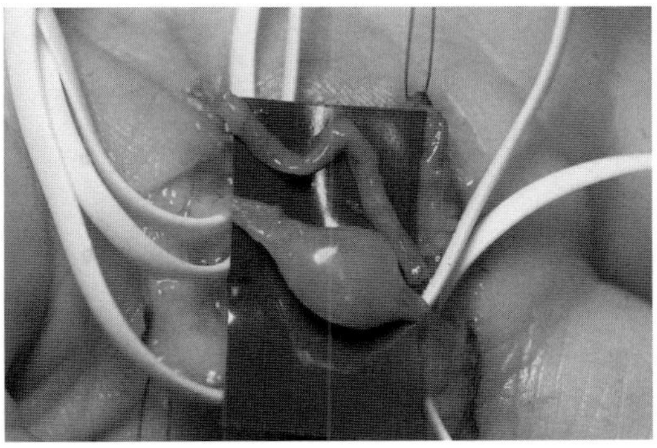

Fig. 4. Nerve and AVNC.

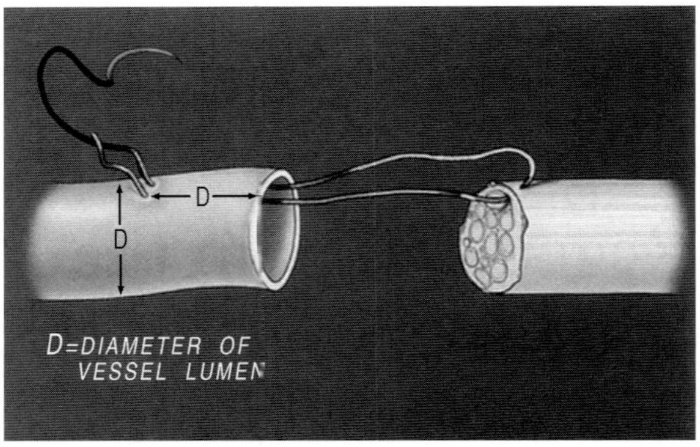

Fig. 5. Telescoping venoneurroraphy. (*From* Tseng CY, Hu G, Ambron RT, Chiu DT. Histologic analysis of Schwann cell migration and peripheral nerve regeneration in the autogenous venous nerve conduit (AVNC). J Reconstr Microsurg 2003;19:331–40; with permission.)

conduits have the obvious advantages of no donor site morbidity, but they tend to be expensive to produce commercially. Their efficacy is still of some concern [9].

Surgical technique

The procedure used for reconstruction of digital nerve defects with AVNCs varies according to the pathology leading to the nerve defect and possible other pathology in that limb. Following is a description of a digital nerve defect including delineation of the defect, harvesting of the donor vein, and placement of the nerve ends inside the AVNC. Figs. 1 through 8 illustrate the specific case. The procedure is performed using at least loupe magnification and preferably an operating microscope.

The digital nerve is found in its usual anatomic location (Fig. 1). If necessary, the nerve ends can be found proximally and distally, out of the zone of pathology. The digital nerve is identified, and in this case a nerve tumor is apparent (Fig. 2). The likely defect in the digital nerve is measured. The dorsum of the hand was chosen in this case as the donor site for the vein harvest; however, several other donor sites can be used for harvesting a vein conduit of up to 3 cm. A transverse incision is used to harvest a longitudinal vein graft (Fig. 3). Fig. 4 shows the generous vein graft that has been harvested before tumor removal. Under high-power magnification, the nerve tumor is excised. The normal fascicles are left intact, and the abnormal fascicles are removed along with the tumor. The cut proximal end of the nerve is placed inside the end of the vein that was distal (in situ) using a telescoping suture shown in Fig. 5 schematically; the specific case is shown in Fig. 6. The same is done to the other end of the nerve after the vein graft is cut to the appropriate length. Fig. 7 shows the end result with the AVNC

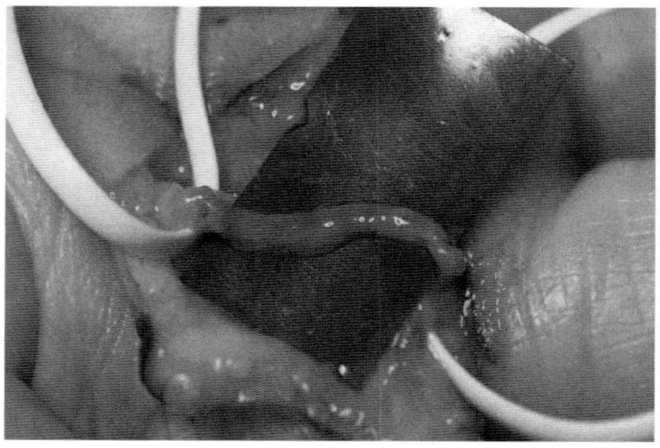

Fig. 6. Proximal end of nerve in AVNC.

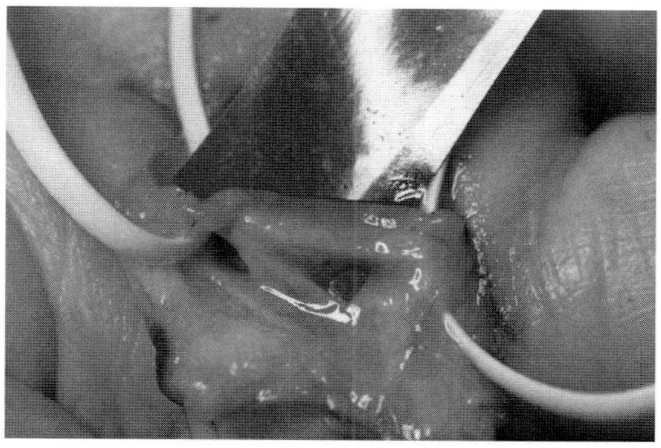

Fig. 7. AVNC next to remaining nerve fascicles.

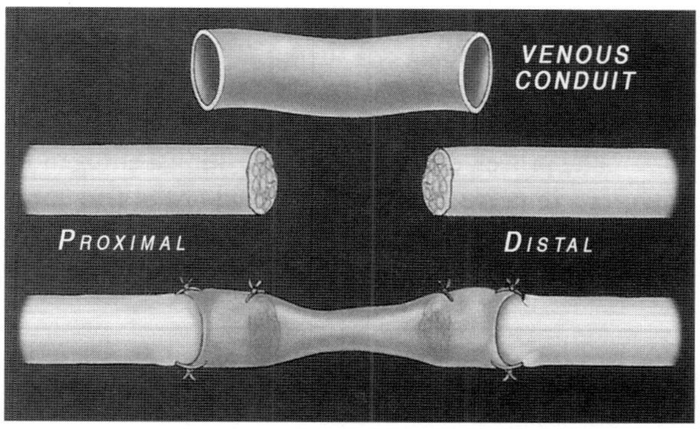

Fig. 8. Schematic AVNC. (*From* Tseng CY, Hu G, Ambron RT, Chiu DT. Histologic analysis of Schwann cell migration and peripheral nerve regeneration in the autogenous venous nerve conduit (AVNC). J Reconstr Microsurg 2003;19:331–40; with permission.)

laying next to the remaining intact nerve fascicles, and Fig. 8 shows the schematic representation. Both wounds are closed in the usual manner. A bulky dressing is applied.

Complications and limitations

There are few reported complications specific to this procedure because it is simple and requires relatively basic microsurgical skills. The donor site for the vein conduit is commonly on the dorsum of the hand, and this can lead to a visible scar. Occasionally, this scar can be painful, and the dorsal cutaneous nerves are at risk of injury, especially if magnification is not used. Authors generally have recommended that the largest defect to be spanned using these techniques should be 3 cm; larger defects probably should be treated with autogenous nerve graft.

Summary

Although autogenous nerve grafting remains the gold standard for reconstruction of nerve defects, the AVNC has been shown to be an excellent option for the reconstruction of digital nerve defects. Its advantages include little donor site morbidity. Animal and clinical studies have proved its efficacy. It is a simple and time-efficient surgical treatment and should be considered for defects in digital nerves of 1 to 3 cm.

References

[1] Gluck T. Ueber neuroplastic auf dem wege de transplantation. Arch Klin Chir 1880;25:606.
[2] Bungnar O. Generations und regenerations: vorgange am nerven nack verletzungen beitr. Pathol Anat 1891;10: 321–93.
[3] Foramitti C. Zur technik der nervennaht. Arch Klin Chir 1904;73:643.
[4] Nageotte J. De processus de la cicatrisation des nerfs. CT Sea NC Soc Biol 1921;78:249.
[5] Chiu DT, Janecka I, Krizek TJ, Wolff M, Lovelace RE. Autogenous vein graft as a conduit for nerve regeneration. Surgery 1982;91:226–33.
[6] Chiu DT, Strauch B. A prospective clinical evaluation of autogenous vein grafts used as a nerve conduit for distal sensory nerve defects of 3 cm or less. Plast Reconstr Surg 1990;86:928–34.
[7] Tseng CY, Hu G, Ambron RT, Chiu DT. Histologic analysis of Schwann cell migration and peripheral nerve regeneration in the autogenous venous nerve conduit (AVNC). J Reconstr Microsurg 2003;19:331–40.
[8] Chiu DTW, Chen L, Smahel J, et al. Neurotropism revisited. Neurol Res 2004;26:381–7.
[9] Meek MF, Coert JH. Clinical use of nerve conduits in peripheral nerve repair: review of the literature. J Reconstr Microsurg 2002;18:97–109.
[10] Al-Qattan MM. Terminolateral neurorrhaphy: review of experimental and clinical studies. J Reconstr Microsurg 2001;17:99–108.

ELSEVIER
SAUNDERS

Atlas Hand Clin 10 (2005) 141–170

Atlas of the
HAND
CLINICS

Neurosensory Pedicled Flaps to the Hand

David J. Slutsky, MD, FRCS(C)*

Private Practice, South Bay Hand Surgery Center, 3475 Torrance Boulevard, Suite F, Torrance, CA 90503, USA

Neurosensory is defined as being of or relating to afferent nerves [1]. For the purpose of this article, a neurosensory flap can be thought of as an innervated flap that provides sensory feedback, either immediately or after a neurorrhaphy. Incorporating a cutaneous nerve in a skin flap provides a means for sensory innervation and may aid the flap circulation because the skin vascularity partly depends on the vessels around these nerves [2]. Noninnervated flaps also may acquire some degree of sensibility through the ingrowth of peripheral nerve fibers, but often to a lesser degree.

Neurosensory flaps have special application to hand injuries [3,4]. Protective sensibility is desirable when providing soft tissue coverage of the dorsum of the hand and palm, but critical sensibility of the digits is important for functional hand use [5]. Moberg [6] stated that precision sensory grip or tactile gnosis requires 2-point discrimination of less than 6 mm, whereas gross sensory grip is possible at 6 to 15 mm. Pedicled neurosensory flaps have certain advantages over free tissue transfer. The arterial supply is often more reliable, which simplifies postoperative monitoring and lends itself to outpatient procedures. Finger flaps may be harvested from the same finger (homodigital) or an adjacent finger (heterodigital). Pedicled flaps may be antegrade or retrograde (reversed flow). Most of these flaps can be dissected under loupe magnification and permit early active motion, a desirable feature in acute injuries. Microvascular technique is helpful but not an absolute prerequisite.

Some general contraindications to pedicled flaps include any cause of massive hand swelling, such as crush-avulsion and wringer injuries, high-energy trauma, or prior arterial injury. Some pitfalls common to pedicled flaps include an inadequate arc of rotation, a short pedicle, vascular insufficiency due to tunneling, or inadequate flap size. It is good practice to add 10% to 15% more to the length and the size of the flap. Incorporating a small skin island along the vascular pedicle simplifies insetting and aids in avoiding skin bridges. Methods of salvaging a failing flap may include suture removal, leech therapy, or conversion to a free flap.

Myriad pedicled neurosensory flaps are described for fingertip and thumb coverage. Flap selection ultimately is based on the size of the defect; the requirements for sensibility; the surgeon's comfort level; and the patient profile, including gender, age, and systemic disease. Knowledge of the skin topography and flap anatomy is integral to the success of any flap. The following discussion focuses on a select number of reliable and relatively easy to dissect flaps. Flap variations and typical sensory recovery are presented.

Hueston flap

The Hueston flap is a local transposition flap for fingertip skin loss that is pedicled on one neurovascular bundle. It was described by Hueston [7] in 1966 and subsequently modified by Souquet and Souquet [8] in 1986 to include both neurovascular bundles.

* 3475 Torrance Boulevard, Suite F, Torrance, CA 90503, USA.
E-mail address: d-slutsky@msn.com

1082-3131/05/$ - see front matter
doi:10.1016/j.ahc.2004.10.003

Anatomy

The flap is an asymmetrical arterial advancement flap based on either the radial or the ulnar neurovascular bundle. It relies on cutaneous perforators from the digital artery. The flap is drained by the venae comitantes and the intact subdermal venous plexus. It receives its innervation from the proper digital nerve. The advancing free edge of the flap is initially insensate, but regains sensibility with time. It has a range of advancement of 12 to 18 mm.

Indications

The flap is used to cover a loss of the pulp tissue of the fingers and thumb. It is indicated in situations in which it is important to preserve bone length to diminish the risks of a hook nail deformity and in which there is no possibility of distal replantation.

Advantages

The flap is homodigital and provides satisfactory texture for resurfacing fingertips. It is simple, it is reliable, and it allows immediate finger motion.

Limitations

The flap cannot be used with injury to a neurovascular bundle. It is not indicated when more than 18 mm of transposition is required.

Surgical technique

The skin is advanced on the side of relatively less functional importance, such as the radial pulp of the thumb and small finger or the ulnar border of the middle digits. An L-shaped incision is made proximal to the fingertip defect. The longitudinal limb extends along the midlateral line, while the transverse limb is placed in the metacarpophalangeal (MCP) or proximal interphalangeal (PIP) flexion crease. The plane of dissection passes superficial to the neurovascular bundle that is closest to the midlateral incision. The contralateral neurovascular bundle is incorporated into the base of the flap, which is advanced obliquely to cover the amputation stump. A proximally based triangle of skin raised along the longitudinal border of the flap can be rotated transversely to cover the donor site [9].

Variations

The flap can be modified by including both neurovascular bundles (Fig. 1). This modification was thought to preserve the sensibility of the flap, at the expense of restricting some distal advancement [8]. The longitudinal incision is made in the same manner as already described, whereas the transverse incision is extended to the opposite midlateral line, ending with a back cut. The plane of dissection proceeds deep to both neurovascular bundles, which are incorporated into the skin flap. The flap is advanced and inset as already described.

Sensory recovery

In Foucher's series [9] of 43 flaps, 2-point discrimination averaged 7 mm in the standard Hueston flap (31 cases) and 6 mm with the modified flap (12 cases).

Complications

The palmar tension pulls on the nail matrix, which causes a tendency toward a parrot beak nail deformity. This tendency can be minimized by skewering the tip of the flap with a transfixing needle. The free edge of the flap can lead to a dog-ear deformity, which can be

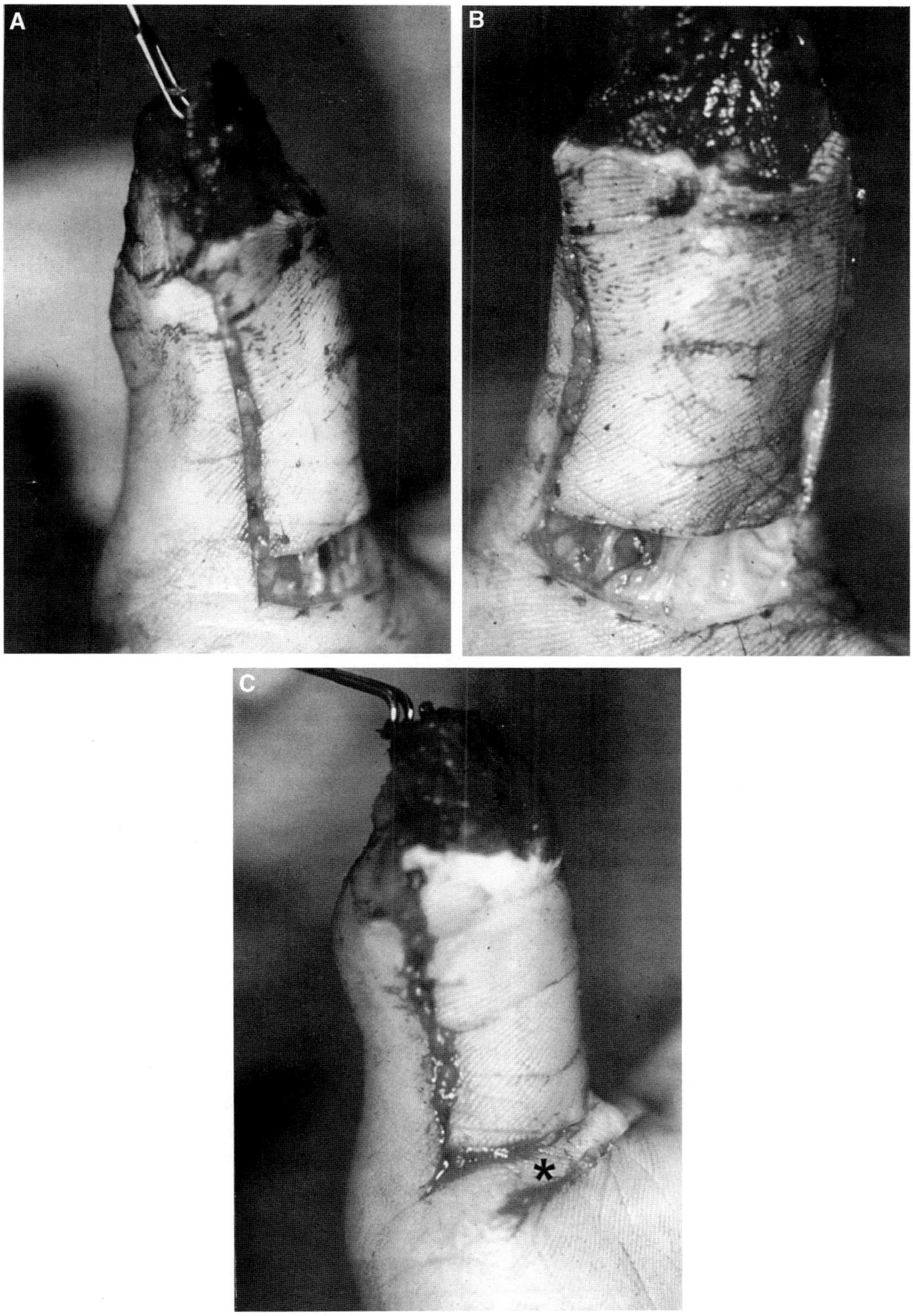

Fig. 1. (*A*) Sideways view of modified Hueston flap for thumb coverage. (*B*) Note amount of advancement based on both neurovascular bundles. (*C*) A proximally based triangle of skin raised along the longitudinal border of the flap is rotated transversely to cover the exposed pedicles (*asterisk*).

corrected by excising a segment of dorsal skin. Cold intolerance is common during the first year and correlates with poorer return of sensation. Persistent fingertip sensitivity may occur secondary to neuroma formation. A contracture of the distal interphalangeal or PIP joint may result if there is excessive joint flexion during flap insetting.

Innervated cross finger flap

More than 50 years after its description, the cross finger flap is still widely in use [10]. In cases in which the dorsal digital networks cannot be used or when elaborate microsurgical procedures are not available, cross finger flaps are still useful for finger coverage distal to the PIP joint. Sensory return is unpredictable, however, and can mar the ultimate functional result. The innervated cross finger flap was developed to improve on this by transferring the dorsal skin over the middle phalanx along with its sensory nerve [11]. A neurorrhaphy is performed between this nerve and one of the severed digital nerve ends of the injured finger.

Anatomy

The initial blood supply of this random pattern flap comes from one of the paired dorsal branches arising from the palmar digital artery at the proximal one third of the middle phalanx [12]. The venous drainage is initially from the venae comitantes and subdermal veins. The superficial branch of the radial nerve (SBRN) and the dorsal cutaneous branch of the ulnar nerve innervate the dorsum of the hand up to the level of the PIP joints. Distal to this, the dorsal skin is innervated by a dorsal sensory branch that arises from the proper digital nerve. This branch most commonly arises proximal to the PIP flexion crease (see Fig. 2). It then crosses superficial or deep to the digital artery to lie just above the extensor mechanism, innervating the dorsum of the middle phalanx [13,14].

The arc of rotation of the cross finger flap is short because the skin is pedicled on the midlateral line of the finger. The flap is left attached to the donor finger until sufficient peripheral arterial and venous anastomoses have occurred, then it is divided.

Indications

The innervated cross finger flap is indicated in cases of full-thickness loss of the entire pulp of an adjacent finger, especially with exposed bone or tendon. The long finger is used for coverage of the thumb pulp.

Advantages

The cross finger flap is extremely reliable and easy to perform. It can be used for larger defects that may not be suitable for homodigital flaps. With the innervated flap, no additional donor finger denervation occurs because the dorsal sensory branch ordinarily is transected when

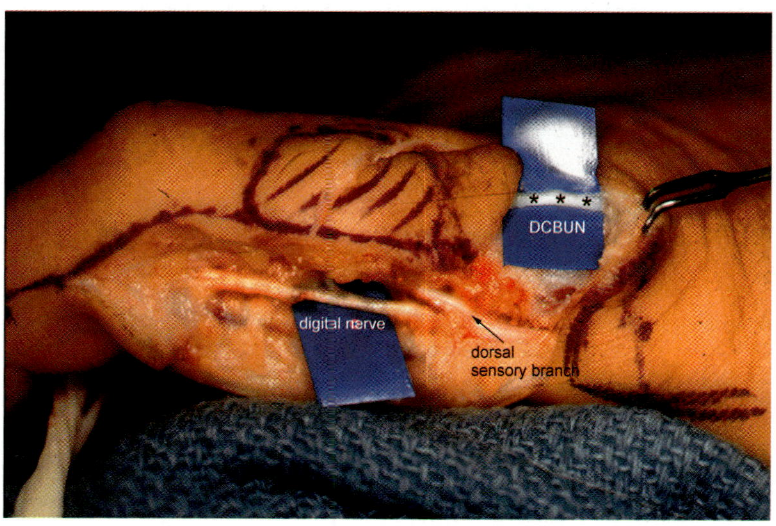

Fig. 2. Dorsal sensory branch arising from the proper digital nerve of the small finger. Asterisks show the dorsal cutaneous branch of the ulnar nerve.

elevating the standard cross finger flap. Suturing this branch to the transected digital nerve in the recipient finger allows reinnervation without any need for cortical reorientation.

Limitations

The innervated cross finger flap cannot be used when there is concomitant injury to adjacent digits. Flap innervation is not possible if there has been damage to either the dorsal sensory branch or the proximal digital nerve. Patients who are older than 40 years old are relatively contraindicated because of the finger stiffness that results from 2 weeks of immobilization to an another digit [15].

Surgical technique

The dissection is performed under tourniquet control [16]. A pattern of the defect is outlined over the dorsum of the middle phalanx of an adjacent finger. Two transverse incisions delineate the proximal and distal extent of the flap. A longitudinal incision is made on the side opposite the injured finger. The incision should not extend volar to the midlateral line to prevent a scar contracture. The dorsal sensory branch is isolated through a separate proximal incision, which extends to the edge of the flap. The nerve is sectioned proximally, leaving a 1.5- to 2-cm tail. The flap is elevated along with the nerve branch. The plane of dissection proceeds superficial to the paratenon of the extensor mechanism. The flap is dissected laterally to the opposite midlateral line, until it can be transposed without acute angulation.

Next the digital nerve end is isolated along the opposite border of the injured digit. The tourniquet is released ensuring flap viability. A full-thickness skin graft is placed over the donor site and secured with a tie-over bolster. The flap is transposed and inset so that the deep surface of the flap lies against the finger defect (Fig. 3). An epineurial repair between the dorsal sensory nerve branch and the digital nerve is performed with 9-0 nylon suture. A finger spica splint or bulky dressing is applied to prevent tension on the suture sites. At the time of flap division 2 weeks later, no special care for the nerve repair is necessary because the nerve junction is on the side opposite the flap base.

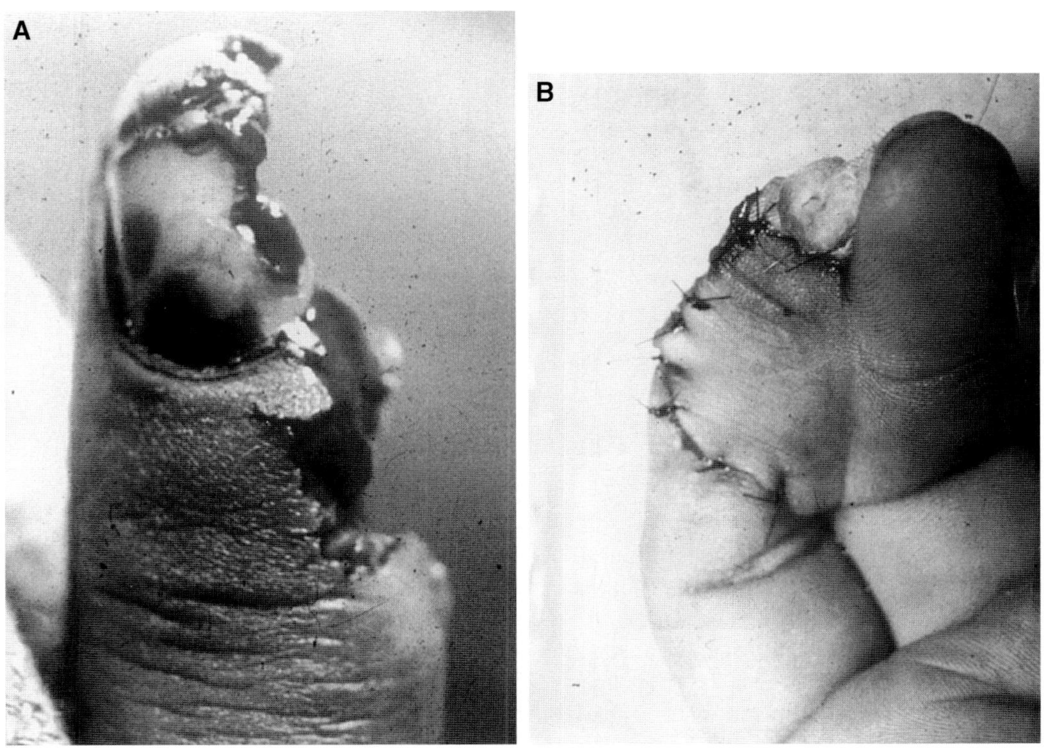

Fig. 3. (*A*) Fingertip saw injury. (*B*) Pedicled cross finger flap.

Variations

Lassner et al [17] have used a bilaterally innervated sensory cross finger flap. First, the contralateral dorsal sensory branch is elevated with the flap at the PIP joint level and sutured to the digital nerve end on the far side of the injured finger. After 3 weeks, when the pedicle is dissected, the remaining dorsal sensory branch is dissected and sutured to the remaining digital nerve of the injured finger. Because the regenerative distance is only 1.5 to 2 cm, there is excellent sensory reinnervation, with 2-point discrimination ranging from 2 to 6 mm.

Gaul [18] described an innervated cross finger flap from the index that provides immediate sensation for resurfacing volar defects of the thumb. The flap is transferred along with the dorsoradial digital nerve to the index, which is a continuation of the major dorsal branch of the superficial radial nerve [19]. This sensory branch is mobilized at the same time the cross finger flap is transposed and transferred subcutaneously to lie under the volar skin envelop of the thumb.

In an effort to improve the ultimate sensibility, Hastings [20] modified this index finger flap by turning it into a dual innervated flap (Fig. 4). The superficial radial sensory nerve is mobilized and transposed as described earlier. The dorsal sensory branch of the proper radial digital nerve of the index is sutured to the severed end of the ulnar digital nerve of thumb. Sensory reinnervation is reported to be rapid and does not require cortical reorientation.

Sensory recovery

In one series of innervated cross finger flaps, seven of eight patients achieved an average 2-point discrimination of 4.8 mm compared with patients with noninnervated cross finger flaps, who achieved a mean value of 9 mm [16].

Complications

Joint stiffness is common. The flap may be hair bearing. Donor finger morbidity includes poor skin graft color match and a visible contour deformity. If only one digital nerve anastomosis is performed, a painful neuroma may develop from the unrepaired digital nerve stump.

The functional outcome of the radial sensory innervated cross finger flap is compromised in some patients by double sensitivity. In this case, sensation from the ulnar side of the flap is interpreted as arising from the dorsum of the index finger, whereas sensation on the radial side of the flap is interpreted as coming from the thumb. Sensory testing shows that after transfer to the thumb, the ulnar side of the flap still receives its innervation from the superficial sensory branch of the radial nerve [21].

Reversed digital artery flap

The reversed digital artery (RDA) flap, described in 1986 by Kojima et al [22], is used for one-stage reconstruction of finger pulp defects. The flap can be innervated by including the dorsal sensory nerve branch.

Anatomy

The RDA flap is harvested from the dorsolateral skin of the proximal phalanx, which derives its blood supply from the opposite digital artery through abundant communicating branches. There are three transverse palmar arches connecting the radial and ulnar digital arteries. The proximal and middle arches are always in association with the limbs of the C1 and C3 pulleys. The distal arch lies just beyond the insertion of the profundus tendon [23].

When the proximal digital artery is ligated, the blood crosses over from the opposite digital artery through the middle and distal transverse palmar arches. The blood flows down the ligated artery in a retrograde fashion (Fig. 5). The RDA flap is designed over the dorsolateral area of the proximal phalanx, which is nourished by a proximal dorsal cutaneous branch. This small

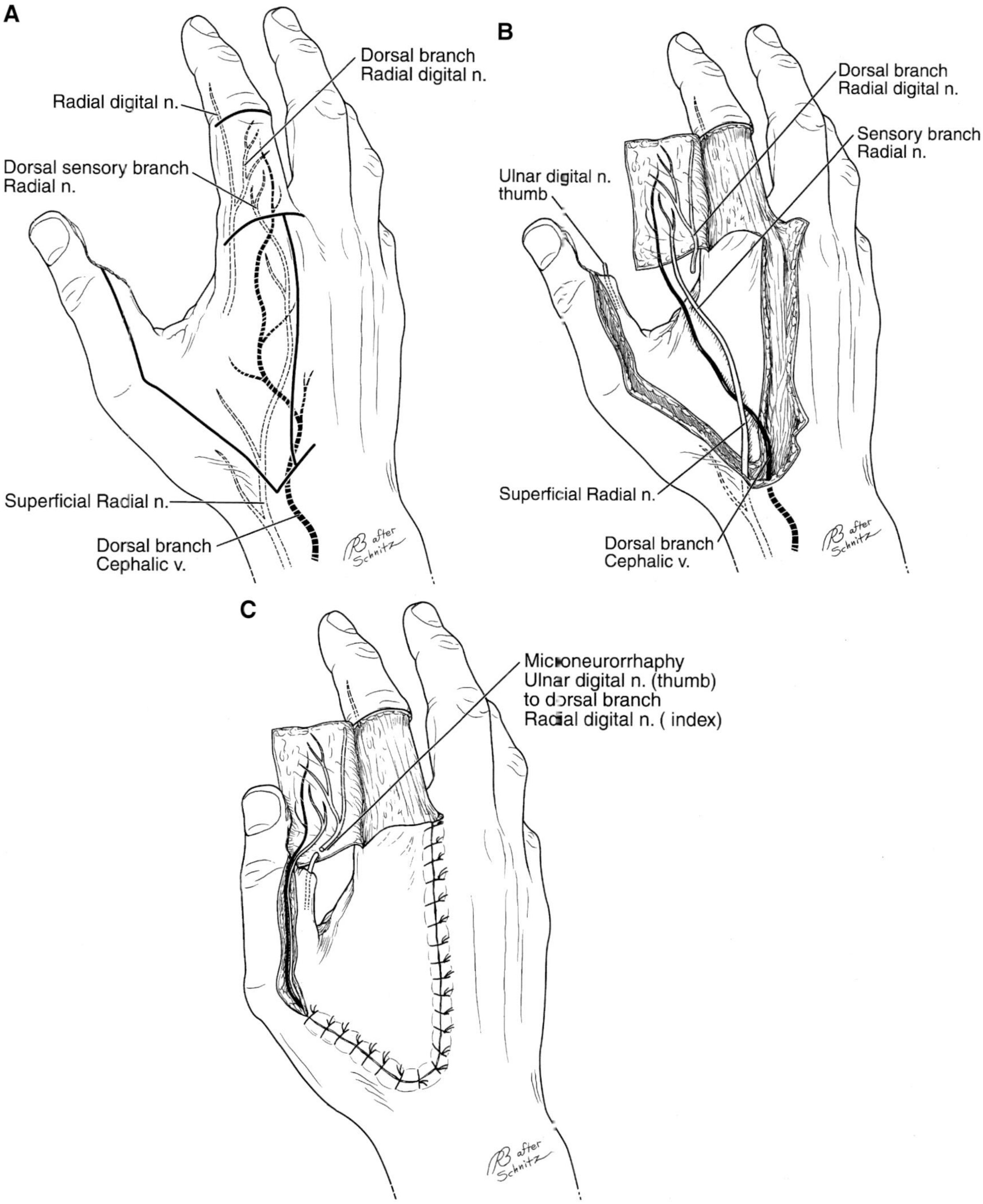

Fig. 4. (*A–C*) Drawing of the surgical technique. (*Adapted from* Hastings H 2nd. Dual innervated index to thumb cross finger or island flap reconstruction. Microsurgery 1987;8:168–72; with permission.)

branch, 0.3 to 0.6 mm in size, arises from the palmar digital artery at the midpoint of the proximal phalanx (Fig. 6) [12]. It passes through Cleland's ligament, running close to the bone, and emerges on the dorsal aspect of the finger. Histologic studies revealed the presence of venules and capillaries in the perivascular fat tissue, which appear to represent adequate channels for venous drainage [13].

The dorsal sensory nerve branch is harvested with the skin flap (see Fig. 2). In the border digits, the terminal branches of the superficial radial nerve or dorsal cutaneous branch of the ulnar nerve also can be transferred. The arc of rotation is around the midpoint of the middle

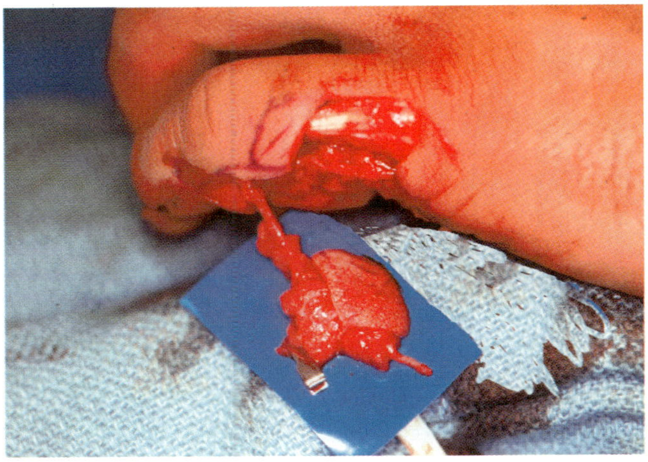

Fig. 5. Retrograde blood flow down the ligated artery (clamp). Note the dorsal sensory nerve branch.

phalanx, which allows the flap to reach the fingertip easily. The digital artery cannot be elevated beyond the middle phalanx for fear of disrupting the distal transverse arch.

Indications

The RDA flap is indicated for coverage of acute and chronic fingertip defects. It can be used for fingertip reconstruction to correct a hooknail deformity (Fig. 7). Some authors recommend the RDA flap for coverage of large defects of the dorsal aspects of the middle and distal phalanx, which cannot be covered with other local digital sensory flaps (Fig. 8) [24]. It also may be useful after release of volar scar contractures of the fingers.

Advantages

This procedure provides a method for a one-stage reconstruction of finger pulp defects. It restores sensation with a good color match, while allowing early finger motion. The RDA flap has great mobility and transfers to the pulp defect without any tension when based on a reverse vascular pedicle. Neurorrhaphy between the dorsal sensory branch and the terminal digital

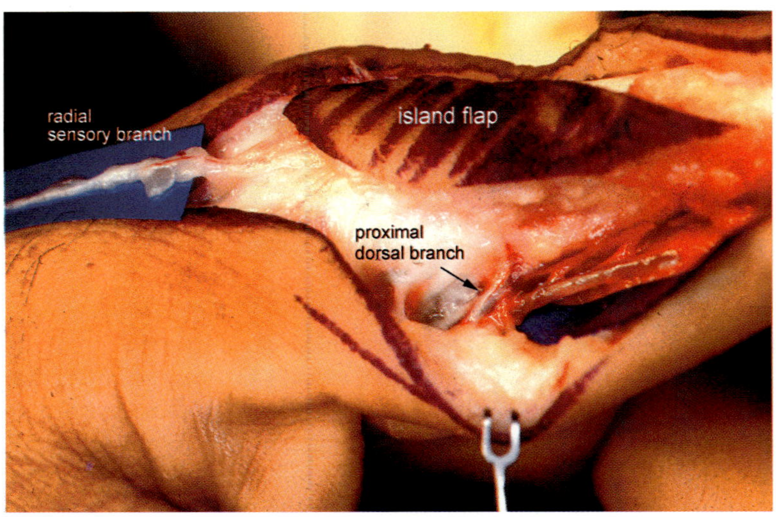

Fig. 6. Proximal dorsal branch supplying a skin island flap of the index finger. Note the proximal tail on the skin flap and terminal branch of the superficial radial sensory nerve.

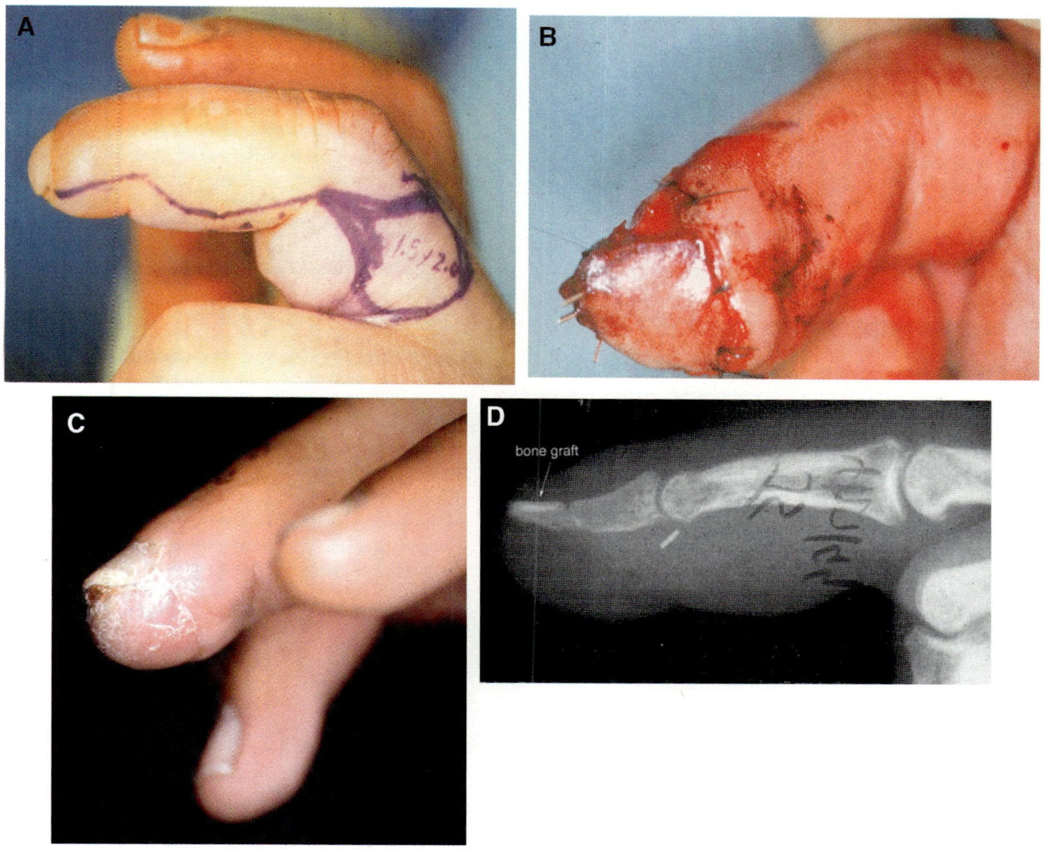

Fig. 7. (*A*) 1.5 × 2 mm RDA flap outlined for hook nail deformity. (*B*) RDA flap transposed to fingertip after bone grafting. (*C*) Good fingertip contour with straight nail plate. (*D*) Bone grafting of distal phalanx.

nerve allows for flap innervation through the normal anatomic pathway so that cortical misinterpretation can be avoided [13].

Limitations

A disadvantage of this procedure is that it sacrifices a digital artery, and a nerve repair is required. The RDA flap cannot be used if there is only one patent digital artery or if there has been an injury to the distal transverse palmar arch.

Surgical technique

A digital Allen's test with or without Doppler is used to ascertain that both digital arteries are intact [25]. Under tourniquet control, the injured tip is débrided, and a pattern of the defect is outlined over the proximal phalanx. The flap margins are incised and elevated, including the subcutaneous tissue and the digital artery. The dorsal sensory branch is identified and divided 10 mm proximal to the flap margin. A midlateral incision is made from the distal flap margin, as far as the midpoint of the middle phalanx. The artery is separated from the digital nerve, leaving as much surrounding fat as possible for venous drainage.

A microvascular clamp is applied to the digital artery proximal to the skin flap, while the tourniquet is released to check the circulation of the finger and the flap. The proximal artery is divided and elevated to the midportion of the middle phalanx.

The skin island is rotated 180° into the fingertip defect, taking care to avoid kinking the pedicle. Leaving a tail on the flap or skin grafting the pedicle can avoid arterial compression. The dorsal sensory nerve branch is sutured to the recipient nerve before insetting. Donor site defects of 2 × 3 cm can be closed primarily. Flaps 5 × 2 cm can be harvested.

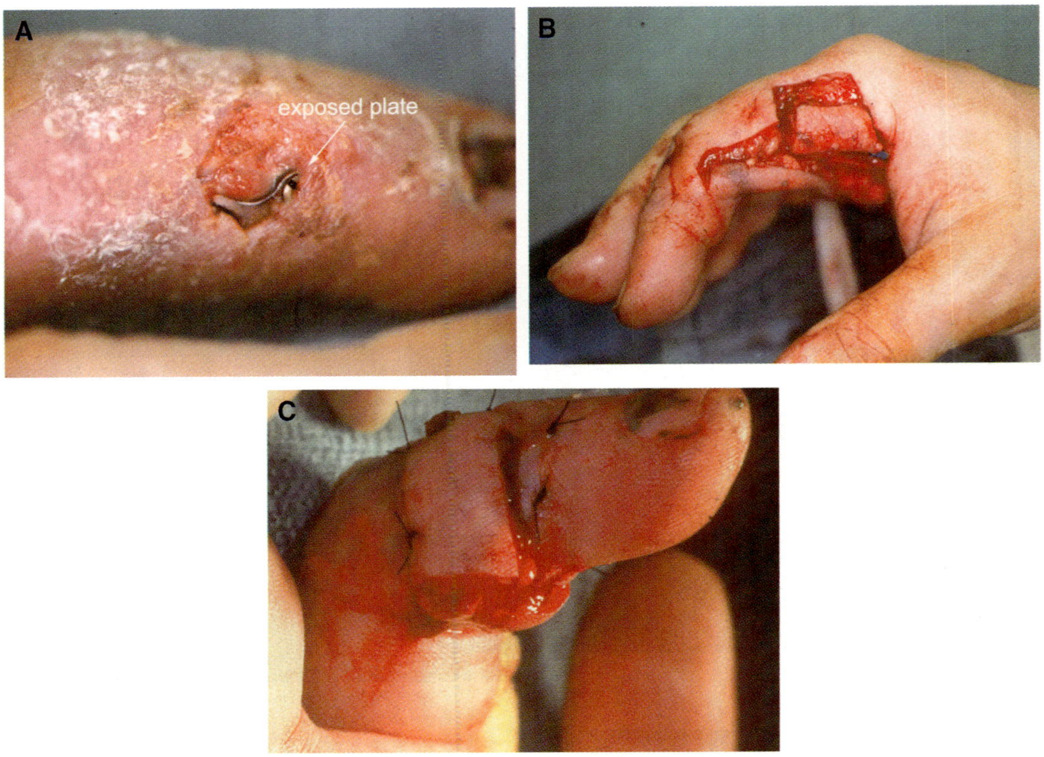

Fig. 8. (*A*) A 56-year-old man status post open reduction with internal fixation of open fracture with exposed plate along ulnar side of index. (*B*) RDA flap raised from radial side of the index finger. (*C*) Flap insetting.

Variations

Lai et al [26] described an extended RDA flap in which the dorsal skin over the MCP joint may be included. This skin extension is a fasciocutaneous flap that survives on the rich anastomosis between the first dorsal metacarpal artery and the digital artery near the metacarpal head [27]. Lai et al [26] noted that the sensory recovery of this skin extension was relatively poor. In an effort to overcome this poor sensory recovery, the dorsal sensory branch from the proper digital nerve and the superficial sensory branch from the corresponding radial or ulnar nerve are sectioned at their proximal ends and included with the RDA flap (see Fig. 2). For bilaterally innervated flaps, these branches are sutured to both digital nerve ends. Static 2-point discrimination of 5 mm was obtained in Lai's series of 3 patients [26].

In cases in which one of the digital arteries has been injured, an innervated RDA cross finger flap harvested from the proximal phalanx of the adjacent finger can be used to cover defects of the middle and distal phalanges. A piece of skin graft is placed over the pedicle, which is divided at 2 weeks [28]. In situations in which the fingertip pulp is lost completely, some authors have included the proper digital nerve in the pedicle, which is sutured to the stump of the opposite proper digital nerve [29].

Sensory recovery

Mean values for 2-point discrimination range from 6 to 10 mm [30]. Noninnervated flaps also have been reported to regain less than 10 mm of 2-point discrimination sensation [31].

Complications

Flap edema secondary to impaired venous drainage from kinking of the pedicle or an inadequate amount of perivascular fat for venous drainage is common. The flap tends to be bulky if applied over subcutaneous tissue rather than bone (Fig. 9). Skin grafting the pedicle at the distal interphalangeal joint may be necessary. Inadequate finger perfusion occurring when

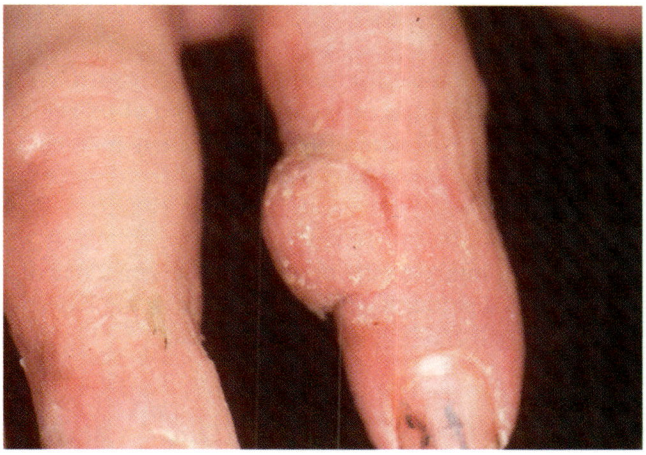

Fig. 9. Note bulkiness of flap when applied directly over bone.

the digital artery proximal to the island flap is clamped may preclude use of this flap. Numbness over the dorsum of the middle phalanx owing to transection of the dorsal sensory branch may be bothersome. If the margin of the flap extends volar to the midaxial line, a PIP flexion contracture can develop. Cold intolerance is a risk, especially for outdoor workers in cold climates.

Dorsoulnar flap of the thumb

The arterial supply of the thumb is different from that of the fingers. Direct or reverse flow volar island flaps centered on only one arterial pedicle, which have been described for the fingers, are not possible for the thumb. Through their anatomic studies, Brunelli et al [32] discovered a consistent artery along the dorsoulnar aspect of the thumb, which they used as the basis for a reverse pedicled skin flap. The flap can be innervated by incorporating the terminal branches of the superficial radial nerve and can be used for coverage of distal thumb defects.

Anatomy

The arteria princeps pollicis divides into two palmar digital arteries at the level of the MCP flexion crease. As a consequence, any pedicled flap of the thumb that is based on the palmar arteries has a short pedicle; this would require marked interphalangeal joint flexion to prevent undue tension on the princeps pollicis. The dorsal arteries of the fingers are extremely segmental, inconstant, and dependent on palmar anastomoses. In the thumb, there is a constant dorsoulnar artery, which originates from the palmar arteries at the neck of the thumb metacarpal and runs along the dorsoulnar side of the thumb. It may be 0.1 mm and travels superficially within the subcutaneous tissue, above the aponeurosis. A similar, but less constant and smaller artery may be found 72% of the time along the dorsoradial aspect of the thumb [33].

The dorsoulnar artery is reinforced by an anastomosis with the palmar digital artery at the neck of the proximal phalanx, approximately 2.3 cm from the nail fold. The artery terminates in a dorsal arcade within 0.7 mm of the nail. Venae comitantes can be present when the artery is of a large size (about 50% of cases). In the remaining cases venous drainage is based on tiny venules in the perivascular fatty tissue (Francesco Brunelli, MD, personal communication). The terminal sensory branch of the superficial radial nerve is located 1 to 2 cm from the median axis of the thumb.

Indications

The dorsoulnar flap is indicated for reconstruction of extensive loss of the thumb pulp. It can be used for coverage of amputation stumps at the interphalangeal joint level or for coverage of dorsal skin loss over the proximal and distal phalanx.

Advantages

The flap provides satisfactory texture for resurfacing fingertips and is homodigital, which allows immediate thumb motion. Because of the distal nature of its pedicle, the flap can reach the tip of the thumb easily. Primary closure of the donor site is possible for smaller flaps.

Limitations

The flap cannot be used with injury to the princeps pollicis or ulnar digital artery. It also is contraindicated when there is a significant soft tissue injury at the base of the thumb.

Surgical technique

The following points are marked first on the skin [34]: (1) the dorsal arcade of the proximal nail fold, 0.9 cm proximal to the nail base; (2) the palmar anastomosis at the level of the neck of the proximal phalanx, 2.5 cm proximally; and (3) the course of the dorsoulnar artery, 1 cm from the median axis of the thumb at the level of the neck of the proximal phalanx (Fig. 10). The flap dimensions are marked out on the dorsoulnar aspect of the MCP joint, centered over the dorsoulnar artery. The flap is raised in a proximal-to-distal direction. The terminal sensory branch of the radial nerve is located and divided 2 cm from the proximal flap edge. A midlateral incision is extended along the ulnar side of the thumb connecting to the distal area of soft tissue loss. This incision is superficial to avoid damaging the arterial pedicle. Two dermoepidermis skin flaps are raised in a dorsal and palmar direction starting from the ulnar incision, taking care not to harm the subcutaneous tissue. A 1-cm-wide, full-thickness strip of subcutaneous tissue is harvested en bloc and centered around the arterial axis of the flap, leaving the extensor aponeurosis in situ. The flap artery may be quite small and is not directly isolated during harvesting to avoid damage. Care should be taken to avoid any tension or compression where the subcutaneous pedicle is reflected on itself.

The flap can be pedicled distally at two levels, which determines the arc of rotation. It can be pedicled at the dorsal nail fold arcade for cases of distal amputation or for loss of palmar or dorsal tissue. Dissection of the pedicle must be limited to 1 cm from the nail base. When used for more proximal amputation stumps, it is pedicled on the palmar anastomosis at the neck of the proximal phalanx. In this case, the dissection should be limited to 2.5 cm from the nail base.

Variations

The flap can be used as a cross finger variant for coverage of skin loss of the fingers. Any part of the hand is accessible to this flap based on the distal end of a mobile thumb [35]. The temporary pedicle, composed of a 1-cm-wide band of skin and subcutaneous tissue, is divided at 15 days after a clamping test confirms that the flap has become autonomous.

The dorsoulnar artery sends several periosteal and osseous branches to the neck of the first metacarpal. Vascularized bone from the metacarpal neck can be harvested with a reversed pedicled dorsoulnar skin flap for reconstruction of combined skin and bone defects of the distal phalanx [36].

Sensory recovery

Sensory recovery is disappointing, ranging from 10 mm to protective sensibility. In Brunelli's series [32], there was no significant difference in sensibility between innervated and non-innervated flaps.

Complications

Raising the flap proximal to the MCP joint may exclude the nutrient artery, resulting in flap failure. Harvesting the terminal radial sensory nerve branch of the thumb leads to sensory loss

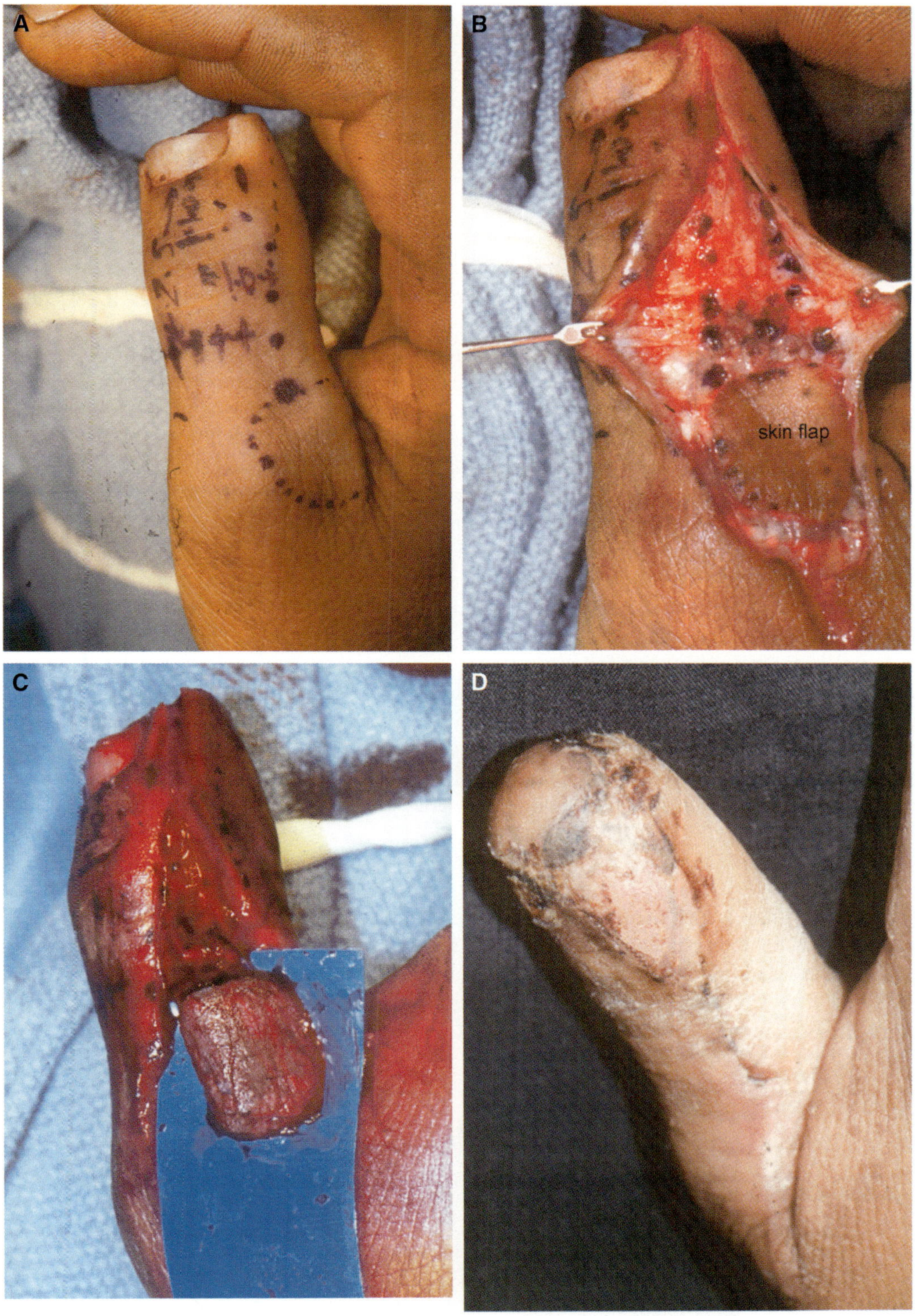

Fig. 10. (*A*) Skin markings for dorsoulnar thumb flap. (*B*) Flap elevated on dorsoulnar artery. (*C*) Skin flap elevated. (*D*) Good color match and contour of distal thumb.

over the dorsum of the thumb and could result in neuroma formation. Harvesting the skin from the dorsoulnar aspect of the thumb MCP can result in a restriction of MCP motion along with a decrease in the first web space span. The donor area is hair bearing, and debulking of the flap may be necessary because of overlap of the pedicle.

First dorsal metacarpal artery flap

The first dorsal metacarpal artery (FDMA) flap is a fasciocutaneous flap first described by Holevich in 1963 [37]. It was modified and used as a neurosensory island flap by Foucher and Braun in 1979 [38]. It is based on the FDMA or its dorsal digital branches. The flap is innervated by terminal sensory branches of the superficial radial nerve.

Anatomy

The FDMA arises from the radial artery just distal to the extensor pollicis longus tendon, before the artery dives between the two heads of the first dorsal interosseous (FDI) muscle (Fig. 11). The FDMA typically measures 1.2 to 1.5 mm in diameter. There is usually more than one accompanying vein. The artery runs superficial to the FDI fascia and divides into three terminal branches: a radial (FDMAr), ulnar (FDMAu), and intermediate branch. The radial branch runs along the thumb metacarpal and becomes or anastomoses with the dorsoulnar artery. The ulnar branch runs along the index metacarpal up to the MCP joint, giving branches to the periosteum and adjacent extensor tendons. It terminates in a plexus over the dorsal fascia of the index (Fig. 12). The intermediate branch runs toward the first web space and anastomoses with branches from the other two. The flap is based on either the radial or the ulnar branch of the FDMA. A proximally based flap is rotated around the point of origin of the artery at the base of the first dorsal interosseous space. The arc of rotation can include the palmar or dorsal thumb, wrist, and palm to the third metacarpal.

The venous drainage is that of the accompanying superficial veins. The superficial branch of the radial nerve becomes subcutaneous after it leaves the brachioradialis, then bifurcates into two major branches 4 cm proximal to the styloid [39]. Both branches pass radial to Lister's tubercle. The major palmar branch passes over the first dorsal wrist compartment, then continues distally to become the dorsoradial digital nerve of the thumb. The major dorsal branch also bifurcates into the dorsoulnar digital nerve to the thumb and the dorsoradial digital nerve to the index, which supplies the adjacent sides of the second web space [19].

Indications

The FDMA flap is indicated for resurfacing either volar or dorsal defects of the distal thumb as far distal as the interphalangeal joint (Fig. 13). It can be used to cover the ulnar surface of the dorsum of the hand and the wrist or the palm up to the third metacarpal. The FDMA flap is useful for first web space reconstruction after contracture, and it can provide soft tissue coverage of the index finger up to the level of the proximal phalanx (see Fig. 13A–C).

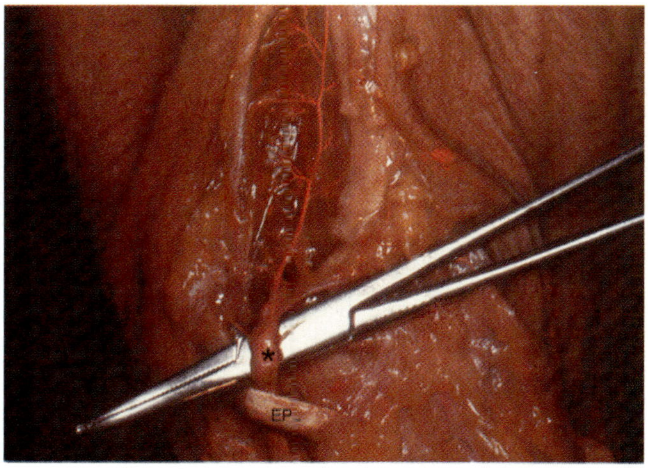

Fig. 11. Cadaver injection studies showing the origin of the FDMA from the radial artery (*). EPL, extensor pollicis longus.

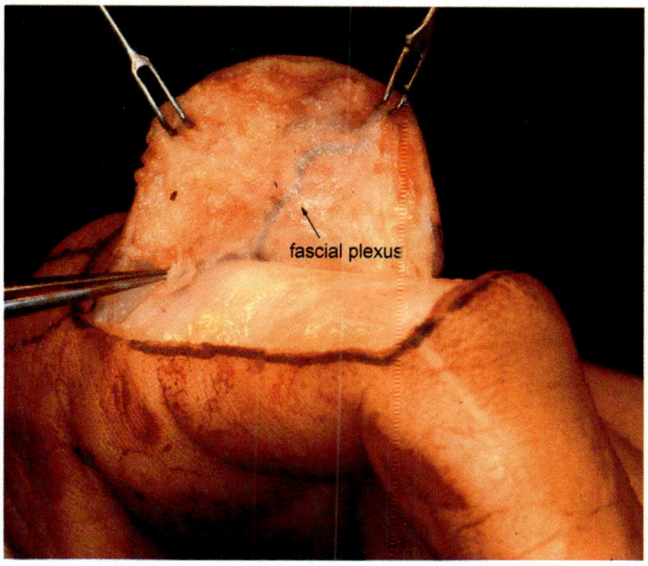

Fig. 12. Demonstration of the FDMAu, which terminates in a plexus over the dorsal fascia of the index.

Advantages

Advantages of this flap are its variable size, stability, and pliability. It provides innervated skin with no major donor site morbidity. Its elevation does not sacrifice a major artery. It can be transferred as a pedicled flap or an island flap. The innervated FDMA flap allows immediate postoperative mobilization and the avoidance of a nerve repair. It restores sensibility, particularly in older patients, in whom nerve repairs of a pedicle or free flaps yield poorer results than in younger patients [40].

Limitations

The flap cannot be used with radial artery injury in the snuffbox. If the skin overlying the firts web space is included in the flap, skin grafting the donor site defect may lead to a secondary contracture. The arterial pedicle is difficult to dissect. The flap is at risk of partial necrosis if pedicled on a nondominant branch.

Surgical technique

Pedicled flap

A Doppler probe may be used to check the pulse of the FDMAr and FDMAu against the first and second metacarpals. The flap is drawn over the dorsum of the index, thumb, or back of the hand according to the skin defect. Under tourniquet, the flap is raised from distal to proximal, in the areolar plane over the extensor paratenon. The skin incision is continued along the radial aspect of the index metacarpal to include a large subcutaneous vein in the pedicle. At the second metacarpal neck, a large perforator is consistently present and should be ligated. The entire interosseous fascia over the FDI is included to avoid a meticulous dissection of the pedicle and to avoid raising the flap on a nondominant branch. A small cuff of muscle of the FDI may be included to ensure the artery is included in the pedicle. Either the palmar or the dorsal branch of the SBRN is incorporated into the flap. The fascia is released from the metacarpal until the flap can reach the defect. If the flap is used for first web space reconstruction, the interosseous fascia is released from the thumb and index metacarpals. The flap is enlarged ulnarly toward the third metacarpal so that the skin extension lies on the first web space, avoiding a first web space contracture [41].

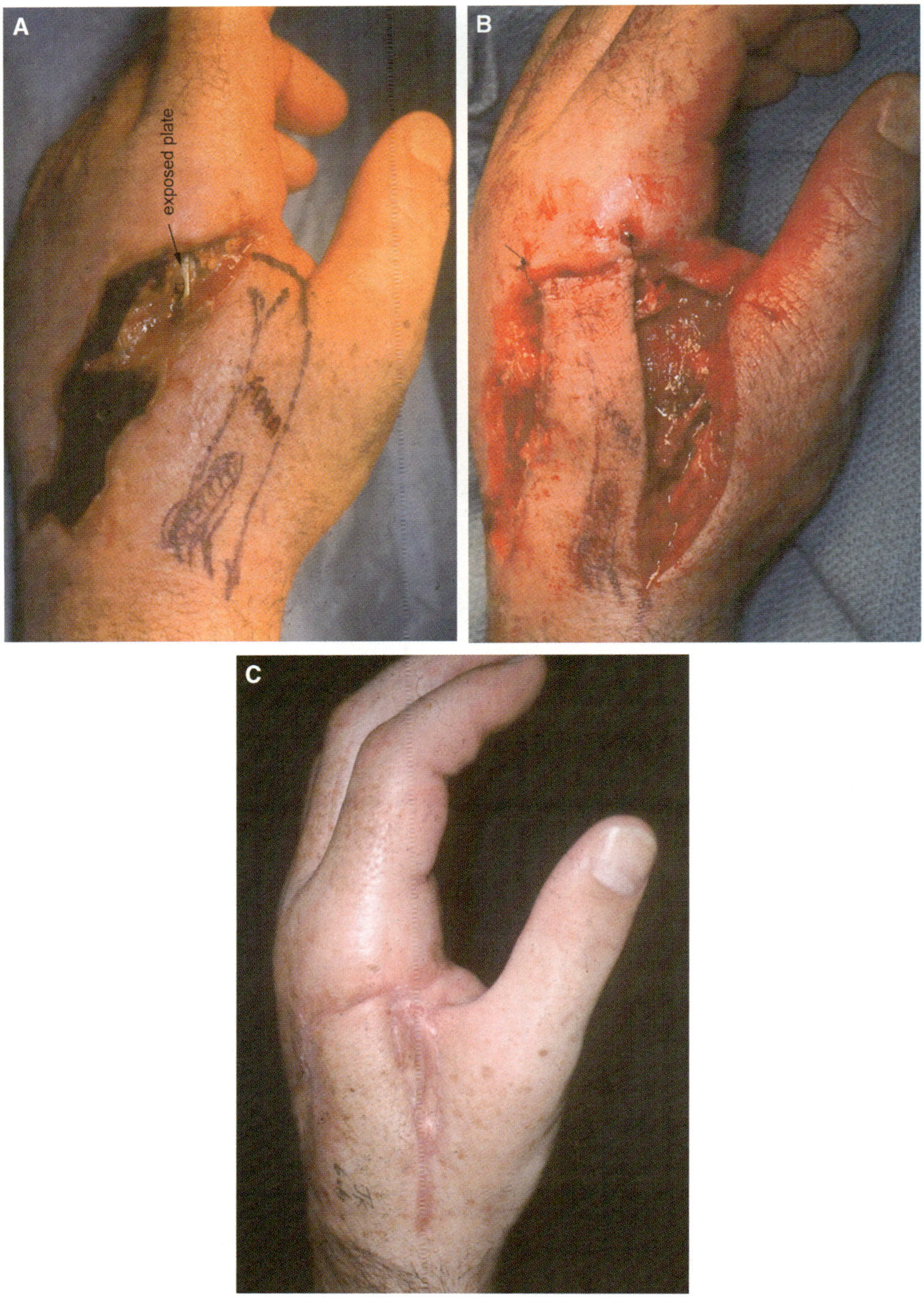

Fig. 13. (*A*) Exposed plate after revascularization for partial hand amputation. (*B*) Flap based on the FDMAr. (*C*) Long-term result.

Island flaps

The flap is pedicled on the FDMAu when used to cover defects over the volar surface of the distal thumb (Fig. 14) [42]. Alternatively the dorsal skin over the proximal phalanx of the thumb, which is supplied by the FDMAr, can resurface the radial side of the index. The flap is outlined over the dorsum of the index proximal phalanx. A proximal longitudinal incision is

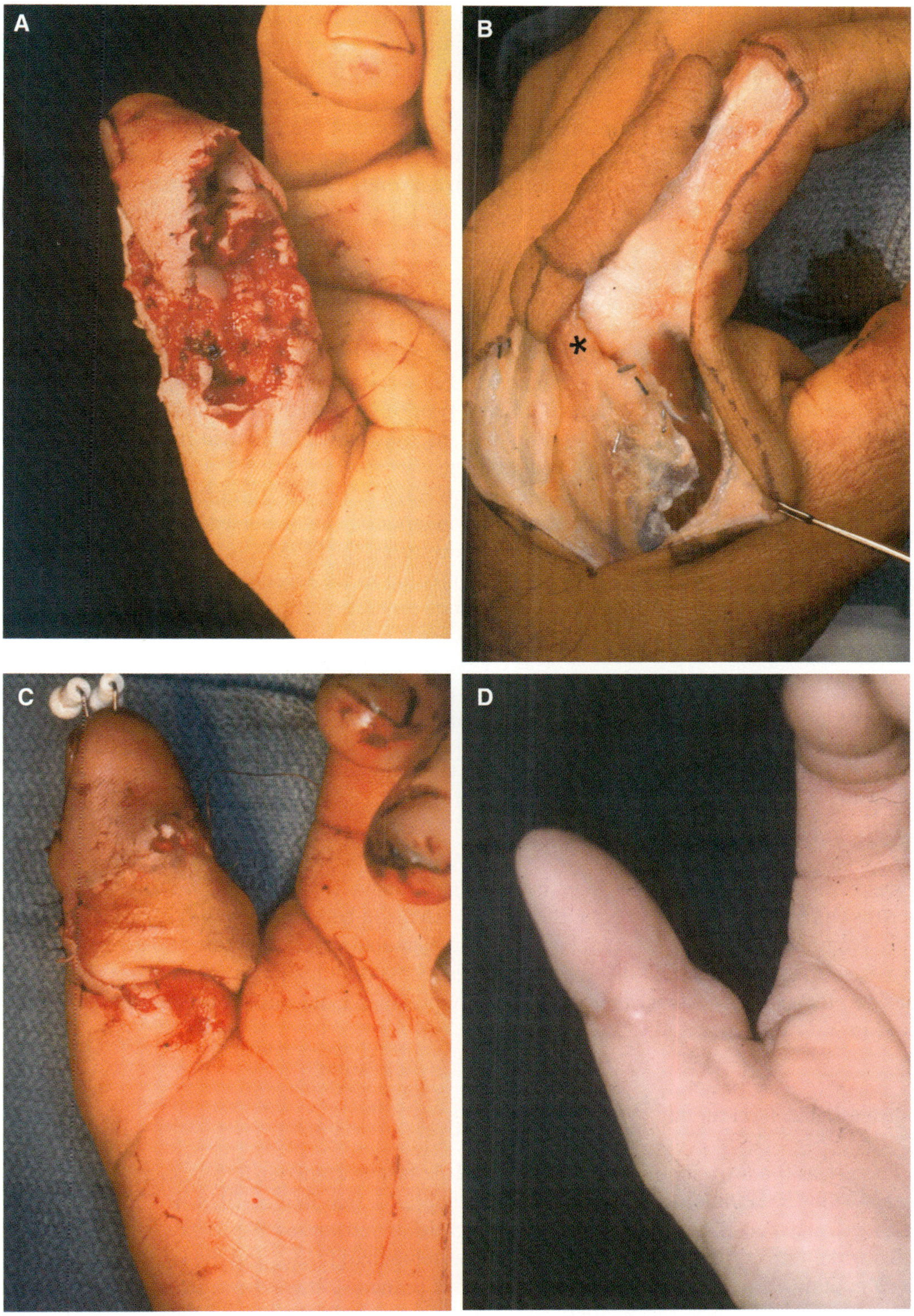

Fig. 14. (*A*) Saw injury to right thumb with destruction of the interphalangeal joint. (*B*) FDMA flap raised from dorsum of index with a proximal skin tail. Note preservation of the continuity of the fascia (*) between the skin island and the interosseous muscle. (*C*) Insetting of flap after interphalangeal joint fusion. (*D*) Long-term result.

made over the FDI muscle. The flap is elevated starting distally, developing the plane between the subcutaneous tissue and the extensor tendon paratenon up to the level of the MCP joint. The dorsoradial branch of the SBRN is harvested with the skin island. The subdermal fascia can be quite thin; care is taken to preserve its continuity with the FDI fascia. Inclusion of a small strip of extensor hood along the radial aspect of the extensor hood is recommended to protect the vascular connection from the pedicle to the skin island [43]. Flap dimensions extend from the base of the proximal phalanx to the PIP extension crease and can be 4 × 2 cm. The pedicle can be 9 cm in length.

The proximally based flap is rotated around the origin of the FDMA at the base of the first web space. It can be rotated and passed through a subcutaneous tunnel, taking care not to compress the pedicle at the thumb interphalangeal joint. Harvesting a proximal tail with the island flap simplifies insetting and avoids the need for tunneling (see Fig. 6). The donor site is skin grafted.

Variations

Harvesting the dorsal skin over the middle phalanx of the index as a random extension allows coverage of larger defects than a standard FDMA flap in a normal-length thumb [44]. Composite flaps include the extensor indicis proprius or communis tendon, which can be transferred as a vascularized tendon graft. An insensate fascial flap also may be used for soft tissue coverage only, but it requires skin grafting.

Reversed flow fascial flaps can be used for coverage of the dorsum of the digits proximal to the PIP joints [41]. This flap variant cannot be innervated. The reversed flow flap can reach as far ulnarly as the fifth metacarpal head. In this variation, the FDMA is ligated at its origin from the radial artery. The interosseous fascia is elevated up to the level of the metacarpal neck. The donor site is skin grafted if primary closure is not possible.

Sensory recovery

In one large series, the average 2-point discrimination was 10.8 mm (range 4–15 mm). There was no difference in patients younger or older than 50 years old. The average loss of 2-point discrimination over the flap area compared with the donor area was 2.7 mm [43].

Complications

Postoperative complications may include flap edema from kinking of the pedicle. Flap necrosis can occur with injury to the thin fascial extension between the index island flaps and the FDI. Numbness over the dorsum of the middle phalanx of the index or hair growth over the volar aspect of the thumb may be an irritation. Loss of index finger motion and poor take of the skin graft over the index extensor tendon are possible. Cold intolerance and dysesthesia can occur in 30% of patients [45].

Pedicled radial forearm flap

The radial forearm flap is a useful and versatile fasciocutaneous flap designed on the radial artery. Yang et al [46] initially developed this flap as a free flap in 1978. It subsequently was described as a pedicled flap using either antegrade or retrograde blood flow [47,48]. The flap includes the volar forearm skin, the underlying antebrachial fascia, and the intermuscular fascia, which contains the radial artery and its cutaneous branches. It can be innervated by the medial and lateral antebrachial cutaneous nerves. With retrograde flaps, neurorrhaphy to the local nerves is required.

Anatomy

The skin of the forearm flexor surface does not have any truly axial artery. An axial pattern flap in effect is created by raising a flap including the fascial and subcutaneous vessels with their longitudinal orientation and interconnections [49]. The entire radial artery from its brachial artery origin to the wrist can be transferred. For most of its course, the radial artery lies under the brachioradialis. The pronator teres, flexor pollicis longus, and pronator quadratus lie deep to the artery. The SBRN is lateral to the artery under the brachioradialis. After giving off the radial recurrent artery near its origin, the radial artery has no named branches until it reaches the wrist. Here it gives off a superficial palmar branch and a palmar carpal branch. Cadaver studies have shown 9 to 17 branches from the radial artery to the fascia along the flexor surface of the forearm. The branches supplying the skin are contained in an intermuscular septum between the brachioradialis and the flexor carpi radialis (Fig. 15). These branches are arranged into a proximal and distal group with corresponding zones of perfusion [50]. In the distal half of the forearm, there are branches every 1 to 2 cm. As elsewhere, one vascular zone can be extended into another. The distal zone vessels can perfuse a fasciocutaneous flap as far proximal as the elbow. In a reverse pedicled flap, the skin blood supply depends on retrograde flow from the ulnar artery through the deep palmar arch.

Venous drainage of the radial forearm flap is by means of the superficial and the deep veins. There are three subcutaneous veins—the cephalic, basilic, and median forearm veins—and the paired deep venae comitantes of the radial artery. A reverse pedicled flap is drained by means of retrograde flow through the venae comitantes. Normally the venous valves prevent backflow. When a distally based flap is raised, the veins are denervated. The veins are kept filled by blood from the wrist and hand, which leads to increased venous pressure after ligation of their proximal ends. The combination of these factors allows reverse flow through the venous valves [50].

The SBRN, brachioradialis, flexor carpi radialis, and palmaris longus tendons are supplied by direct branches and branches off cutaneous vessels. The medial and lateral antebrachial cutaneous nerves enter the proximal margin of the flap and supply sensibility to the volar forearm.

The radial artery gives off at least two periosteal branches of 0.2 to 0.5 mm in size along the lateral aspect of the radius, immediately distal to the pronator teres insertion. These branches are accompanied by two small venae comitantes and pass along the fascial layer deep to the extensors carpi radialis longus and brevis. Musculoperiosteal vessels form a constant source of blood supply over the anterior aspect of the distal shaft. They are fed by branches of the radial artery supplying the flexor pollicis longus and pronator quadratus [51].

Over the distal volar forearm, the flap is thin with little fat, but it leaves a poor bed for skin grafting, consisting of tendons covered only by paratenon. A proximal flap is hair bearing and thicker because it has more subcutaneous fat. The donor site contains muscle bellies, which is more favorable for skin grafting. The skin can be innervated by including the medial or lateral antebrachial cutaneous nerve. The flap can include the entire volar forearm skin from the subcutaneous border of the ulna around to the radial dorsum of the forearm, extending as far proximal as the antecubital fossa. Forearm flaps measuring 35 × 15 cm have been reported.

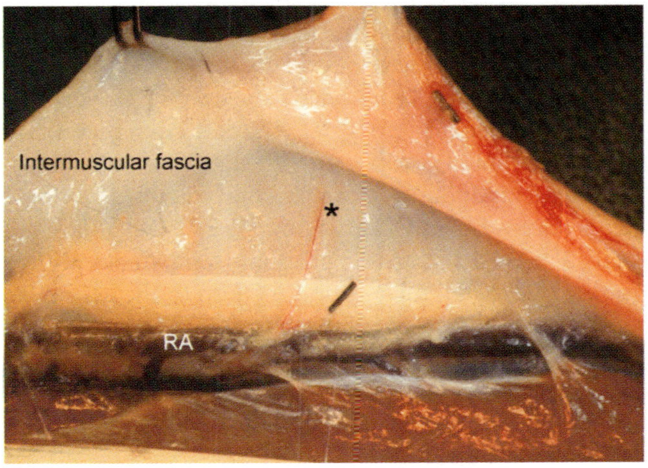

Fig. 15. Demonstration of cutaneous branches (*) arising from the radial artery (RA) coursing through the intermuscular septum.

Indications

The flap is useful for thumb reconstruction (Fig. 16). It can be used for coverage of the palm or extensor surface of the carpus, with or without vascularized tendon (Fig. 17). It provides a durable surface for coverage of amputation stumps (Fig. 18).

Advantages

Distally based radial forearm flaps designed on the proximal forearm can reach the dorsal and palmar surfaces of the hand easily. They can include vascularized tendon and bone. Pedicle lengths of 15 cm are possible. If the flap is less than 6 cm in width, the donor site can be closed primarily.

The flap arc of rotation can be increased by freeing the radial artery in the snuffbox and passing the flap underneath the thumb extensors; this allows the flap to reach as far as the thumb tip [38]. The forearm flap permits postoperative elevation and early mobilization of the injured limb. Proximally based flaps can be used to resurface defects well above the elbow joint [52]. These flaps are directly innervated by including the medial or lateral cutaneous nerve of the forearm.

Limitations

Underdevelopment of the radial artery or injury to the superficial and deep palmar arches would preclude the use of this flap, as would the absence of a connection between the radial and ulnar arteries. In Coleman and Anson's [53] dissection of 650 cadaver arms, only 3.2% had no communication between the radial and ulnar artery, and 3% had an incomplete deep arch. If both of these variations are present, the thumb is dependent on the radial artery (approximately 1 in 1100). This situation can be identified by a preoperative Allen's test [54]. Vein graft reconstruction of the radial artery would be necessary in these cases. Care should be exercised in acute trauma when hematoma extends to the snuffbox.

Surgical technique

The course of the radial artery is marked [25]. Using a pattern from the recipient site, the size of the defect is outlined on the proximal forearm. If the flap is outlined over the proximal ulnar forearm, it is thinner and less hair bearing. A thin skin island can be left over the course of the radial artery to prevent the need for skin grafting the pedicle later on and to avoid an overlying skin bridge. The flap is incised down to the deep fascia. Veins are harvested along the proximal medial border of the flap; this allows an easier anastomosis with local veins when the flap has been rotated 180°. The medial or lateral antebrachial cutaneous nerve is identified, then a proximal extensile incision is made for a longer nerve pedicle. The SBRN should be protected to preserve sensation to the radial aspect of the hand.

A plane is developed deep to the radial artery at the wrist, and the intermuscular septum is found between the flexor carpi radialis and the brachioradialis. The deep fascia is incised over the flexor carpi radialis muscle belly, well medial to the intermuscular septum. The interval between the deep fascia and the muscle is dissected. The deep fascia is sutured to the skin flap to minimize shear on the septocutaneous perforators. The dissection is continued deep to the radial artery on both sides of the septum. The fascia superficial to the radial artery is left undisturbed because it contains the septocutanous perforators that supply the skin flap. After the flap dissection is complete, a microvascular clamp is applied to the proximal radial artery before releasing the tourniquet. If there is adequate perfusion to the flap and the thumb, the artery is divided. The flap is raised, ligating all the perforators deep to the artery. The flap is transposed to the dorsum of the hand. If desired, a venous anastomosis is performed before insetting the flap (see Fig. 16D).

Variations

The radial forearm flap can be raised as a composite skin flap including vascularized bone and tendon for thumb reconstruction [55]. A purely fascial radial forearm flap can be used to

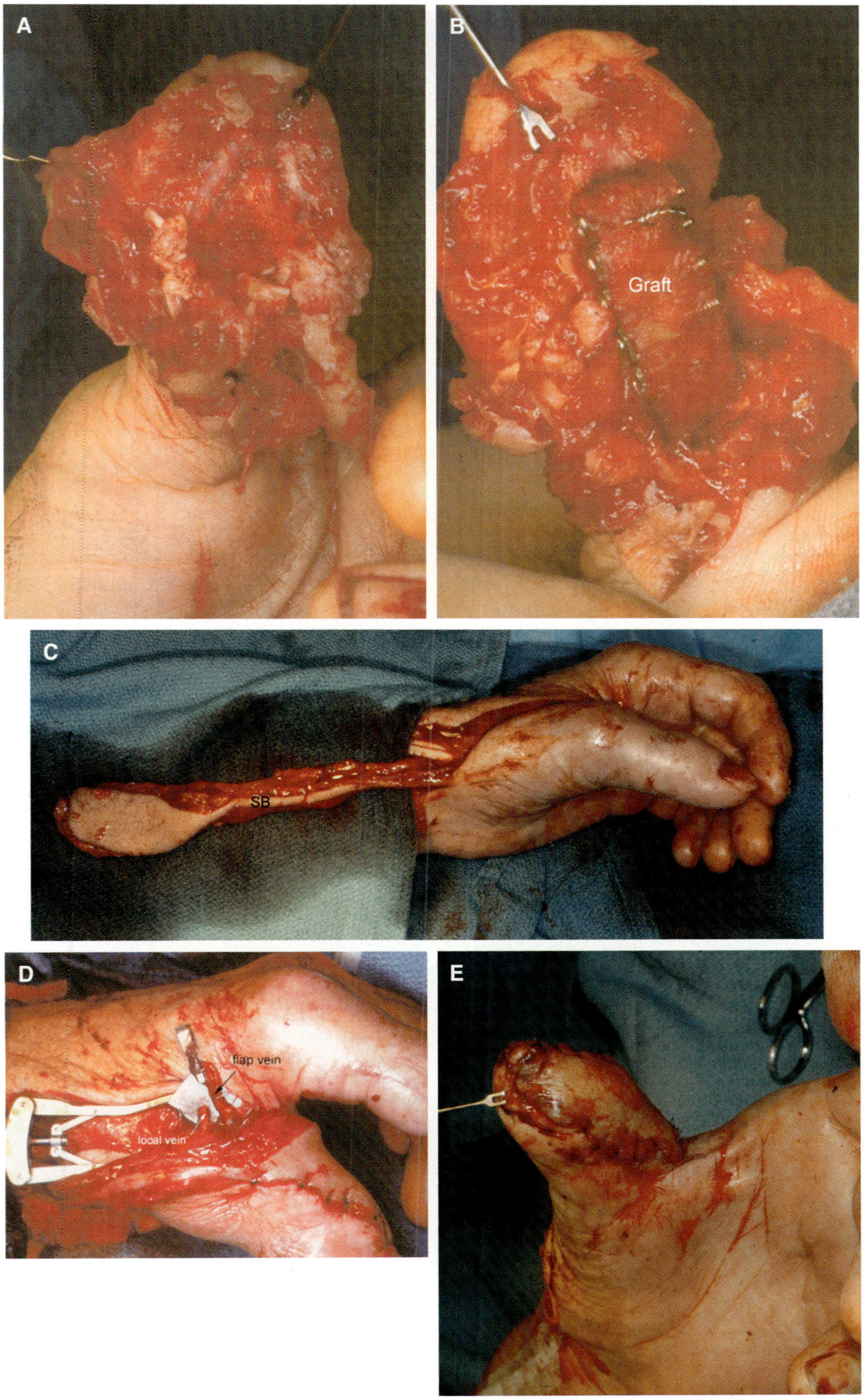

Fig. 16. (*A*) Saw injury with skin and bone loss of distal thumb. (*B*) Bone reconstruction using iliac crest graft and minicondylar plate. (*C*) Pedicle reversed flow radial forearm flap. Note skin bridge (SB) over the pedicle. (*D*) Supplemental venous anastomosis. (*E*) Insetting of flap. (*F*) Long-term result.

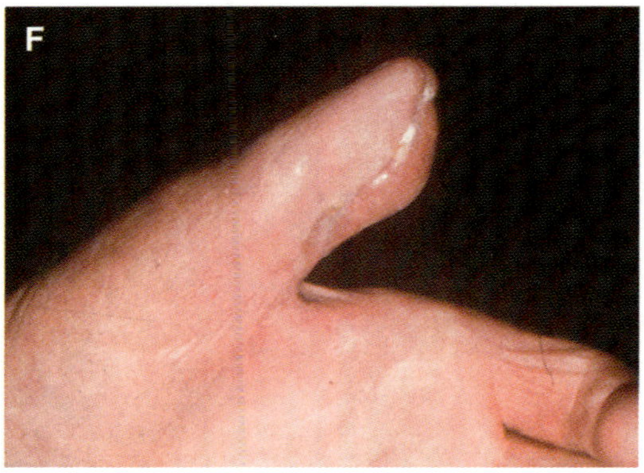

Fig. 16 (*continued*)

cover exposed tendons on the dorsum of the hand, but it has to be skin grafted, and innervation is not possible [56]. A reverse radial fascial-fat flap preserves the radial artery and has been used to cover a scarred median nerve [57,58].

Vascularized bone dissection

The vascularized bone graft does not carry an intact blood endosteal supply, but instead survives on the periosteal branches. The lateral half of the radius from the insertion of the pronator teres to the metaphyseal flare of the distal radius can be harvested; 10 cm of slightly curved, mostly cortical bone, constituting half the circumference of a circle, is obtained. The perforators deep to the radial artery along the length of the desired bone graft are preserved. Dissection is carried out medial to the intermuscular fascia over the radius. The pronator teres, sublimis muscle, and flexor pollicis longus muscle are divided directly on top of the midline of

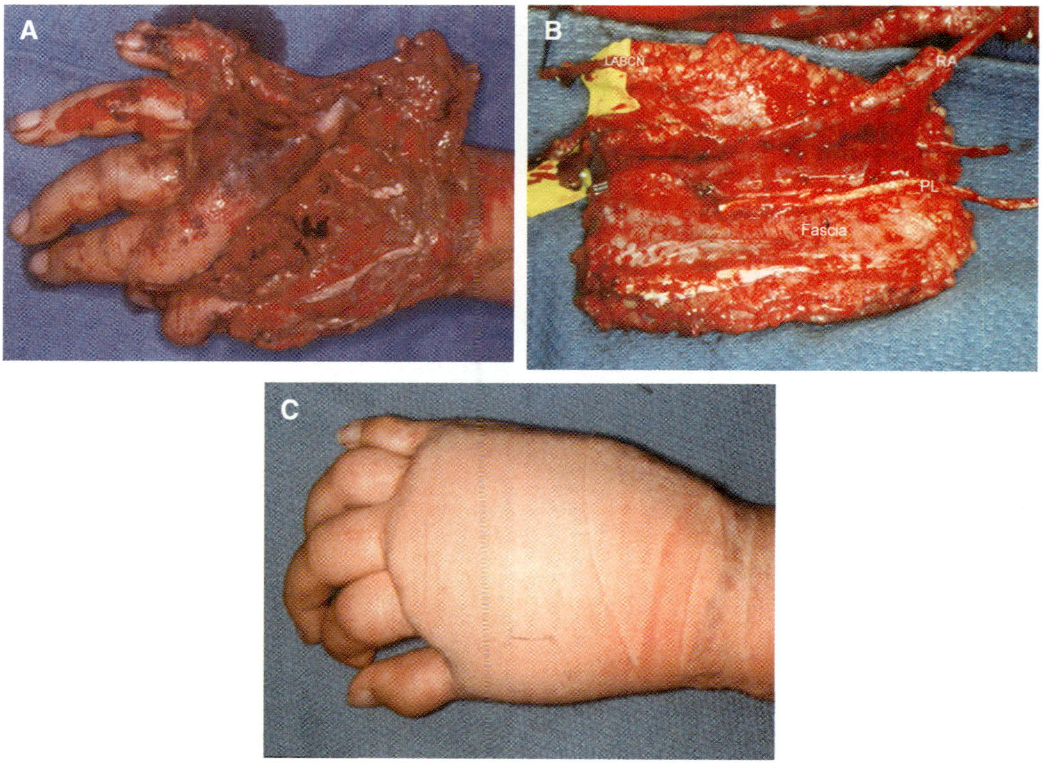

Fig. 17. (*A*) Rollover crush injury with devitalized skin, extensor tendon loss, and multiple open fractures. (*B*) Pedicled retrograde flap based on the radial artery (RA). Note the vascularized palmaris longus tendon (PL) and the lateral antebrachial cutaneous nerve (LABCN). (*C*) Long-term result.

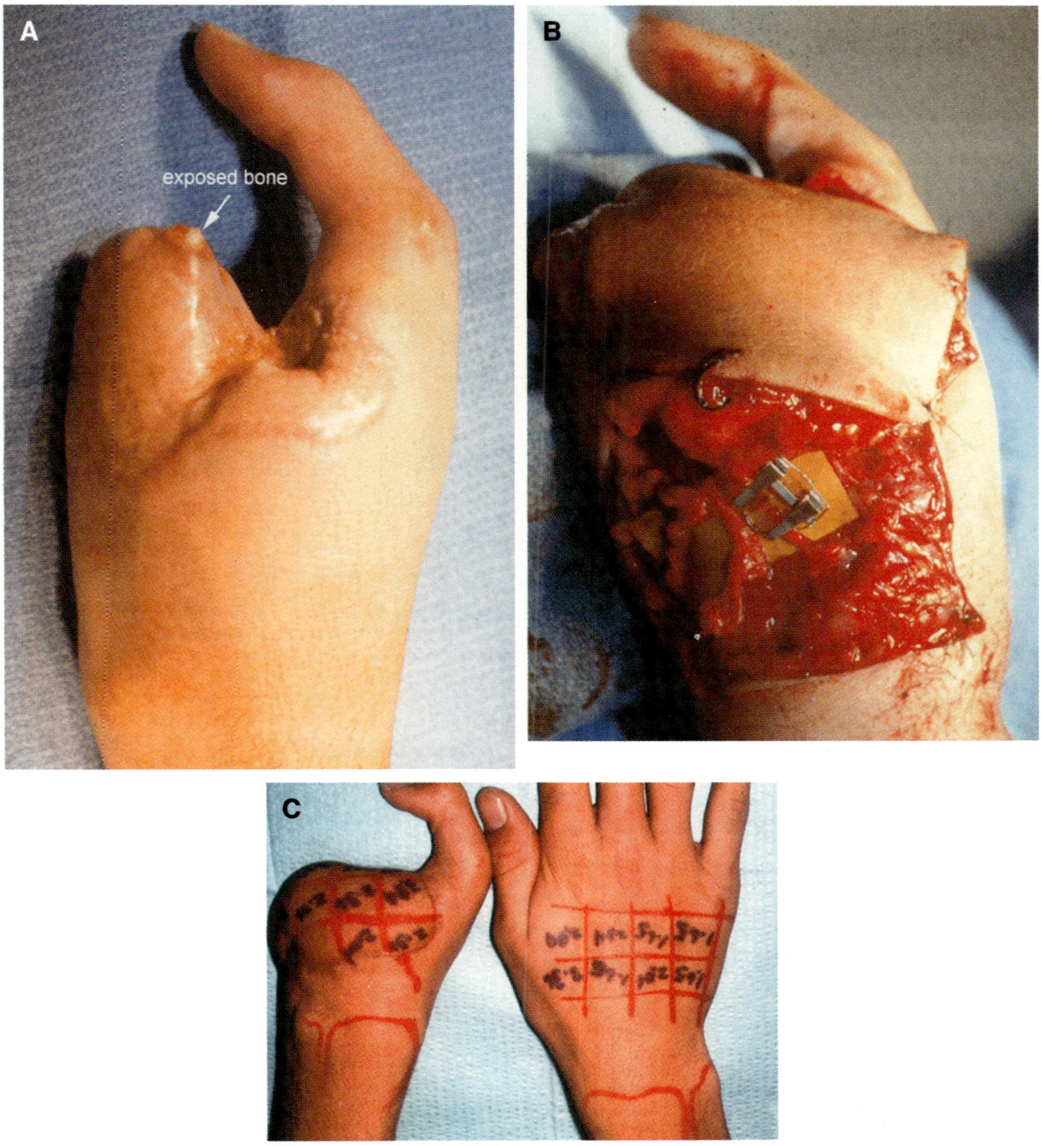

Fig. 18. (*A*) Transmetacarpal amputation with unstable stump. (*B*) Reversed pedicled forearm flap with venous anastomosis. (*C*) Sensibility testing with Semmes-Weinstein filaments is comparable to other side.

the bone; this preserves the musculoperiosteal branches to the bone graft. The osteotomy site is predrilled before performing the osteotomy. The proximal and distal corners are beveled to decrease stress risers and to diminish the risk of postoperative fracture.

Fascial flap dissection

A purely fascial flap is raised in a similar manner to the fasciocutaneous flap. The plane of dissection proceeds between the deep fascia and the skin, which divides all the cutaneous branches.

The reverse radial fascial-fat flap survives on retrograde blood flow through perforating vessels coming off the radial artery. These perforators are found within 1.5 to 7 cm from the radial styloid and run directly upward from the radial artery into the fascia (Fig. 19). The fascia serves as a viable supporting membrane for perfusion of the fat on its surface [57]. The most proximal perforators are sacrificed for retrograde orientation of this flap. The fat and deep fascia are developed as a long, distally based rectangular flap. The interval between the fat and fascia is not violated. The lateral antebrachial cutaneous nerve and SBRN are preserved. After elevation, the flap is turned distally 180° and simultaneously twisted 90° to place the vascularized fat layer directly over the median nerve (Fig. 20). The donor site is closed primarily.

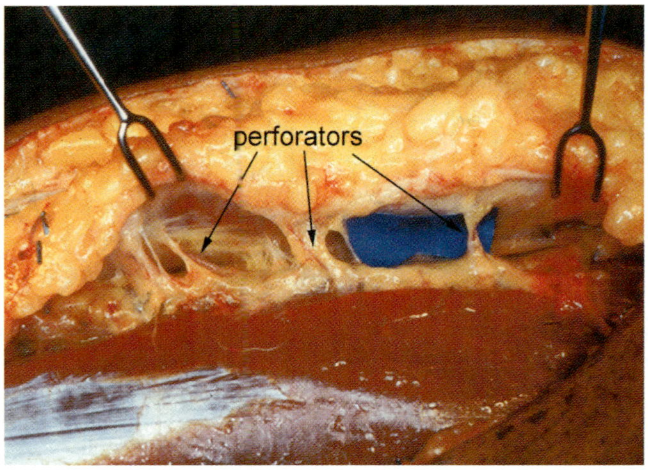

Fig. 19. Demonstration of perforating vessels supplying the deep fascia.

Sensory recovery

In one series, the moving 2-point discrimination averaged 13.2 mm. This was more sensitive than the donor forearm, and it was postulated that the sensory return depended more on the recipient nerve than the donor nerve [59]

Complications

Postoperative complications include flap edema, unstable skin graft over tendons, hand swelling, and superficial radial nerve injury. Flap edema is common because of associated forearm injury or impaired venous drainage. Additional venous anastomoses help minimize this edema. Skin graft failure is most likely to occur over tendons, especially the flexor carpi radialis. Even when they have successfully taken on tendons, skin grafts may experience recurrent breakdown. Avoidance of the distal forearm as a donor site and covering the tendons with adjacent muscle fibers from portions of the brachioradialis, flexor digitorum superficialis, and flexor carpi ulnaris provide a better skin graft bed. Unmeshed skin grafts can be used to maximize the bridging phenomenon. Preoperative tissue expansion also can be used [60].

The donor site defect is quite noticeable. The flap is hair bearing and often bulky. A radial shaft fracture can occur after harvest of vascularized one; above-elbow casting or splinting for up to 8 weeks is recommended. Although digital temperature comparisons show an average 2.5% decrease after the use of the radial forearm flap, cold intolerance is often transient [61].

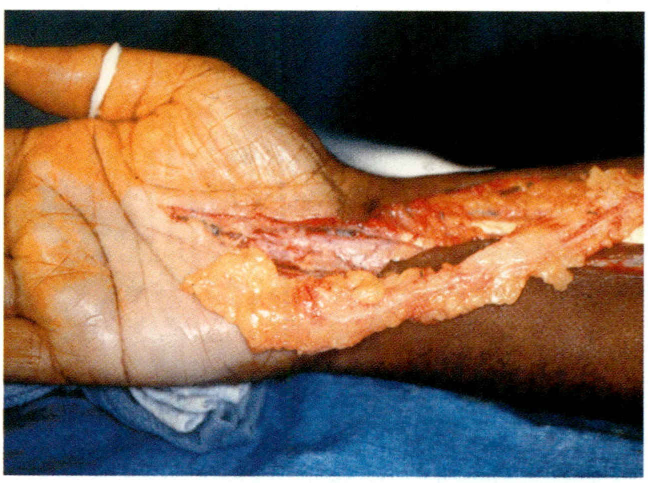

Fig. 20. Pedicled fascial forearm flap used to cover median nerve after neurolysis.

Innervated groin flap

The groin flap, introduced by McGregor and Jackson [62] in 1972, was one of the first axial pattern flaps. It was revolutionary because it allowed greater potential for reconstruction of difficult upper extremity wounds. Despite the wide variety of pedicle flaps, the groin flap still has a place in cases in which there are inadequate vessels for a free flap or in which there has been an injury to the carpal arch that precludes the use of a pedicled forearm flap. Joshi [63] modified the flap to include branches of the lateral cutaneous branch of the subcostal nerve (12th thoracic nerve). This modification facilitates sensory innervation of the flap after neurorrhaphy to local donor nerves.

Anatomy

The groin flap is supplied by either the superficial circumflex iliac artery (SCIA) or the superficial epigastric artery (SEA). Taylor and Daniel [64] found the SCIA to be present and greater than 1 mm in diameter 98% of the time. The SCIA and SEA usually arise separately off the femoral artery, although a common arterial trunk was found in 29% of specimens in one series [65]. Either the common trunk or the SCIA is used as the pedicle, unless the SEA is larger.

The SCIA arises from the anterolateral aspect of the femoral artery, 2 to 3 cm below the inguinal ligament. It runs laterally in a line parallel to the inguinal ligament superficial to the iliacus fascia, enveloped by the fatty lymphatic tissue in the femoral triangle. At the medial border of the sartorius muscle, it usually divides into a superficial and deep branch. The superficial branch continues laterally, above the sartorius fascia to supply the skin surrounding the anterior superior iliac spine (ASIS). The deep branch runs underneath the sartorius fascia. It pierces the fascia at the lateral border of the sartorius, 1 to 4 cm below the ASIS, giving off cutaneous and muscular branches. If a long groin flap is required, the deep branch must be included in the pedicle. The vascular network lateral to the ASIS is quite extensive, allowing elevation of a large random pattern skin extension of the flap.

The SEA arises in a similar fashion to the SCIA, then runs laterally, superficial and superior to the inguinal ligament. It remains medial to the ASIS to supply an area of skin above the territory of the SCIA. The territories of these vessels overlap.

The venous drainage is quite variable. The groin area is drained by the superficial epigastric vein, the superficial circumflex iliac vein, and the associated venae comitantes. These veins drain into either the saphenous bulb or the femoral vein. The superficial epigastric vein and superficial circumflex iliac vein lie superficial to their respective arteries and to Scarpa's fascia. They frequently form a common trunk measuring greater than 2 mm [66].

The sensory supply of the lateral half of the groin flap corresponds to nearly the entire distribution of the lateral cutaneous branch of the subcostal nerve. This branch exits between the internal and external oblique muscles. It descends over the iliac crest about 5 cm behind the ASIS, before supplying the skin over the front part of the buttocks. This nerve branch is separate from the lateral cutaneous nerve of the thigh, which arises from the lumbar plexus (L2 and L3), then travels behind the inguinal ligament.

Indications

The groin flap is indicated for cases requiring massive soft tissue coverage of the hand. It provides a means for the resurfacing of large soft tissue defects—15 × 30 cm. This flap may be used for thumb reconstruction or for limb salvage after a failed free or pedicled flap. It may be useful in selected pediatric cases in which the donor site defect from other pedicled or free flaps may be substantial.

Advantages

The flap anatomy is reliable, and microvascular technique is not a prerequisite to raising the flap. This flap can be used in situations in which inadequate vessels or patient factors (age,

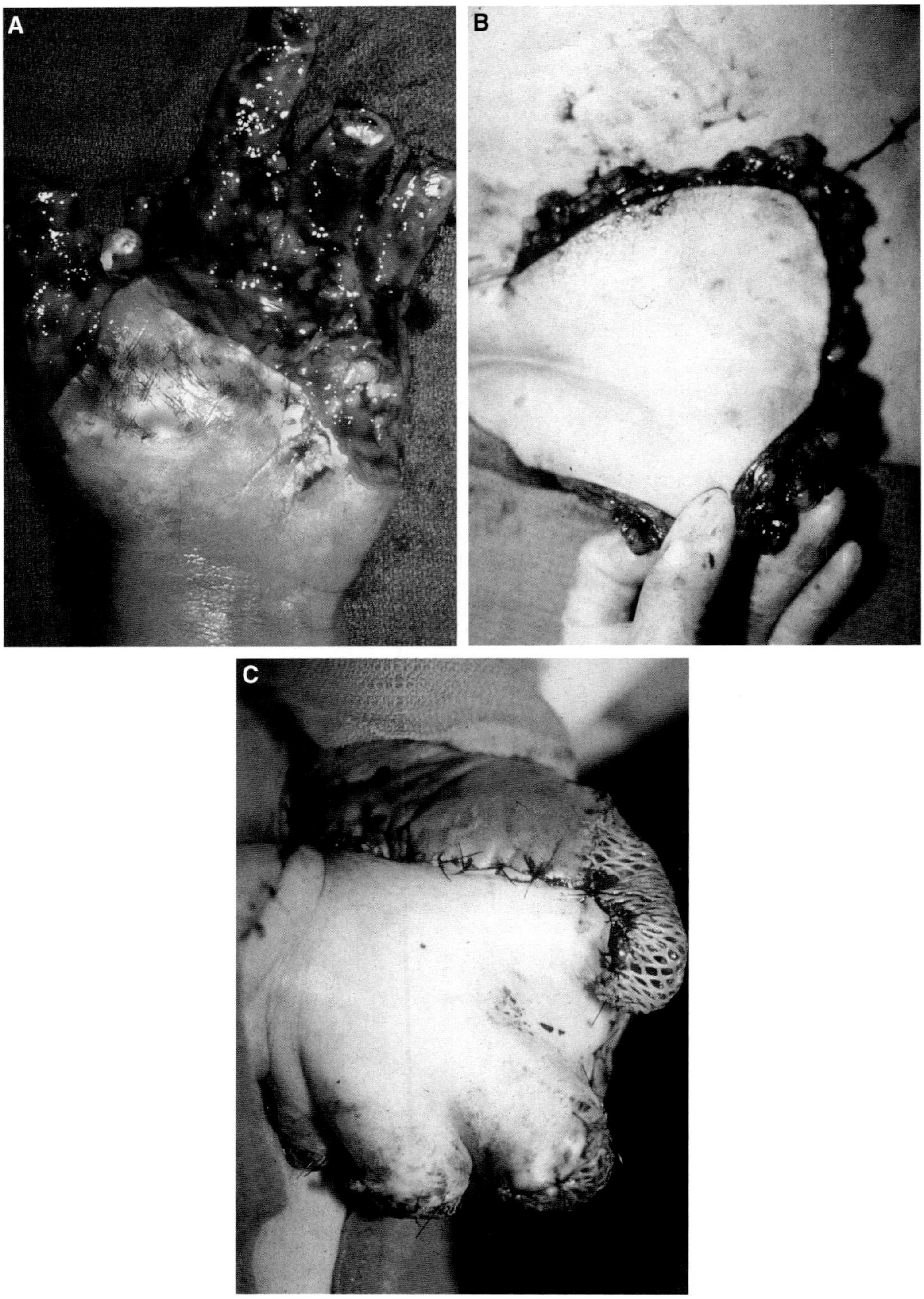

Fig. 21. (*A*) Degloving hand injury. (*B*) Elevation of groin flap. (*C*) Resurfacing of palm.

systemic illness, atherosclerotic vessels) preclude the use of a free flap. It may be useful when there is an injury to the superficial and deep palmar arch that precludes the use of a reversed pedicled radial forearm flap (Fig. 21). The donor site scar can be closed primarily and is hidden by a bathing suit. Because regional nerves are used, there is no problem with cortical reorientation.

Limitations

A history of lymphadenitis or previous surgery in the groin, including hernia repairs, lymph node biopsies, or vein stripping, may preclude use of this flap for fear of prior injury to the vascular pedicle. Patients with marked limb edema, patients with shoulder or elbow contractures, and patients who cannot tolerate prolonged upper extremity immobilization for psychological reasons may not be appropriate candidates.

Surgical technique

The patient is positioned supine with a sand bag under the ipsilateral buttock. The amount of skin that can be removed while still allowing direct closure can be estimated by flexing the hip and approximating the skin edges manually. The pubic tubercle, inguinal ligament, and ASIS are drawn along with a pattern taken from the tissue defect. The most dependable approach is to approximate the flap axis through the center of both vascular territories by drawing a line 2 cm distal to the inguinal ligament that extends past the ASIS.

The flap is elevated from lateral to medial to allow identification of the SCIA or SEA. The flap is based on the larger of the two arteries at the time of dissection. A thin layer of subcutaneous fat is harvested with the skin lateral to the ASIS because this represents a random pattern flap extension of the flap. When the ASIS is encountered, however, the entire width of the subcutaneous fat must be harvested to include the arterial pedicle. The interval between the tensor fascia lata and the sartorius is delineated. The deep branch of SCIA courses from a deep to a superficial plane as it passes through the sartorius fascia to reach the subcutaneous tissue. The fascia and the subcutaneous tissue are elevated carefully from the lateral border of the muscle to prevent injury to the SCIA. If the SCIA is not visible, transilluminating the flap may be helpful.

The subcostal nerve emerges from the oblique muscles and spreads into two branches just below the iliac crest. The nerve is divided at the iliac crest region so that it remains ensheathed in the layers of the groin flap. The two branches are available for suture to donor nerves in the hand, with the pedicle entering on one end and the nerve exiting the other end of the flap [63]. The hand is placed in the groin, and the flap is sewn over the soft tissue defect. Shoulder range-of-motion exercises are emphasized until the flap is divided at 3 to 4 weeks.

Variations

If the flap is tubed for thumb reconstruction (Fig. 22), one side of the flap is cut longer than the other and diagonal closure of the donor site and the flap is performed. This diagonal closure increases the circumference of the tube at the base of the flap, reducing the risk of vascular compression. Diagonal closure also produces a spiral in the tube. The direction of the spiral can be controlled to facilitate closure of defects on the palm or dorsum of the hand [67]. The use of a pedicled, osteocutaneous groin flap to reconstruct a composite interpositional bone loss of the thumb has been described (Fig. 23) [68]. Taylor et al [69] showed the superiority of the deep circumflex iliac vessels when harvesting vascularized bone with the groin flap.

Sensory recovery

In Joshi's series [63] of four patients, the innervated groin flap provided protective sensation or better. The maximum return of sensation occurred by 4 months compared with 18 months for a noninnervated flap.

Complications

The flap carries pubic hair on its medial aspect. The flap is bulky, and a secondary procedure for defatting may be necessary. Shoulder stiffness is common, especially in elderly patients. Partial fat necrosis, seroma, infection, and complications related to bed rest can complicate the results.

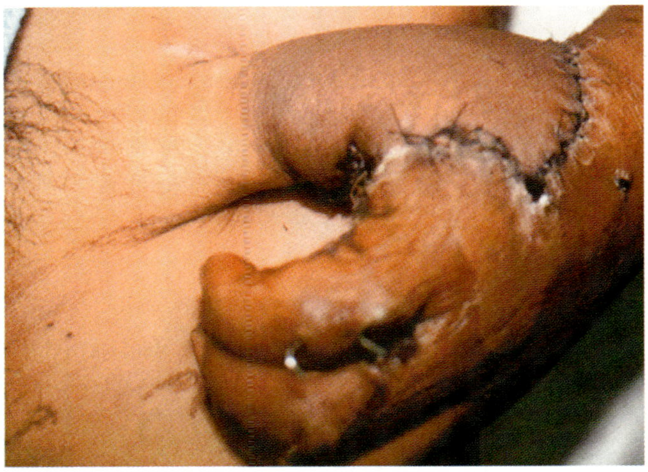

Fig. 22. Tubed groin flap for thumb reconstruction.

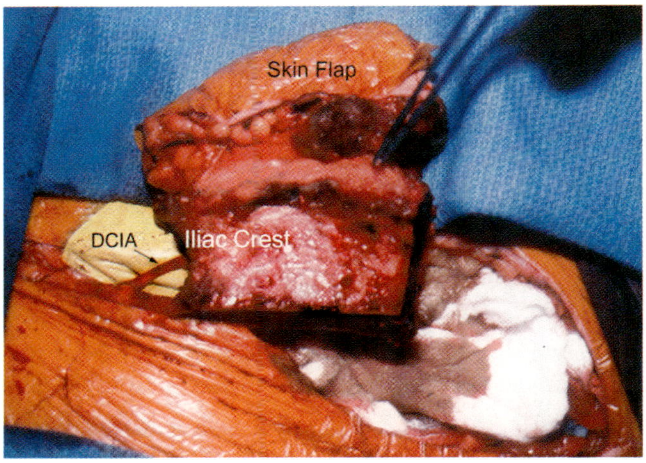

Fig. 23. Osteocutaneous groin flap pedicled on the deep circumflex iliac artery (DCIA).

Summary

Any particular soft tissue defect of the hand can be managed in a variety of ways. Often the simplest procedure with the fewest potential complications suffices. Soft tissue coverage is merely one component in the management of complex hand injuries, which also may require bony stabilization, neurovascular repair, and tendon reconstruction. Although not specifically addressed, the role of aggressive hand therapy with edema control, early active motion, and functional retraining cannot be overemphasized. Providing stable soft tissue coverage with the potential for sensibility expands the subsequent reconstructive options and enhances the ultimate functional result. Through an intimate understanding of the neurovascular anatomy, innovative hand surgeons undoubtedly will continue to find new applications for established techniques, limited only by their imagination.

References

[1] Merriam-Webster's Online Dictionary. Springfield, MA: Merriam-Webster Inc.

[2] Bertelli JA, Catarina S. Neurocutaneous island flaps in upper limb coverage: experience with 44 clinical cases. J Hand Surg [Am] 1997;22:515.

[3] Slutsky DJ. Vascularized pedicled flaps of the forearm and hand. Presented at American Society for Surgery of the Hand 53rd Annual Meeting. Minneapolis, September 1998.

[4] Slutsky DJ. Vascularized pedicled flaps of the forearm and hand. Presented at American Society for Surgery of the Hand 54th Annual Meeting. Boston, September 1999.
[5] Swartz WM. Restoration of sensibility in mutilating hand injuries. Clin Plast Surg 1989;16:515.
[6] Moberg E. Aspects of sensation in reconstructive surgery of the upper extremity. J Bone Joint Surg Am 1964;46:817.
[7] Hueston J. Local flap repair of fingertip injuries. Plast Reconstr Surg 1966;37:349.
[8] Souquet R, Souquet JR. The actual indications of cross finger flaps in finger injuries. Ann Chir Main 1986;5:43.
[9] Foucher G, Dallaserra M, Tilquin B, et al. The Hueston flap in reconstruction of fingertip skin loss: results in a series of 41 patients. J Hand Surg [Am] 1994;19:508.
[10] Cronin TD. The cross finger flap: a new method of repair. Am Surg 1951;17:419.
[11] Berger A, Meissl G. [Reestablishment of sensation in the distal phalanges using innervated flaps or grafts]. Handchirurgie 1975;7:169.
[12] Endo T, Kojima T, Hirase Y. Vascular anatomy of the finger dorsum and a new idea for coverage of the finger pulp defect that restores sensation. J Hand Surg [Am] 1992;17:927.
[13] Lai CS, Lin SD, Chou CK, et al. A versatile method for reconstruction of finger defects: reverse digital artery flap. Br J Plast Surg 1992;45:443.
[14] Tellioglu AT, Sensoz O. The dorsal branch of the digital nerve: An anatomic study and clinical applications. Ann Plast Surg 1998;40:145.
[15] Kleinert HE, McAlister CG, MacDonald CJ, et al. A critical evaluation of cross finger flaps. J Trauma 1974;14:756.
[16] Cohen BE, Cronin ED. An innervated cross-finger flap for fingertip reconstruction. Plast Reconstr Surg 1983;72: 688.
[17] Lassner F, Becker M, Berger A, et al. Sensory reconstruction of the fingertip using the bilaterally innervated sensory cross-finger flap. Plast Reconstr Surg 2002;109:988.
[18] Gaul JS Jr. Radial-innervated cross-finger flap from index to provide sensory pulp to injured thumb. J Bone Joint Surg Am 1969;51:1257.
[19] Abrams RA, Brown RA, Botte MJ. The superficial branch of the radial nerve: an anatomic study with surgical implications. J Hand Surg [Am] 1992;17:1037.
[20] Hastings H 2nd. Dual innervated index to thumb cross finger or island flap reconstruction. Microsurgery 1987;8: 168.
[21] Walker MA, Hurley CB, May JW Jr. Radial nerve cross-finger flap differential nerve contribution in thumb reconstruction. J Hand Surg [Am] 1986;11:881.
[22] Kojima T, Hayashi Y, Sakurai N, et al. Eleven cases of vascular pedicle island flap for difficult skin defects on the hand. J Jpn Soc Surg Hand 1986;3:350–4.
[23] Strauch B, de Moura W. Arterial system of the fingers. J Hand Surg [Am] 1990;15:148.
[24] Oberlin C. A reversed digital artery island flap for the treatment of fingertip injuries. J Hand Surg [Am] 1994;19:342.
[25] Slutsky DJ. Cadaver dissections: vascularized pedicled flaps of the forearm and hand. Presented at Videotape Theater, American Society for Surgery of the Hand 53rd Annual Meeting. Minneapolis, September 1998.
[26] Lai CS, Lin SD, Chou CK, et al. Innervated reverse digital artery flap through bilateral neurorrhaphy for pulp defects. Br J Plast Surg 1993;46:483.
[27] Earley MJ, Milner RH. Dorsal metacarpal flaps. Br J Plast Surg 1987;40:333.
[28] Lai CS, Lin SD, Tsai CC, et al. Reverse digital artery neurovascular cross-finger flap. J Hand Surg [Am] 1995;20: 397.
[29] Karacalar A, Sen C, Ozcan M. A modified reversed digital island flap incorporating the proper digital nerve. Ann Plast Surg 2000;45:67.
[30] Han SK, Lee BI, Kim WK. The reverse digital artery island flap: clinical experience in 120 fingers. Plast Reconstr Surg 1998;101:1006.
[31] Sapp JW, Allen RJ, Dupin C. A reversed digital artery island flap for the treatment of fingertip injuries. J Hand Surg [Am] 1993;18:528.
[32] Brunelli F, Pegin Z, Cabral J. Dorsal arterial supply to the thumb: new surgical possibilities for palmar skin coverage. Surg Radiol Anat 1991;13:240.
[33] Pistre V, Pelissier P, Martin D, et al. Vascular blood supply of the dorsal side of the thumb, first web and index finger: anatomical study. J Hand Surg [Br] 2001;26:98.
[34] Brunelli F, Vigasio A, Valenti P, et al. Arterial anatomy and clinical application of the dorsoulnar flap of the thumb. J Hand Surg [Am] 1999;24:803.
[35] Kumar VP, Satku K, Liu J. The Brunelli reversed flow pedicle flap from the thumb. Plast Reconstr Surg 1996;98: 1298.
[36] Cavadas PC. Reverse osteocutaneous dorsoulnar thumb flap. Plast Reconstr Surg 2003;111:326.
[37] Holevich J. A new method of restoring sensibility to the thumb. J Bone Joint Surg Br 1963;45:496.
[38] Foucher G, Braun JB. A new island flap transfer from the dorsum of the index to the thumb. Plast Reconstr Surg 1979;63:344.
[39] Steinberg BD, Plancher KD, Idler RS. Percutaneous Kirschner wire fixation through the snuff box: an anatomic study. J Hand Surg [Am] 1995;20:57.
[40] Chiu HY, Shieh SJ, Hsu HY. Multivariate analysis of factors influencing the functional recovery after finger replantation or revascularization. Microsurgery 1995;16:713.
[41] Sherif MM. First dorsal metacarpal artery flap in hand reconstruction: II. Clinical application. J Hand Surg [Am] 1994;19:32.
[42] Slutsky DJ. The first dorsal metacarpal artery flap. In: Wrist Arthroscopy 2000 Course Videotapes. Chicago: American Society for Surgery of the Hand; 2000.

[43] Trankle M, Sauerbier M, Heitmann C, et al. Restoration of thumb sensibility with the innervated first dorsal metacarpal artery island flap. J Hand Surg [Am] 2003;28:758.
[44] El-Khatib HA. Clinical experiences with the extended first dorsal metacarpal artery island flap for thumb reconstruction. J Hand Surg [Am] 1998;23:647.
[45] Ege A, Tuncay I, Ercetin O. Foucher's first dorsal metacarpal artery flap for thumb reconstruction: evaluation of 21 cases. Isr Med Assoc J 2002;4:421.
[46] Yang G, Chen B, Gao Y, et al. Forearm free skin flap transplantation. Natl Med J China 1981;61:139.
[47] Muhlbauer W, Herndl E, Stock W. The forearm flap. Plast Reconstr Surg 1982;70:336.
[48] Song R, Gao Y, Song Y, et al. The forearm flap. Clin Plast Surg 1982;9:21.
[49] Cormack GC, Lamberty BG. A classification of fascio-cutaneous flaps according to their patterns of vascularisation. Br J Plast Surg 1984;37:80.
[50] Timmons MJ. The vascular basis of the radial forearm flap. Plast Reconstr Surg 1986;77:80.
[51] Cormack GC, Duncan MJ, Lamberty BG. The blood supply of the bone component of the compound osteo-cutaneous radial artery forearm flap—an anatomical study. Br J Plast Surg 1986;39:173.
[52] Fatah MF, Davies DM. The radial forearm island flap in upper limb reconstruction. J Hand Surg [Br] 1984;9:234.
[53] Coleman SS, Anson BJ. Arterial patterns in the hand based upon a study of 650 specimens. Suvr Med (Sofiia) 1961; 113:409.
[54] Gelberman RH, Blasingame JP. The timed Allen test. J Trauma 1981;21:477.
[55] Biemer E, Stock W. Total thumb reconstruction: a one-stage reconstruction using an osteo-cutaneous forearm flap. Br J Plast Surg 1983;36:52.
[56] Reyes FA, Burkhalter WE. The fascial radial flap. J Hand Surg [Am] 1988;13:432.
[57] Braun RM, Rechnic M, Neill-Cage DJ, et al. The retrograde radial fascial forearm flap: surgical rationale, technique, and clinical application. J Hand Surg [Am] 1995;20:915.
[58] Tham SK, Ireland DC, Riccio M, et al. Reverse radial artery fascial flap: A treatment for the chronically scarred median nerve in recurrent carpal tunnel syndrome. J Hand Surg [Am] 1996;21:849.
[59] Yamauchi T, Yajima H, Kizaki K, et al. Sensory reconstruction in sensate radial forearm flap transfer. J Reconstr Microsurg 2000;16:593.
[60] Liang MD, Swartz WM, Jones NF. Local full-thickness skin-graft coverage for the radial forearm flap donor site. Plast Reconstr Surg 1994;93:621.
[61] Kleinman WB, O'Connell SJ. Effects of the fasciocutaneous radial forearm flap on vascularity of the hand. J Hand Surg [Am] 1993;18:953.
[62] McGregor IA, Jackson IT. The groin flap. Br J Plast Surg 1972;25:3.
[63] Joshi BB. Neural repair for sensory restoration in a groin flap. Hand 1977;9:221.
[64] Taylor GI, Daniel RK. The anatomy of several free flap donor sites. Plast Reconstr Surg 1975;56:243.
[65] Harii K, Omori K, Torii S, et al. Free groin skin flaps. Br J Plast Surg 1975;28:225.
[66] Harii K, Ohmori K, Torii S, et al. Microvascular free skin flap transfer. Clin Plast Surg 1978;5:239.
[67] Schlenker JD. Important considerations in the design and construction of groin flaps. Ann Plast Surg 1980;5:353.
[68] Button M, Stone EJ. Segmental bony reconstruction of the thumb by composite groin flap: a case report. J Hand Surg [Am] 1980;5:488.
[69] Taylor GI, Townsend P, Corlett R. Superiority of the deep circumflex iliac vessels as the supply for free groin flaps. Plast Reconstr Surg 1979;64:595.

ELSEVIER
SAUNDERS

Atlas Hand Clin 10 (2005) 171–185

Atlas of the
HAND
CLINICS

Neurosensory Free Flaps

Bradon J. Wilhelmi, MD[a,*], W.P. Andrew Lee, MD[b]

[a]*Plastic Surgery Institute, Southern Illinois University School of Medicine, 747 North Rutledge, P.O. Box 19653, Springfield, IL 62702, USA*
[b]*University of Pittsburgh Medical School, 3550 Terrace Street, Scaife Hall 690, Pittsburgh, PA 15261, USA*

In reconstructing hand defects, the ultimate goal is not only to provide durable coverage, but also to restore protective sensation. In addition to soft tissue coverage, reconstruction of the hand may necessitate tendon reconstruction to achieve skeletal mobility. An insensate hand is prone to further injury, however, and less likely to be functional than a hand that is sensate and stiff. Reconstruction with sensate soft tissue can be extremely important in hand reconstruction.

Conventional techniques of sensory restoration

The most appropriate means of providing sensory restoration is dictated by the location and size of the defect. Small superficial defects sometimes can heal by secondary intention without significant loss of sensibility [1]. This approach is most appropriate for children and elderly patients [2,3]. Children have a capacity to heal wounds by granulation, contraction, and epithelialization more quickly than adults. Elderly patients potentially can experience complications such as stiffness, failure to regenerate nerve repairs, or inability for cortical reorientation. Another conventional approach to soft tissue restoration includes skin grafting. Skin grafts tend to result in a worse recovery of sensibility than sensory flaps. Some re-innervation of skin grafts can occur over time, but this can take 1 year or more [4–11]. Full-thickness skin grafts have been found to reinnervate more quickly than split-thickness skin grafts [12]. Reconstructing a finger tip defect with a split-thickness graft can minimize the area of decreased sensation through wound contraction [13].

When healing by secondary intention or skin grafting is not suitable, a local sensory flap can be considered. Local flaps are preferred when structures such as bone are exposed or digital shortening is to be avoided. Local flap options for finger wounds include the Atasoy volar V-Y or Kutler bilateral V-Y advancement flaps [14,15]. These flaps are limited in application to small finger wounds because of restricted arc of motion [14,15]. Small thumb tip defects can be reconstructed with the Moberg rectangular advancement flap based on both neurovascular bundles [16]. The Moberg flap has limited mobility and is useful only for 1.5-cm transverse or dorsally directed thumb tip defects. The Moberg flap is discouraged for the fingers because of the risk of dorsal skin necrosis and flexion contracture deformities [17]. Local neurovascular island flaps can provide coverage for larger defects. Littler's neurovascular island flap [18] from the dorsoulnar side of the middle finger is discouraged for older patients because of difficulty with cortical reorientation and flexion contractures of the skin-grafted donor finger [19,20]. The first dorsal metacarpal artery flap is a flap harvested from the dorsum of the index finger over the proximal phalanx with an arc of rotation that provides coverage of larger thumb defects. This flap is sensate with the inclusion of the superficial radial nerve to the dorsum of the index finger. The first dorsal metacarpal artery flap can be complicated, however, with stiffness of the grafted donor index finger and difficulty with cortical reorientation. Cortical reorientation with

* Corresponding author.
E-mail address: bwilhelmi@siumed.edu (B.J. Wilhelmi).

doi:10.1016/j.ahc.2004.10.002

these local neurovascular flaps can be avoided by coapting the nerve within the flap to the proper digital nerve to the wounded digit [21]. The cross finger flap can be modified by coapting the nerve to the flap with the proper digital nerve to the wounded area [22–25]. The disadvantage of the cross finger flap is the 2 weeks of immobilization required before flap division, which can result in joint stiffness, especially in elderly patients. Successful application of a local sensory flap depends on a favorable anatomy of the injured digit. In general, larger defects are more challenging to reconstruct with sensate local tissue transfer.

Indications for neurosensory free flaps

With the development of microsurgery and free tissue transfer, neurosensory flaps became a useful technique for sensory restoration to the injured upper extremity [26–29]. The innervation of the free flap is reestablished by coapting the nerve in the flap to a nerve in the recipient site. Because free flap procedures require extensive surgery and risk entire flap embarrassment, criteria need to be met when this option is considered [30,31]:

1. The potential regenerating axons at the area of tissue loss are insufficient or at too great a distance for local spontaneous sensory neurotization to occur reliably.
2. Sensate tissue coverage cannot be achieved by local or regional tissue transfer.
3. Sensory restoration to the injured part is crucial for hand function, such as with volar thumb. The palm of the hand, dorsum, or web spaces are less important as a fine tactile surface, although a large insensate area would be prone to further injury and could benefit from sensory restoration. The pulp of the index finger is less deserving of a free sensate flap if the middle finger is intact because the index finger would be bypassed for the sensate middle finger [32].

Donor selection for neurosensory flaps

Several neurosensory free flaps have been described. Appropriate flap selection requires an understanding of the sensory receptors in the recipient site and donor skin. Cutaneous sensory receptors convert mechanical stimuli into impulses transmitted by peripheral nerve fibers to the central nervous system [8]. Most sensory receptors are unencapsulated free nerve endings. Unencapsulated free nerve endings are responsible for the sensation of pain and temperature. Additionally, there are four types of encapsulated mechanoreceptors: Meissner and pacinian corpuscles, Merkel cell neurite complexes, and Ruffini end organs. Meissner and pacinian corpuscles are quickly adapting receptors that sense low-frequency (Meissner) and high-frequency (pacinian) vibration. The Merkel cell neurite complexes and Ruffini end organs are slowly adapting receptors that sense constant touch (Merkel) and skin stretch (Ruffini).

The glabrous skin of the hand and feet has the highest density of peripheral nerves, which provides for fine tactile sensation. The ultimate sensibility of the flap depends on the number of cutaneous sensory receptors in the neurosensory flap. Because the glabrous skin has a high density of sensory receptors, it provides the best discriminatory sensation [33]. Another desirable characteristic of a neurosensory flap is for the skin to be thin and malleable, similar to the skin of the hand [31,34,35]. A pedicle with large-caliber vessels and predictable anatomy and a consistent and axial nerve supply, which facilitates flap dissection and the microsurgical repairs, are other appealing features of a neursosensory flap. Donor site functional and esthetic morbidity must be considered, however, against the benefit of the neurosensory flap reconstruction.

In selecting the most appropriate neurosensory flap, it is important to delineate between critical sensibility and protective sensibility in the hand [36]. Critical sensibility is needed for reconstruction of the digital pulp and distal amputation stump. Protective sensibility is required when reconstructing the dorsal or palmar aspect of the hand. The best tissue for discriminatory sensory reconstruction is glabrous skin from the hand and feet. The selection of a neurosensory flap depends on the location and size of the defect versus the potential donor morbidity.

Options for critical sensory restoration

First web space flap

The gold standard neurosensory flap is the first web space flap. The first web space flap is harvested from the lateral aspect of the great toe and the medial aspect of the second toe (Fig. 1). The general dimensions of the flap are 6 cm transversely and 3 cm longitudinally. This flap usually is based on the first dorsal metatarsal artery, which is a branch of the dorsalis pedis artery. It also can be based on the first plantar metatarsal artery, but the dorsal branch usually is used because of difficulty with exposure of the first plantar metatarsal artery. If more pedicle length is required, the arterial dissection can be extended to include the dorsalis pedis artery. The venous drainage of the first web space flap is reliable because either or both the venae comitante and saphenous system can be used. Usually the flap is harvested with the saphenous vein system because of its large caliber and easier dissection.

Anatomic variations of the first dorsal metatarsal artery exist. In a cadaver study, the first dorsal metatarsal artery was found to arise from the dorsalis pedis artery dorsal to the mid-metatarsal axis in 78% of dissections. In the other 22% of dissections, the first metatarsal artery originated from the dorsalis pedis artery volar to the mid-metatarsal axis and deep to the interosseous muscle (Fig. 2) [37]. The anatomy of the first metatarsal artery can be determined by preoperative angiogram specifically with a lateral view of the foot. When the first dorsal metatarsal artery arises at an acute angle, as is seen in type II, the arterial pedicle can be kinked at insetting.

The nerve supply to the first web space flap is by two branches, the deep peroneal nerve dorsally and the medial plantar nerve volarly. When this flap is used to restore sensation to the ulnar aspect of the thumb, the deep peroneal nerve is coapted to the superficial radial nerve dorsally, and the plantar digital branches are coapted to the residual median nerve branches volarly. This flap also is useful to reconstruct the first web space of the hand, with cutaneous extensions onto the ulnar aspect of the thumb and radial aspect of the index finger. When this flap is used for the volar aspect of the thumb, the flap nerves can be repaired to median nerve branches. In reconstructing the first web space of the hand, the ipsilateral foot is used. The flap is harvested based on the first lateral dorsal digital artery to the great toe and the second medial dorsal digital artery to the second toe. The corresponding nerves to the toes are harvested with this flap. Because the first web space donor site on the foot is covered with a split-thickness skin graft, the paratenon on the extensor hallucis longus and the hemipulp from the great and second toe are preserved.

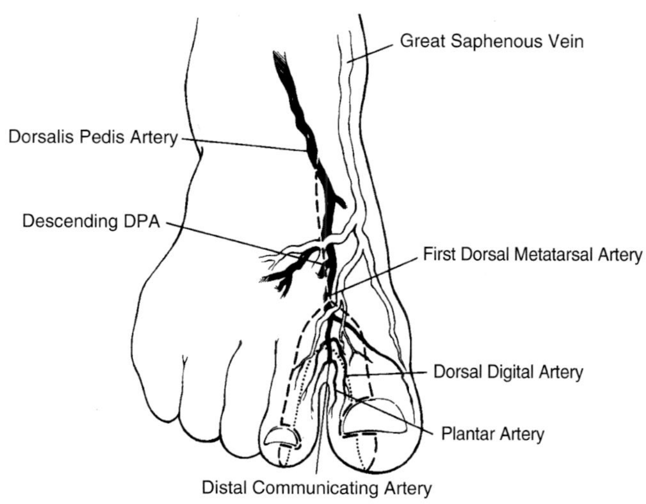

Fig. 1. The first web space flap usually is based on the first dorsal metatarsal artery, a branch of the dorsalis pedis artery. A superficial vein of the saphenous system is often used for venous drainage. DPA, dorsalis pedis artery. (*From* Orgel MG. Innervated free flaps and free vascularized nerve grafts in the hand. In: McCarthy JG, May JW Jr, Littler JW, editors. Plastic surgery. Philadelphia: WB Saunders; 1990. p. 4864; with permission.)

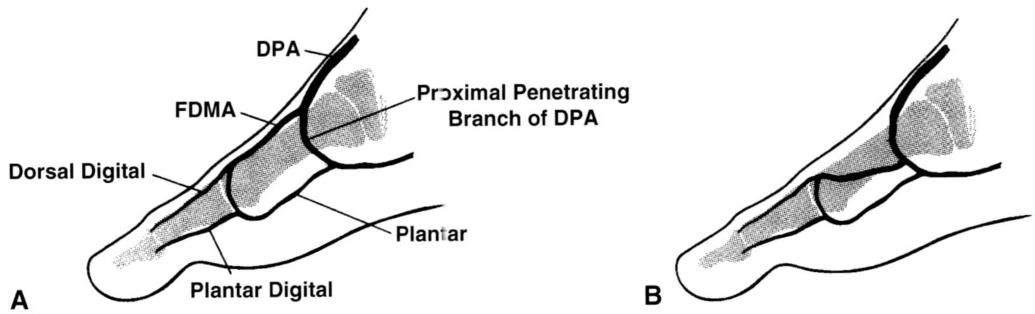

Fig. 2. Anatomic variations of the first dorsal metatarsal artery (FDMA) on the lateral view. (*A*) In type I (78%), FDMA arises from the dorsalis pedis artery (DPA) dorsal to the mid-metatarsal axis. (*B*) In type II (22%), FDMA arises from DPA volar to the mid-metatarsal axis. (*From* May JW Jr. Microvascular great toe to hand transfer for reconstruction of the amputated thumb. In: McCarthy JG, May JW Jr, Littler JW, editors. Plastic surgery. Philadelphia: WB Saunders; 1990. p. 5165; with permission.)

The thin glabrous skin of the flap and its high density of sensory receptors make it a superior choice for sensory restoration. An in situ study of 50 patients showed this flap to provide better 2-point discrimination than that in other neurosensory flap donor options [37]. This study found the 2-point discrimination to be 11 to 16 mm on the plantar surface and 18 to 24 mm on the dorsum. Accordingly the ipsilateral foot is used for ulnar thumb sensory restoration [37]. In general, after transfer, 2-point discrimination in the flap is usually half that of the donor. Other investigators have observed improved sensibility in the flap after transfer to the hand and a 2-point discrimination of 3 to 8 mm [38,39] The reason for this improved 2-point discrimination of this neurosensory flap after transfer is not understood. Increased cortical representation of the nerves in the hand and postoperative sensory reeducation is a better explanation than is growth of sensory receptors [40,41].

There are several advantages to the use of the first web space flap for sensory restoration of the hand. The first web space flap provides a sensate glabrous surface similar to sensate glabrous defects of the hand (Fig. 3). The flap has a relatively constant vascular and neural anatomy. The donor site usually can be covered with a split-thickness skin graft with minimal donor morbidity and minimal disturbance of foot mechanics.

Toe pulp transfers

Another option for critical sensory restoration is the toe pulp transfer, which is a modification of the first web space flap. This flap is applicable to small defects of the digital volar pads. The toe pulp flap is based on the plantar digital artery and vein, which can be dissected into the plantar arch or the dorsal inflow if greater pedicle length is required. The corresponding plantar nerve is harvested with this flap. Clinical series have reported this flap to provide 2-point discrimination of 3 to 7 mm [38,42]. The advantage of this flap is the minimal donor disfigurement because it allows for skin grafting or direct closure.

Wraparound flap

When the defect requires near-circumferential digital reconstruction including the nail, a wraparound flap can be considered. A wraparound flap includes the entire soft tissue envelope of the great or second toe, excluding a strip of medial skin around the toe tip [43]. The flap dimensions are 7cm transversely and 6 cm longitudinally. This flap includes the nail, which provides for pulp stability and improved esthetics. The wraparound flap is based on the first dorsal metatarsal artery and plantar digital nerves. Similar to the first web space flap, the pedicle can be lengthened with extension to include the dorsalis pedis artery and saphenous superficial vein to provide a pedicle length of 6 to 10 cm. Harvesting this lengthened pedicle requires the preservation of the distal communication of the dorsalis pedis artery to the plantar system digital arteries by the deep communicating artery to the first plantar metatarsal artery.

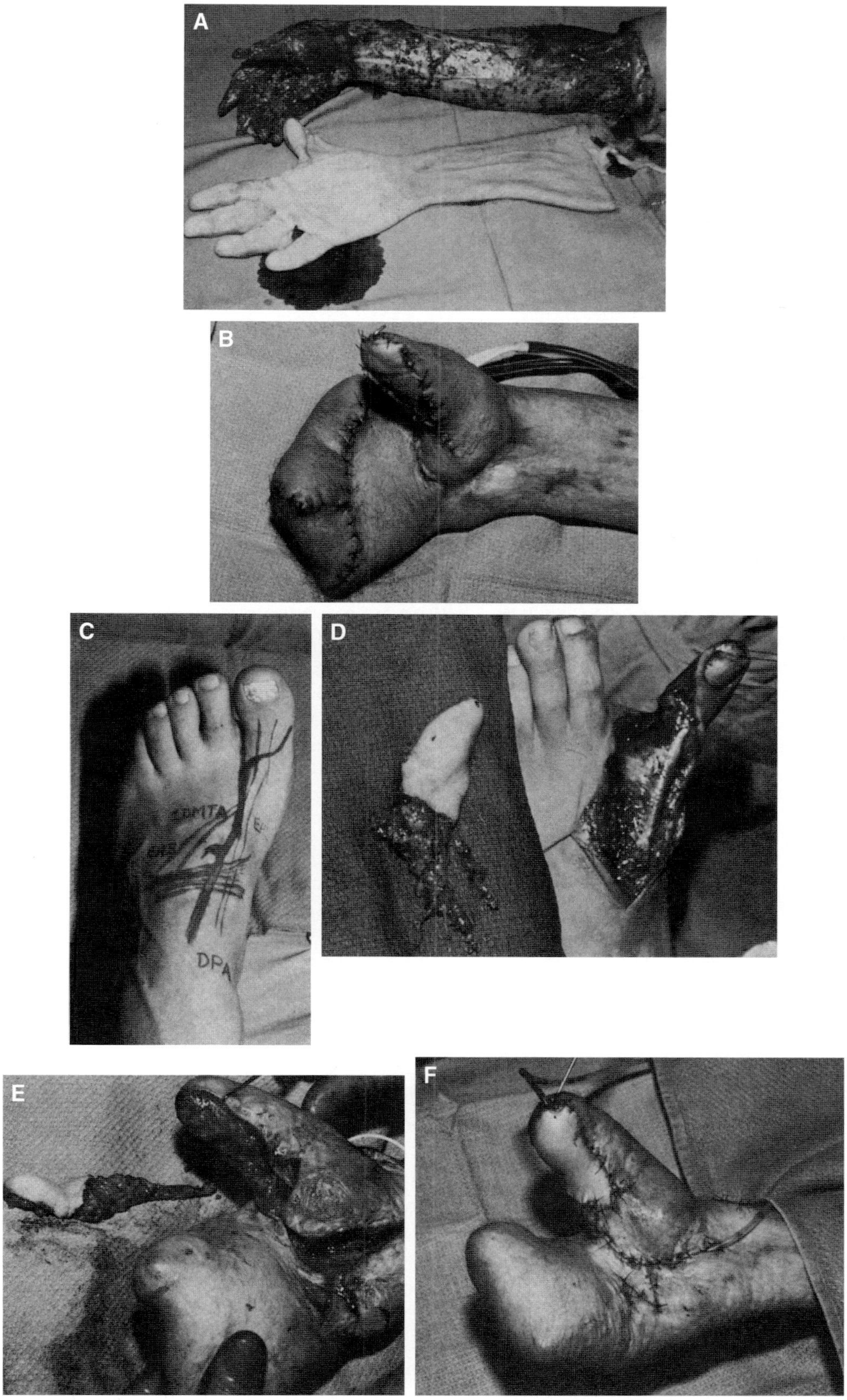

Fig. 3. (*A*) Degloving injury of the hand and forearm. (*B*) Initial coverage with a groin flap. (*C*) Design of the first web space neursensory free flap. (*D*) Flap harvested from the donor site. (*E*) Flap before microneurovascular repair to the hand. (*F*) Flap inset to the thumb pulp. (*G*) Prehensile unit with a 2-point discrimination of 12 mm in the pulp. (*From* Lee WPA, May JW Jr. Neurosensory free flaps to the hand indications and donor selection. Hand Clin 1992;8:469–70; with permission.)

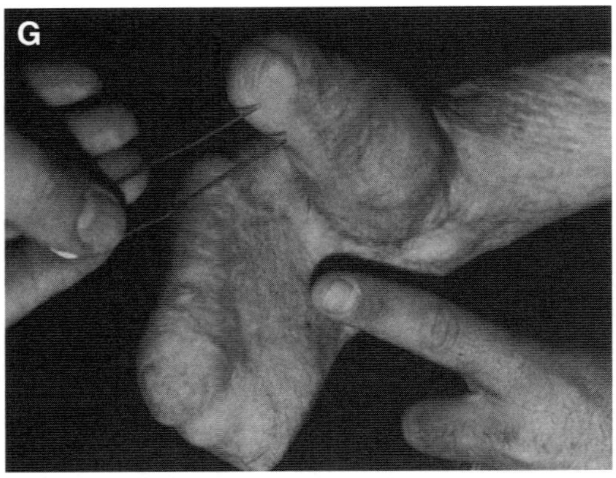

Fig. 3 (*continued*)

Lengthening the pedicle of this flap allows for repair of the dorsalis pedis artery end to side to the larger caliber radial artery in the snuffbox. Pulp sensibility is supplied by the medial and lateral plantar digital nerves.

The wraparound flap is most suitable for reconstruction of combined digital volar pad and nail loss. When reconstructing the thumb, the ipsilateral great toe is preferred to avoid an incision on the ulnar aspect of the thumb. This flap also can be used to reconstruct the whole thumb in conjunction with an iliac bone graft, preserving the great toe, although a simpler technique of total thumb reconstruction is with an entire toe transfer [44–47]. The great toe can be preserved by covering the donor wound with a skin graft, or alternatively the volar great toe pad can be reconstructed with a cross toe flap from the dorsum of the second toe and the dorsum of the great toe and second toe covered with a skin graft. Skin graft take can be optimized by allowing the wound to granulate for 2 weeks before grafting. The wraparound flap provides a return of 2-point discrimination of 6 to 10 mm after transfer [48]. The advantage to the use of the wraparound flap is that it provides similar tissue in reconstructing circumferential digital defects with sensate glabrous tissue and a viable nail.

Plantar flap

The medial plantar flap is a glabrous fasciocutaneous flap that can be used for neurosensory restoration of hand defects. Plantar skin, with its concentration of mechanoreceptors, can provide tactile discrimination. The plantar fasciocutaneous flap can be harvested based on the medial or lateral plantar artery or both. Use of the medial plantar artery flap allows for potential of primary closure of the donor site. Small finger tip wounds can be reconstructed with the medial plantar free flap [49]. The venous return from this flap is through the venae comitante with the artery. The pedicle is 3 to 5 cm long with a vessel diameter of 1 to 2 mm [49,50]. The pedicle can be extended to include the posterior tibial artery to the bifurcation of the medial and lateral plantar artery. The innervation of this flap is by cutaneous branches from the medial plantar nerve. The 2-point discrimination of this flap has been reported to be 5 to 20 mm [49,50]. The disadvantage of this flap is that it can be bulky, and separation of the cutaneous branches of the medial plantar nerve may be difficult, often requiring sacrifice of the common digital nerve of the second web space. Another potential problem is donor morbidity with the risk of developing hyperkeratosis and unstable scar at the donor site. The medial plantar flap is considered a second-choice option for glabrous defects.

Spare parts—index finger

Special circumstances may allow for use of spare parts to restore sensation to glabrous hand and finger defects. An example includes a multiple-digit injury, such as a thumb and index finger, whereby a devascularized index finger can be used as a free neurosensory flap to reconstruct a volar thumb soft tissue defect, through microsurgical repair of vessels and nerves (Fig. 4) [51–53].

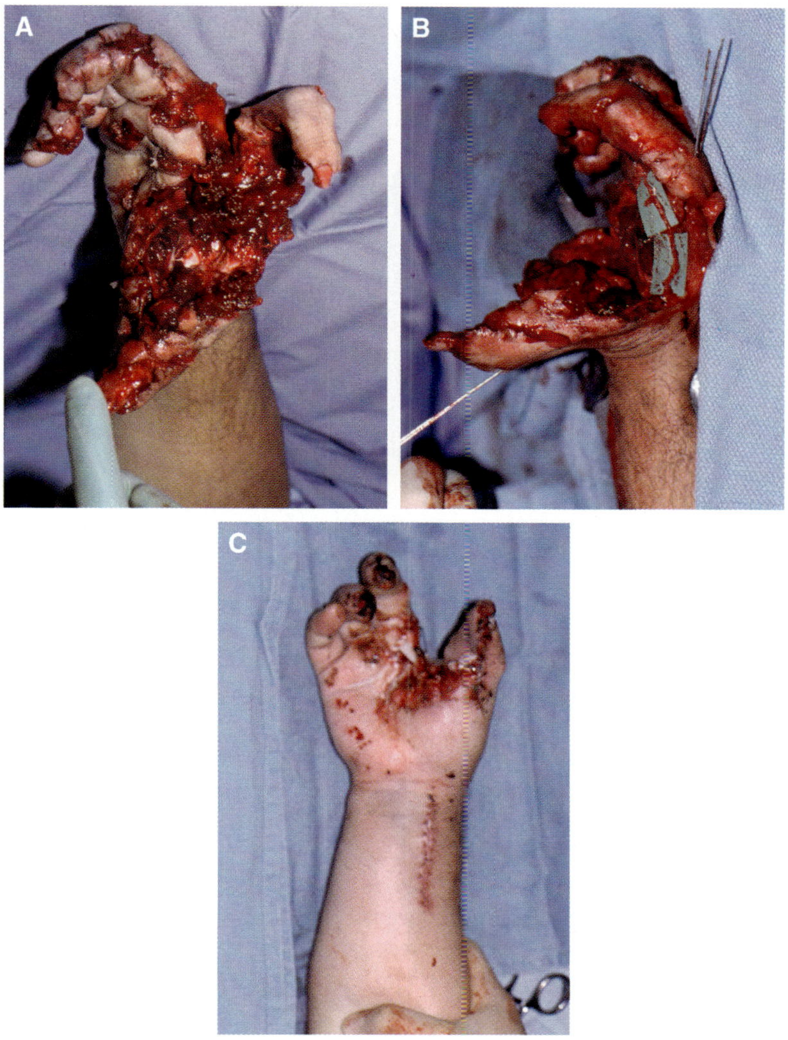

Fig. 4. (*A–C*) This patient had a firework explode in his hand, which resulted in a defect of volar thumb and mutilating devascularizating injury of the index finger. The index was used as a neurosensory flap to restore tactile discrimination to the thumb.

Options for protective sensation restoration

Neurosensory flaps from thin, sometimes hair-bearing areas other than the glabrous skin can be used to restore sensation to the denervated hand. Although these neurosensory flaps do not contain the same concentration of cutaneous sensory receptors, these flaps are capable of providing protective sensibility.

Dorsalis pedis flap

The dorsalis pedis flap first was described in 1975, and this was a commonly used neurosensory flap [26,28,29,54]. The flap is based on small branches from the dorsalis pedis artery and the first dorsal metatarsal artery (Fig. 5). Patent posterior tibial artery circulation to the foot is necessary to allow for the use of this flap. An angiogram should be obtained preoperatively. During harvesting of this flap, it is crucial to avoid separation of the skin from the arterial pedicle [55]. If a longer pedicle is required, the artery can be extended proximally under the extensor retinaculum. The superficial saphenous veins or deep venae comitante are used for venous drainage of the flap. This flap also can be harvested with the underlying extensor tendons and second metatarsal if needed [56,57]. The superficial peroneal nerve innervates the dorsum of the foot. Studies have shown the in situ 2-point discrimination of the

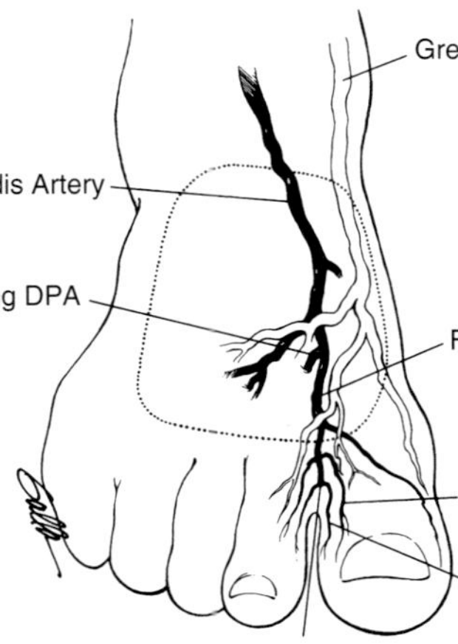

Fig. 5. The dorsalis pedis flap is based on the dorsalis pedis artery and either its venae comitantes or a superficial saphenous vein. DPA, dorsalis pedis artery. (*From* Orgel MG. Innervated free flaps and free vascularized nerve grafts in the hand. In: McCarthy JG, May JW Jr, Littler JW editors. Plastic surgery. Philadelphia: WB Saunders; 1990. p. 4863; with permission.)

dorsalis pedis flap averages between 32 mm and 34 mm [37,58]. After transfer, flap 2-point discrimination is usually half that of the donor. This flap is inferior to the first web space flap because it is unable to provide fine discriminatory sensation after transfer. This flap is most suitable to reconstruct areas requiring only protective sensation, especially an area such as the dorsum of the hand when tendon and bone also is needed. The flap dimension is 15 cm × 12 cm. Because of the multifascicular nature of the superficial peroneal nerve, however, which makes its innervation unpredictable, electrophysiologic sensory mapping is needed for precise determination of the flap's neural boundary [26]. An additional disadvantage for this flap is donor morbidity. It is crucial with flap dissection to preserve the underlying paratenon to provide a bed for skin grafting of the donor site. Even with paratenon preservation, however, prolonged healing and unstable scarring are common complications of this donor site [26,28].

Radial forearm flap

The radial forearm flap is similar to the dorsalis pedis flap. This flap involves harvesting volar forearm skin based over septocutaneous branches of the radial artery (Fig. 6). Venous drainage of this flap is through the basilic or cephalic vein or venae comitante. The flap dimensions are 25 cm × 12 cm of skin innervated by the lateral and medial cutaneous nerves of the forearm. The 2-point discrimination of this volar forearm skin has been measured in situ at 15 to 25 mm [59]; however, 2-point discrimination of this innervated flap after transfer has been reported at 22 to 32 mm [60]. This flap does not provide fine discriminatory sensation [61,62]. Provided that the patient has a satisfactory Allen test, a preoperative angiogram usually is not required to confirm adequate collateral flow to the hand through the ulnar artery before sacrificing the radial artery. Intraoperatively the radial artery can be clamped temporarily and the tourniquet deflated to confirm that the hand is adequately perfused through the ulnar artery. The large caliber of the vessels to the radial forearm flap makes this an attractive free flap to use.

The skin paddle to the radial forearm flap can be proximal or distal. Placing the skin paddle distally allows for the advantage of a longer pedicle, but risks potential exposure of tendons and a less favorable donor site. A proximal skin territory design sometimes can allow for primary closure of the donor but results in a shorter pedicle. With this proximal skin paddle, the flap can be based on retrograde circulation, but this compromises venous return and mandates use of the less reliable venae comitante system. The antegrade design is more practical when using the radial forearm flap for free tissue transfer. This flap also can be based distally as a pedicled flap through retrograde flow across the deep palmer arterial arch if it is patent. When used as a retrograde pedicle flap, the problem of nerve coaptation can be avoided by turning the flap over the dorsal web space, positioning the proximal portion of the flap for coaptation to appropriate

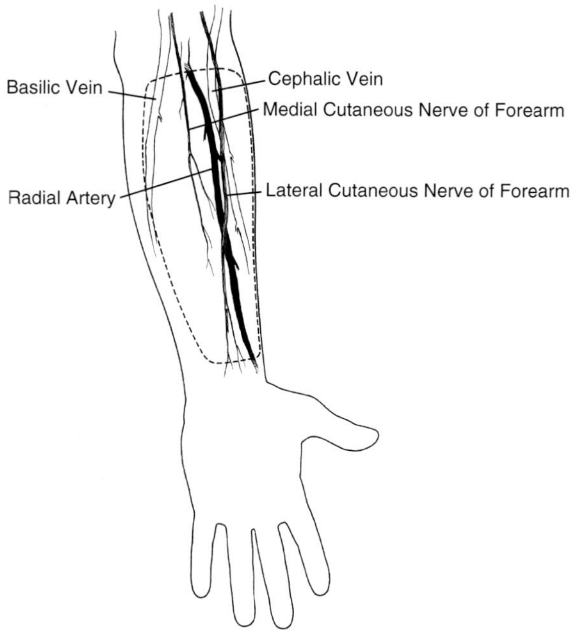

Fig. 6. The radial forearm flap is based on the radial artery, cephalic or basilic vein, and the lateral and medial cutaneous nerves of the forearm. (*From* Orgel MG. Innervated free flaps and free vascularized nerve grafts in the hand. In: McCarthy JG, May JW Jr, Littler JW, editors. Plastic surgery. Philadelphia: WB Saunders; 1990. p. 4869; with permission.)

recipient nerves in the hand [36]. Part of the radius also can be included in the radial forearm flap [59]. Another disadvantage to the use of this flap in addition to higher 2-point discrimination and an unsightly donor is the sacrifice of a major artery to the hand, the radial artery. Arterial reconstruction of the radial artery can be considered, but some of this graft is less protected under the skin graft within the donor site. The side-by-side nerve supply to this flap makes sensory return unpredictable without the aid of neuromapping or preoperative nerve block study. Caution must be exercised when a sensate radial arm flap innervated by the lateral antebrachial cutaneous nerve is raised because sometimes this nerve innervates the radial side of the thumb. This flap provides protective sensory restoration at best.

Lateral upper arm flap

The cutaneous territory of the lateral arm septocutaneous flap includes the skin over the longitudinal axis from the deltoid insertion to the lateral epicondyle. The flap dimensions are 6 cm transversely and 12 cm longitudinally. The lateral arm flap is supplied by the posterior radial collateral artery, a branch of the profunda brachii artery (Fig. 7). The posterior radial collateral artery can be found to arise along the lateral intramuscular septum; after coursing through the lateral intermuscular septum, it terminates in a fascial and subdermal vascular network [63]. The arterial pedicle can be 4 to 8 cm long with a vessel diameter of 1.5 to 2 mm [64]. The venous return of this flap is from two systems—the superficial veins draining the cephalic vein and the deep venae comitante. The artery is accompanied by the posterior cutaneous nerve of the arm, which is a branch of the radial nerve and the innervation to the flap. This flap can provide thin sensate skin to reconstruct upper extremity defects. In obese patients, this flap can be bulky, however. The 2-point discrimination of this flap has been reported at 30 mm [65]. This flap can provide protective sensation only and not tactile discrimination. The lateral arm flap is a suitable option for reconstruction of palmar defects with soft tissue and requiring protective sensation. Another disadvantage of the lateral arm flap is the loss of sensation in the superolateral forearm provided by the posterior cutaneous nerve. Advantages with this flap are that it can be harvested under tourniquet control, with bone, and if the flap design is 6 cm in width, the donor site can be closed primarily.

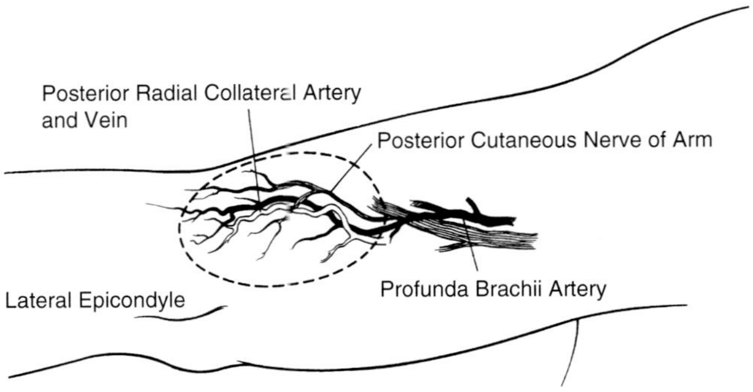

Fig. 7. The lateral upper arm flap is supplied by the posterior radial collateral artery and vein and the posterior cutaneous nerve of the arm. (*From* Orgel MG. Innervated free flaps and free vascularized nerve grafts in the hand. In: McCarthy JG, May JW Jr, Littler JW, editors. Plastic surgery. Philadelphia: WB Saunders; 1990. p. 4868; with permission.)

Medial upper arm flap

The medial arm flap is a 6 cm × 12 cm fasciocutaneous flap based on either the superior ulnar collateral artery or a direct fasciocutaneous branch from the brachial artery or both [66]. There are no direct fasciocutaneous branches from the superior ulnar collateral artery in 20%. If no direct fasciocutaneous branches from the superior ulnar collateral artery are found, dissection in the proximal direction facilitates a direct fasciocutaneous branch from the brachial or profunda brachii artery. The venous drainage of this flap is either the superficial basilic vein or the deep venae comitante. The length of the vascular pedicle is 4 to 5 cm with vessel diameter of 1 to 2 cm. Because the pedicle enters the mid-portion of the flap, the functional length of the flap makes the microanastomosis awkward. The innervation of the medial arm flap is the medial brachial cutaneous nerve, which provides sensory feedback from the distal one third of the medial arm. One advantage of the medial arm flap is the inconspicuous donor site, which can be closed primarily if it is less than 6 cm in width. The variability of the blood supply to the medial arm flap and short pedicle make this a less reliable and a secondary option for neurosensory restoration.

Deltoid flap

The deltoid flap is a fasciocutaneous flap harvested from the posterolateral deltoid muscle based on the posterior circumflex humeral artery. The posterior circumflex humeral artery is a branch from the third portion of the axillary artery. The venous drainage of this flap is by two venae comitante with the artery. This flap s pedicle length is 6 to 8 cm with a vessel diameter of 2 to 4 mm. The innervation of the deltoid flap is the lateral brachial cutaneous nerve, the terminal sensory branch of the axillary nerve [67]. The neurovascular bundle exits the quadrangular space. The neurovascular pedicle can be located preoperatively with the patient in an upright position at the intersection of a line drawn from the acromion to the medial epicondyle and the deltoid triceps groove [68]. This skin territory of the deltoid flap is large (24 cm × 34 cm). The nerve innervates on average a 15 cm × 10 cm portion of the flap centered over the deltoid triceps groove. The 2-point discrimination of this flap has been reported at 20 mm or more after flap transfer. This flap does not provide tactile discrimination. This flap is thin and is an occasional option for providing sensate skin to the glabrous palm. The disadvantage of this flap is that the arterial supply to the skin is inconsistent, which can result in partial necrosis. The donor site is can be unacceptable, especially in women. Sometimes the donor can be closed primarily if less than 7 cm in width.

Tensor fascia lata flap

The tensor fascia lata flap is a myocutaneous flap based on the small tensor fascia lata muscle. This flap can provide 40 cm × 15 cm of sensate skin for reconstruction [69,70]. The arterial supply to the tensor fascia lata flap is the transverse branch of the lateral femoral circumflex artery. The venous drainage of this flap is venae comitante traveling with this artery. The cutaneous territory of the tensor fascia lata flap is innervated by two distinct sensory nerves—the lateral cutaneous branch of T12 proximally and the lateral cutaneous nerve of the thigh L2-L3 distally. The 2-point discrimination of this flap after transfer has been reported to be poor at 40 to 50 mm [35]. In thin patients, this flap is bulky, especially with the inclusion of the muscle. Accordingly, this flap is not commonly used to reconstruct the hand. The bulk of this flap makes it more appropriate for restoring protective sensibility to the forearm or upper limb amputation stump.

Anterolateral thigh flap

The anterolateral thigh flap is a fasciocutaneous flap based on cutaneous perforators of the descending branch of the lateral femoral circumflex vessels. The arterial pedicle is 8 to 12 cm in length with vessel diameter of 2 mm. This flap can provide a large skin quantity (12 cm × 38 cm). The anterolateral thigh flap is innervated by the lateral femoral cutaneous nerve [71]. The venous drainage of this flap is the venae comitante that travel with the artery. Similar to the tensor fascia lata flap, the anterolateral thigh flap can be bulky and hair bearing and result in an unacceptable donor site scar; it has a limited role in upper extremity reconstruction.

Saphenous flap

The saphenous flap is a cutaneous flap over the medial aspect of the knee based on the saphenous artery (Fig. 8). The saphenous artery is a terminal branch of the descending genicular artery that arises from the medial side of the femoral artery 15 cm above the knee just proximal to where the femoral artery passes through the adductor hiatus. This flap has two venous drainage systems superficial through the saphenous vein and deep by venae comitante with the artery. The pedicle of this flap is 15 cm long and 1.5 to 2 mm in diameter [72]. The saphenous artery can be absent in 5% of patients [72]. The saphenous flap is innervated proximally by the medial femoral cutaneous nerve and distally by the saphenous nerve. The numbness of the donor site after skin grafting can be bothersome. The donor site can be closed primarily if less than 7 cm in width but is still unacceptable in women. The flap is thin and can provide a variable size skin paddle from 2 cm × 3 cm to 8 cm × 29 cm. A 2-point discrimination of 9 to 14 mm after transfer has been reported in one case [72]. The advantage of this flap is that it is a thin flap with a long pedicle. The donor site appearance and numbness can be unacceptable, however, and there is little experience reported on the recovery of sensation with this flap. The dissection is technically difficult and sometimes necessitates division of the sartorius muscle.

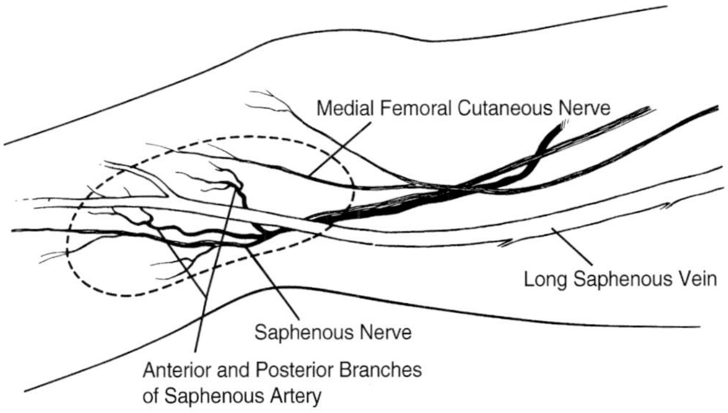

Fig. 8. Based on the saphenous branches of the descending genicular artery, the saphenous flap is innervated proximally by the medial femoral cutaneous nerve and distally by the saphenous nerve. (*From* Orgel MG. Innervated free flaps and free vascularized nerve grafts in the hand. In: McCarthy JG, May JW Jr, Littler JW, editors. Plastic surgery. Philadelphia: WB Saunders; 1990. p. 4870; with permission.)

Posterior calf flap

The posterior calf flap is a fasciocutaneous flap based on either a descending fasciocutaneous branch of the popliteal artery or the lateral sural artery (Fig. 9). The dominant axial artery originates from either the popliteal (50%) or the lateral sural artery (45%) and can be identified in the interval between the posterior midline of the calf and the fibular head [73]. Sometimes the dominant blood supply to the flap is via the medial sural artery (4%). The venous drainage of this fasciocutaneous flap is more reliable by the two venae comitante that course deep with the artery into the fascia than by the lesser saphenous vein, which drains the subcutaneous tissue and not fascia. This flap is innervated by the lateral sural nerve or medial sural nerve, but there is much variability with the innervation of the posterior calf skin, which makes flap dissection tedious. When the flap is based on the medial sural artery, the lateral sural nerve is preserved, and the medial sural nerve can be preserved when the flap is based laterally. One series reported 6 to 12 mm of 2-point discrimination with this flap [74]. This flap can provide a large skin territory, but because the innervation is unpredictable, this flap is less useful for sensory restoration. Significant donor morbidity, such as prolonged lower extremity edema, hematoma formation, graft loss, and loss of sural nerve sensation, has been reported with this flap.

Posterior interosseus flap

The posterior interosseous flap is a septocutaneous flap. The maximal flap dimensions are 10 cm × 6 cm [75]. The flap is based on the posterior interosseous artery, a branch of the common interosseous artery. The arterial pedicle is short, and the vessel diameter is only 0.8 to 1.2 mm. The common interosseous artery arises from the ulnar artery at the level of the radial tuberosity and divides into posterior and anterior branches. The posterior interosseous artery courses with the posterior interosseous nerve under the superficial portion of the supinator.

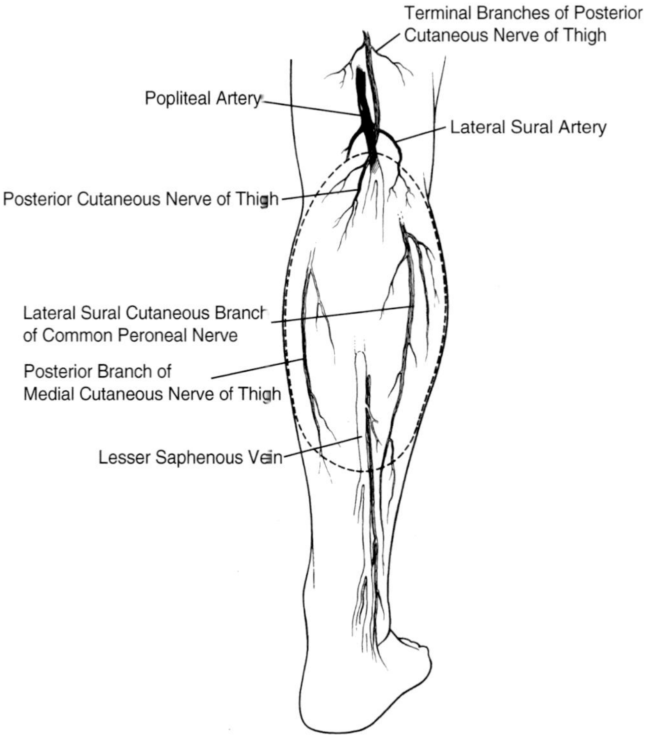

Fig. 9. The posterior calf flap is supplied by branches of the popliteal or lateral sural artery and their venae comitantes Its sensory innervation comes from multiple cutaneous nerves. (*From* Orgel MG. Innervated free flaps and free vascularized nerve grafts in the hand. In: McCarthy JG, May JW Jr, Littler JW, editors. Plastic surgery. Philadelphia: WB Saunders; 1990. p. 4871; with permission.)

After exiting the supinator, the posterior interosseous artery enters the septum between the extensor digiti minimi and extensor carpi ulnaris. Along its course, the posterior interosseous artery gives off several cutaneous arteries (7–14). The largest of these perforating branches is proximal. The posterior artery travels with the posterior interosseous nerve to the mid-wrist along a longitudinal vector from the lateral epicondyle to the dorsal midline of the wrist at the distal radioulnar joint. Because the posterior interosseous nerve has motor and sensory components, it has to be preserved in harvesting this flap to avoid denervation of the wrist and finger extensors.

The posterior interosseous flap can be designed as an antegrade or retrograde flap. The retrograde arterial flow to the posterior interosseous artery is by anastomoses at the wrist with the perforating branch of the anterior interosseous artery, the dorsal carpal arch, and the vascular plexus surrounding the ulnar head. The venous drainage of this flap is more reliable when an antegrade design is used. For the antegrade flap, the venous drainage is best by local superficial veins and not venae comitante. When basing the flap on retrograde flow, however, the venae comitante have to be used. The retrograde design can be used as a pedicle flap for reconstructing hand defects. The antegrade flap can be used as a free flap or as pedicle to reconstruct distal elbow defects.

This flap can be used as a sensate flap. The flap is named after its arterial supply and not innervation. The sensory component of the posterior interosseous nerve is to the wrist. The innervation of this cutaneous territory is the medial antebrachial cutaneous nerve. The donor site can be closed primarily if the flap width is less than 3 cm; otherwise a skin graft is used. The 2-point discrimination achieved with free transfer of this flap was 15 mm in one report [75]. These authors discouraged its use to restore tactile discrimination. Other disadvantages of the free posterior interosseous flap are the tedious dissection, short pedicle, narrow vessels, bulky flap, and hair-bearing skin not suitable for palmar reconstruction.

Other flaps

Other neurosensory flaps that have been described include the distal ulnar artery flap, transverse cervical flap, sensate superior gluteal artery perforator flap, sensate deep inferior epigastric musculocutaneous flap, sensate myocutaneous latissimus flap, sensate osteocutaneous fibula flap, and lateral intercostal flap [66,76–84]. Many of these flaps have been reported to provide protective sensation to other areas, such as the head and neck, breast, or other areas, and not enough clinical experience has been obtained to establish their usefulness in sensor reconstruction of the hand.

Summary

Neurosensory free flaps can provide sensibility, vascularity, and soft tissue coverage to an injured hand. In determining the most suitable means of reconstructing a defect, the benefit of the reconstruction has to outweigh the risk of donor morbidity. Appropriate selection of a neurosensory flap is based primarily on the need for tactile discrimination or protective sensation. Because of its thin, glabrous skin, constant vascular and neural anatomy, minimal donor morbidity, and in situ 2-point discrimination, the first web space flap of the foot (or its variants) is considered to be the best choice for restoration of critical sensibility to the digital tips or first web space of the hand. Several other neurosensory flaps have been described that can be used to restore protective sensation for other areas on the hand. The return of sensation with these other flap options is variable, and it is crucial to scrutinize the individual reports on the use of these flaps to determine appropriately the chance for long-term sensory ability in selecting a donor neurosensory flap.

References

[1] Louis DS, Palmer AK, Burney RE. Open treatment of digital tip injuries. JAMA 1980;244:697.
[2] Illingworth CM. Trapped fingers and amputated fingertips in children. J Pediatr Surg 1974;9:853.

[3] Rosenthal LJ, Reiner MA, Bleicher MA. Nonoperative management of distal fingertip amputations in children. Pediatrics 1979;64:1.
[4] Adeymo O, Wyburn GM. Innervation of skin grafts. Transplantation 1957;4:152.
[5] Porter RW. Functional assessment of transplanted skin volar defects of the digits: a comparison between free grafts and flaps. J Bone Joint Surg Am 1968;50:955.
[6] Terzis JK. Functional aspects of reinnervation of free skin grafts. Plast Recosntr Surg 1976;58:142.
[7] Terzis JK, Dykes RW, Turnbull BG. Properties of mechanoreceptive fibers serving skin grafts transferred to the hands of adult baboons. J Physiol 1984;357:1.
[8] Terzis JK, Michelow BJ. Sensory receptors. In: Gelberman RH, editor. Operative nerve repair and reconstruction, vol. 1. Philadelphia: JB Lippincott; 1991. p. 85.
[9] Davis L. The return of sensation to transplanted skin. Surg Gynecol Obstet 1934;59:533.
[10] Mannerfelt L. Evaluation of functional sensation of skin grafts in the hand area. Br J Plast Surg 1962;15:136.
[11] Maquieira NO. An innovative full thickness skin graft to restore sensibility to fingertips and heels. Plast Reconstr Surg 1974;53:568.
[12] Williams WG, Cameron A, Robson MC, Hendon DN, Phillips LG. A model for assessment of sensory recovery of skin. Ann Plast Surg 1999;43:397.
[13] Beasley RW. Reconstruction of amputated fingertips. Plast Reconstr Surg 1969;44:349.
[14] Atasoy E, Iakimidis E, Kasdan ML, et al. Reconstruction of the amputated finger tip with a triangular flap. J Bone Joint Surg Am 1970;52:921.
[15] Kutler W. A new method for finger tip amputation. JAMA 1947;133:29.
[16] Moberg E. Aspects of sensation and reconstructive surgery of the upper extremity. J Bone Joint Surg Am 1964;46: 817.
[17] Snow JW. The use of a volar flap for repair of fingertip amputations: a preliminary report. Plast Reconstr Surg 1967;40:163.
[18] Littler JW. Neurovascular pedicle transfer of tissue in reconstructive surgery of the hand. J Bone Joint Surg Am 1956;38:917.
[19] Markley JM. The preservation of close two point discrimination in the interdigital transfer of neurovascular island flaps. Plast Reconstr Surg 1977;59:812.
[20] Muray JF, Ord JVR, Gavelin GE. The neurovascular island pedicle flap: an assessment of late results in sixteen cases. J Bone Joint Surg Am 1967;49:1285.
[21] Hentz VR. Reconstruction of individual digits. Hand Clin 1985;1:335.
[22] Adamson JE, Horton CE, Crawford HH. Sensory rehabilitation of the injured thumb. Plast Reconstr Surg 1967;40: 53.
[23] Cohen BE, Cronin ED. An innervated cross finger flap for fingertip reconstruction. Plast Reconstr Surg 1983;72: 688.
[24] Gaul JS. Radial innervated cross finger flaps from index to provide sensory pulp to injured thumb. J Bone Joint Surg Am 1969;51:1257.
[25] Walker MA, Hurley CB, May JW Jr. Radial nerve cross finger flap differential nerve contribution in thumb reconstruction. J Hand Surg [Am] 1986;11:881.
[26] Daniel RK, Terzis J, Midgley RD. Restoration of sensation to an anesthetic hand by a free neurovascular flap from the foot. Plast Reconstr Surg 1976;57:275.
[27] Daniel RK, Terzis J, Schwartz G. Neurovascular free flaps: a preliminary report. Plast Reconstr Surg 1975;56:13.
[28] Ohmori K, Harii K. Free dorsalis pedis sensory flap to the hand with microneurovascular anastomoses. Plast Reconstr Surg 1976;58:546.
[29] Robinson DW. Microsurgical transfer of the dorsalis pedis neurovascular island flap. Br J Plast Surg 1976;29:209.
[30] Hing DN, Buncke HJ, Alpert BS, et al. Free flap coverage of the hand. Hand Clin 1985;1:741.
[31] Orgel MG. Innervated free flaps and free vascularized nerve grafts in the hand. In: McCarthy JG, May JW Jr, Littler JW, editors. Plastic surgery, vol. 7. Philadelphia: WB Saunders; 1990. p. 4859.
[32] Lee WPA, May JW Jr. Neurosurgery free flaps to the hand. Hand Clin 1992;8:465.
[33] Dellon AL. Evaluation of sensibility and reeducation of sensation in the hand. Baltimore: Williams & Wilkins; 1981.
[34] Gilbert A, Morrison WA, Tubiana R. Transfer sur la main d'un lambeau libre sensible. Chirurugie 1973;101:691.
[35] Strauch B, Greenstein B. Neurovascular flaps to the hand. Hand Clin 1985;1:327.
[36] Swartz WM. Restoration of sensibility in mutilating hand injuries. Clin Plast Surg 1979;16:170.
[37] May JW Jr, Chait LA, Cohen BE, et al. Free neurosensory vascular flap from the first web of the foot in hand reconstruction. J Hand Surg 1977;2:238.
[38] Buncke HJ, Rose EH. Free toe to fingertip neurovascular flaps. Plast Reconstr Surg 1979;63:607.
[39] Bucke HJ, Strauch B. Sensory rehabilitation of the hand utilizing free microneurovascular flaps from the foot. In: Omer GE, Spinner M, editors. Management of peripheral nerve problems. Philadelphia: WB Saunders; 1980.
[40] Brown CJ, McKinnon SE, Dellon AL, et al. The sensory potential of free flap donor sites. Ann Plast Surg 1989;23: 135.
[41] Strauch B, Tsur H. Restoration of sensation to the hand by a free neurovascular flap from the first web space of the foot. Plast Reconstr Surg 1978;62:361.
[42] Foucher G, Merle M, Maneaud M, et al. Microsurgerical free partial toe transfer in hand reconstruction: a report of 12 cases. Plast Reconstr Surg 1980;65:616.
[43] Morrison WA, O'Brien BM, MacLeod AM. Thumb reconstruction with free neurovascular wraparound flap from the big toe. J Hand Surg 1980;5:575.
[44] Leung P-C, Ma F-Y. Digital reconstruction using the toe flap: report of 10 cases. J Hand Surg 1982;7:366.

[45] Tsai TM, Falconer D. Modified great toe wrap for thumb reconstruction. Microsurgery 1986;7:193.
[46] May JW Jr. Microvascular great toe to hand transfer for reconstruction of the amputated thumb. In: McCarthy JG, May JW Jr, Littler JW, editors. Plastic surgery, vol. 8. Philadelphia: WB Saunders; 1990. p. 5153.
[47] May JW Jr, Daniel RK. Great toe to hand transfer. Clin Orthop 1978;133:140.
[48] Kato H, Ogino T, Minami A, et al. Restoration of sensibility in fingers repaired with free sensory flaps from the toe. J Hand Surg Am 1989;14:49.
[49] Lee HB, Tark KC, Rar DK, Shin KS. Pulp reconstruction of fingers with very small sensate medial plantar free flap. Plast Reconstr Surg 1998;101:999.
[50] Narsete TA. Anatomic design of a sensate plantar flap. Ann Plast Surg 1997;38:538.
[51] May JW Jr, Gordon L. Palm of hand free flap for forearm length preservation in nonreplantable forearm amputation: a case report. J Hand Surg 1980;5:377.
[52] Rohrich RJ, Ehrlichman RJ, May JW Jr. Sensate palm of hand free flap for forearm length preservation in nonreplantable forearm amputation: long term follow-up. Ann Plast Surg 1991;26:469.
[53] Wilhelmi BJ, Lee WPA, Pagenstert IG, May JW Jr. Replantation in the mutilated hand. Clin Hand Surg 2003;19:89.
[54] McCraw JB, Furlow LT. The dorsalis pedis arterialized flap: a clinical study. Plast Reconstr Surg 1975;55:177.
[55] Man D, Acland RD. The microarterial anatomy of the dorsalis pedis flap and its clinical applications. Plast Reconstr Surg 1980;65:419.
[56] Taylor GI, Townsend PLG. Composite free flap and tendon transfer: an anatomical study and clinical technique. Br J Plast Surg 1979;32:170.
[57] Zuker RM, Manktelow RT. The dorsalis pedis free flap technique of elevation, foot closure, and flap application. Plast Reconstr Surg 1986;77:93.
[58] Morrison WA, O'Brien BM, MacLeod AM, et al. Neurovascular free flaps from the foot for innervation of the hand. J Hand Surg 1978;3:235.
[59] Foucher G, van Genechten F, Merle N, et al. A compound radial artery forearm flap in hand surgery: an original modification of the Chinese forearm flap. Br J Plast Surg 1984;37:139.
[60] Muhlbauer W, Herndl E, Stock W. The forearm flap. Plast Reconstr Surg 1982;70:336.
[61] Song R, Gao Y, Song Y, et al. The forearm flap. Clin Plast Surg 1982;9:21.
[62] Soutar DS, Tauner NSB. The radial forearm flap in the management of soft tissue injuries for the hand. Br J Plast Surg 1984;37:18.
[63] Song R, Song Y, Yu U, et al. The upper arm free flap. Clin Plast Surg 1982;9:27.
[64] Katsaros J, Schusterman M, Beppu M, et al. The lateral upper arm flap: anatomy and clinical applications. Ann Plast Surg 1984;12:489.
[65] Katsaros J, Tan E, Zoltie N, et al. Further experience with the lateral arm free flap. Plast Reconstr Surg 1991;87: 902.
[66] Newsom HT. Medial arm free flap. Plast Reconstr Surg 1981;67:63.
[67] Franklin JD. The deltoid flap: anatomy and clinical applications. In: Buncke HJ, Furnas DW, editors. Symposium on clinical frontiers in reconstructive microsurgery, vol. 24. St. Louis: CV Mosby; 1983. p. 63.
[68] Russell RC, Guy RJ, Zook EG, et al. Extremity reconstruction using the free deltoid flap. Plast Reconstr Surg 1985; 76:586.
[69] Hill HL, Nahai F, Vasconez LO. The tensor fascia lata myocutaneous free flap. Plast Reconstr Surg 1978;61:517.
[70] Nahai F, Hill HL, Hester TR. Experiences with the tensor fascia lata flap. Plast Reconstr Surg 1978;63:788.
[71] Pribaz JJ, Orgill DP, Epstein MD, et al. Anterolateral thigh free flap. Ann Plast Surg 1995;34:585.
[72] Acland RD, Schusterman M, Godina M, et al. The saphenous neurovascular free flap. Plast Reconstr Surg 1981;67: 763.
[73] Walton RL, Bunkis J. The posterior calf fasciocutaneous free flap. Plast Reconstr Surg 1984;74:76.
[74] Walton RL, Petry JJ. Follow-up on the posterior calf fasciocutaneous free flap. Plast Reconstr Surg 1985;76:149.
[75] Chen HC, Tang YB, Chuang D, Wei FC, Noordhoff MS. Microvascular free posterior interosseous flap and a comparison with the pedicled posterior interosseous flap. Ann Plast Surg 1996;36:542.
[76] Badran HA, El Helaly MS, Safe I. The lateral intercostals neurovascular free flap. Plast Reconstr Surg 1984;73:17.
[77] Morris RL, Dillman D, McCabe JS, et al. The transverse cervical neurovascular free flap. Ann Plast Surg 1983;10: 90.
[78] Woerdeman LA, Chaplin BJ, Griffioen FM, et al. Sensate osteocutaneous fibula flap anatomic study of the innervation pattern of the skin flap. Head Neck 1998;20:310.
[79] Wei FC, Chuang SS, Yim KK. The sensate fibula osteoseptocutaneous flap: a preliminary report. Br J Plast Surg 1994;47:544.
[80] Mawera G, Kalangu KK, Muguti GI. The sensate deep inferior epigastric musculocutaneous flap and the twelfth thoracic nerve. Br J Plast Surg 1995;48:455.
[81] Blondeel PN. The sensate free superior gluteal artery perforator (S-GAP) flap: a valuable alternative in autologous breast reconstruction. Br J Plast Surg 1999;52:185.
[82] Schultes G, Karcher H, Gaggl A. Sensate myocutaneous latissimus dorsi flap. J Reconstr Microsurg 1998;14:541.
[83] Muguti GI, Mawera G, Kalangu KK. The sensate deep inferior epigastric musculocutaneous flap: details of the operative technique. Cent Afr J Med 1997;43:340.
[84] Mawera G, Kalanu KK, Muguti GI. The sensate deep inferior epigastric musculocutaneous flap and the twelfth thoracic nerve. Br J Plast Surg 1995;48:455.

ELSEVIER
SAUNDERS

Atlas Hand Clin 10 (2005) 187–197

Atlas of the
HAND
CLINICS

The Peripheral Nerve Allograft: a Decade of Advancement

Peter J. Evans, MD, PhD, FRCSC

Cleveland Combined Hand Fellowship and Peripheral Nerve Center, Hand, Elbow & Shoulder Surgery, Department of Orthopaedic Surgery, Cleveland Clinic Foundation, A40, Crile Building, 9500 Euclid Avenue, Cleveland, OH 44195, USA

There has been a renewed interest in peripheral nerve allografts, and great progress in the understanding of their neuroimmunologic consequences has led to their subsequent clinical implementation. Since the last comprehensive reviews of nerve allografting in the 1990s [1–3], many advances in the understanding of transplant immunobiology have led to new strategies to prevent graft rejection, while imparting less severe side effects to the recipient [4–6]. This article highlights these successes and outlines the challenges that are still to be met before peripheral nerve allografting becomes a routine surgical procedure clinically.

Need

Despite advances in motor vehicle and industry safety, significant numbers of peripheral nerve injuries occur annually. Smaller injuries typically are treated with traditional methods of neurolysis, neurorrhaphy, and nerve autografting when there is a segmental loss. Autografting trades a sensory deficit for a potential motor/sensory gain in a more important body region. Donor site neuromas can develop and cause pain in addition to the loss of sensation, leaving a patient despondent with at best half the motor/sensory recovery in the recipient limb and a painful donor site. In addition, there is often not enough expendable donor graft available to reconstruct long or segmental nerve injuries. The need exists for a readily available source of grafts of various lengths and diameters that can be implemented in an elective manner, with minimal risks and with the potential to provide regenerative results equal to autografts. With the advent of broad immunosuppression [7,8], nerve allografts have been shown to provide equivalent regeneration, but now the focus has shifted to strategies of minimizing recipient drug-related morbidity for this non–life-threatening reconstructive procedure.

Allograft rejection

Nerve allografts seem to differ when compared with solid-organ (eg, lung) allografts and composite tissue (eg, whole hand) allografts (CTAs). CTAs have many different types of tissue of variable antigenicity complicating immunosuppressive regimens, whereas solid-organ allografts are more amenable to fixed protocols optimized for the particular organ used. Nerve allografts may be "privileged," and immunosuppressive protocols may be required only during the time needed for recipient (host) axons to grow across the donor graft and reinnervate the motor or sensory target [9–11]. Nevertheless, the initiation of the host immune response must be blocked to prevent acute allograft rejection. Successful nerve allografting requires the optimization of all interdependent steps in the transplantation process, many of which have seen great advances since the 1990s (Fig. 1). An understanding of the highlights of the immune

E-mail address: evansp2@ccf.org

doi:10.1016/j.ahc.2004.09.004

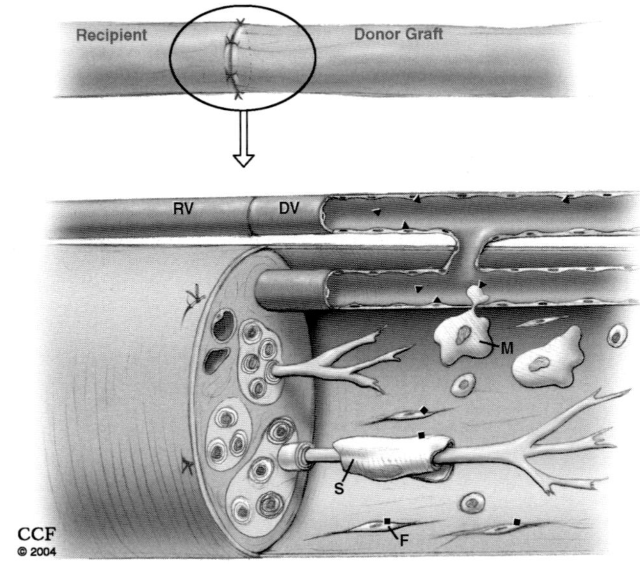

Fig. 1. Overview of nerve allograft events. After neurorrhaphy, recipient (RV) and donor (DV) vessels connect within 72 hours via inosculation permitting passenger lymphocytes entry to recipient circulation and host lymphocytes and macrophages (M) entry to the graft. Schwann cells (S) and fibroblasts (F) within the donor graft begin active relationship with regenerating recipient axons. Foreignness is expressed via donor (*triangles*) and recipient (*squares*) antigens.

response to allograft tissue is paramount to understanding the advances and future direction of transplantation immunotherapy.

Briefly, the host immune response to an allograft proceeds in three phases: (1) allorecognition, (2) clonal expansion of host T-cell and B-cell lines, and (3) a resulting effector response predominantly cell mediated (activated T cells and B cells) and humoral (antibody) leading to graft destruction [1,3]. Allorecognition begins after graft revascularization when circulating host T cells recognize differences between host and donor tissue major histocompatibility complex (MHC) loci (Fig. 2). *Direct recognition* refers to host T-cell recognition of donor MHC (with or without processed peptide in the MHC binding site) [12]. *Indirect recognition* refers to host T-cell recognition of donor MHC peptide, processed and presented by host antigen presenting cell (APC) in the context of host MHC. Two T-cell subsets—T helper (Th) cells ($CD4^+$) and cytotoxic T lymphocytes (CTLs) ($CD8^+$)—preferentially interact with antigen associated with MHC class II and I.

Class II mechanisms are considered more important, and Th cell activation requires two signals (Fig. 3). *Signal 1* involves the recognition of processed donor MHC peptide by host APC in the context of host MHC. This binding is stabilized by nonspecific intercellular adhesion molecular pairs (ICAM/LFA, VCAM/VLA, and others); this stimulates the calcium-calmodulin complex and induces expression of CD154 on the surface of the Th cell. *Signal 2* involves the engagement of CD154 with CD40 on APCs, initiating the *coactivation* of the Th cell. *Signal 2* up-regulates costimulatory molecules B7-1 and B7-2 on APCs, which bind to CD28 and CTLA 4 complex, completing the *costimulation* process and fully activating the Th cell. The Th cell secretes numerous cytokines (including interleukin [IL]-2), which initiate a molecular and cellular cascade leading to progressive infiltration into the graft of immunocompetent cells. Another cytokine generated, interferon-γ, further up-regulates class II MHC expression in the allograft, propagating the process. The rejecting allograft is infiltrated by Th cells and CTLs (and other cells, such as macrophages) and receives insults from cytotoxic cells and secondary mediators of inflammation, especially to graft endothelial cells leading to occlusion of microvasculature, ischemic injury, and ultimately graft necrosis.

Transplantation strategies

Conventional methods of preventing nerve allograft rejection employed immunosuppressive drug regimens that globally suppressed the immune system. Advances in research led to

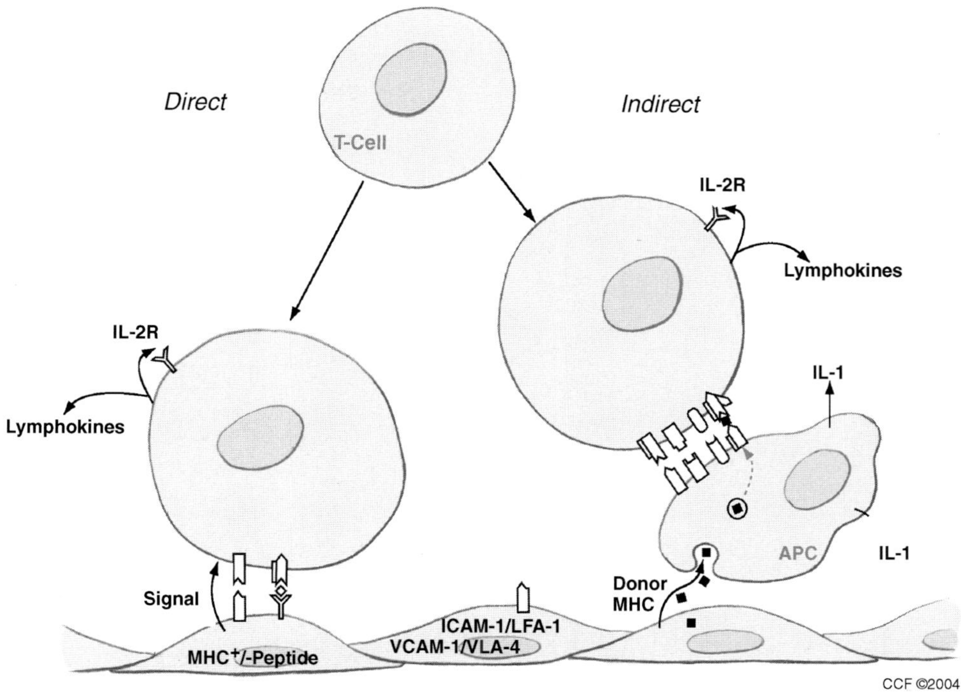

Fig. 2. Cell-mediated immune response to nerve allografts. Allorecognition begins when circulating host T cells recognize differences between host and donor tissue MHC loci. *Direct recognition* refers to host T-cell recognition of donor MHC (with or without processed peptide in the MHC binding site). *Indirect recognition* refers to host T-cell recognition of donor MHC peptide, processed and presented by host APC in the context of host MHC.

optimized protocols using cyclosporine, which blocks IL-2 production by the Th cell (Fig. 3). More recently, cyclosporine has been supplanted by tacrolimus (FK506), which works via similar mechanisms, but has an added advantage of enhancing nerve regeneration (see later). As a result of general immunosuppression, however, both drugs carry increased risks of infection, fracture, malignancy, permanent end-organ damage, and metabolic effects. The increased risk of these complications generates practical and ethical issues and fuels the search for less morbid means of immunosuppression. Other aspects in the immune response to allografts have been discovered and targeted in recent years and are reviewed in the context of the steps required to perform nerve transplantation (see Fig. 1).

Donor harvest

After a potential donor is identified by the transplant team, the process is initiated, and elective operating time is coordinated for the recipient within 6 to 8 days. Although not delineated yet, putative *suppressor agents* and donor MHC-binding or other *antigen-binding agents* (eg, anti-CD40L monoclonal antibody; see later) could be centrally perfused in a subset of donors in whom circulatory arrest has not occurred. Nerve grafts would be harvested of various lengths and diameters and immersed in a transport medium. Donor bone marrow (stem cells), spleen cells, and peripheral blood cells would be harvested for *tolerance induction* protocols, which are one form of donor-specific immunosuppression. Since its conception more than 50 years ago [13], the success of tolerance protocols has been greatest in murine models, progressively less in rodent, large animal, and nonhuman primates, and limited in humans. Donor-specific tolerance (DST) is ideal and refers to a host's ability to accept allogeneic material from a specific, immunologically disparate donor, but remain otherwise immunocompetent to other foreign antigens. Many strategies to induce tolerance have been tried, and a review of these in the context of CTA has been published (Fig. 4) [3].

One method of DST requiring donor tissue involves host presensitization to donor antigen by portal venous infusion of ultraviolet B–irradiated donor antigen (eg, spleen cells) 7 days before

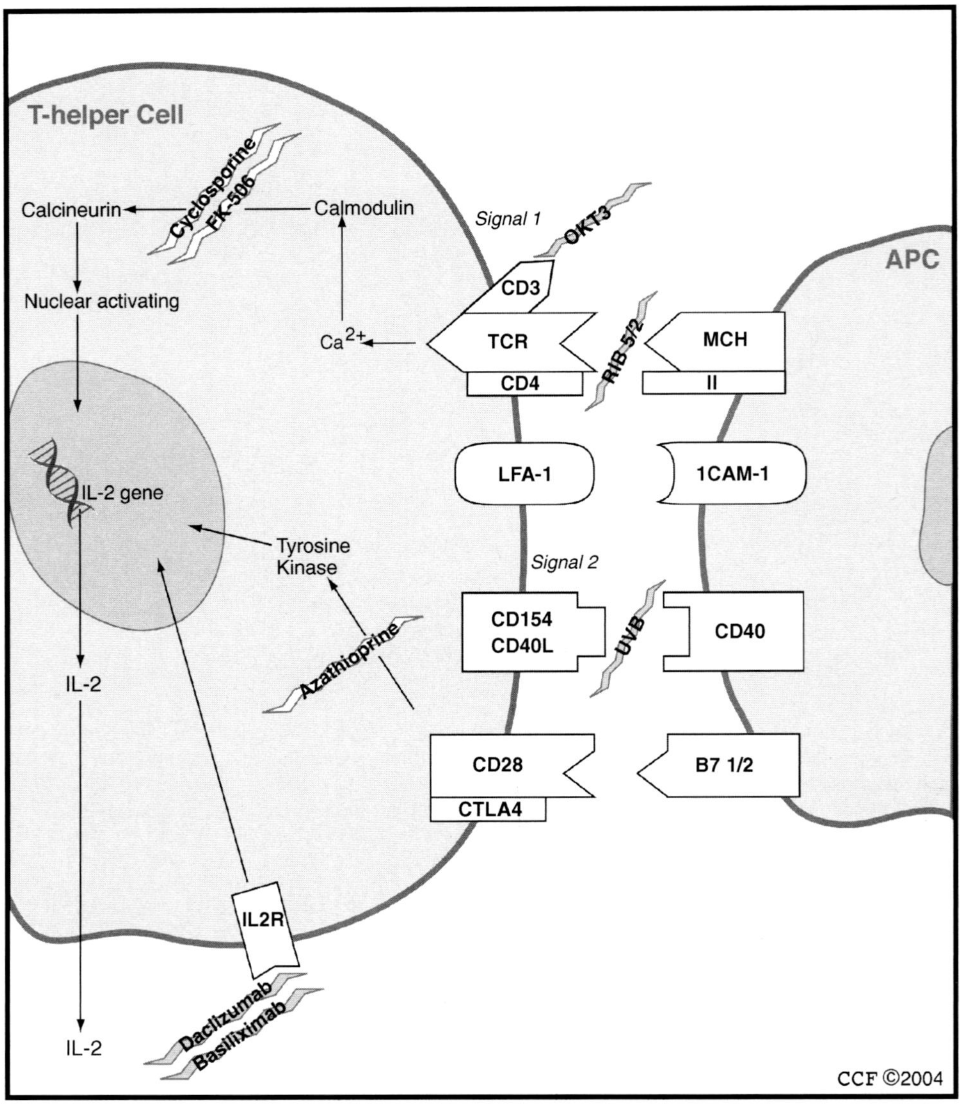

Fig. 3. Indirect allorecognition of nerve allografts. MHC class II mechanisms are considered more important, and Th cell activation requires two signals. *Signal 1* involves the recognition of processed donor MHC peptide by host APC in the context of host MHC. This binding is stabilized by nonspecific intercellular adhesion molecular pairs (ICAM/LFA, VCAM/VLA, and others); this stimulates the calcium-calmodulin complex and induces expression of CD154 on the surface of the Th cell. *Signal 2* involves the engagement of CD154 with CD40 on APCs, initiating the *coactivation* of the Th cell. *Signal 2* up-regulates costimulatory molecules B7-1 and B7-2 on APCs, which then bind to CD28 and CTLA 4 complex, completing the *costimulation* process and fully activating the Th cell. The Th cell secretes numerous cytokines (including IL-2), which initiate a molecular and cellular cascade, leading to progressive infiltration into the graft of immunocompetent cells.

allograft transplantation. Donor antigen is phagocytosed by host Kupffer cells and presented in the context of host MHC to circulating host T cells, which affects the host T-cell CD28 costimulatory pathway (*signal 2*). This activity functionally down-regulates MHC class II antigen expression on the T cell, causing a decreased immune responsiveness and clinical tolerance of the donor allograft. In a series of studies using this method with donor alloantigen (splenocytes) alone [14,15] or combined with anti-ICAM-1/anti-LFA-1 monoclonal antibodies [16] or anti-CD4 monoclonal antibody (mAB) (eg, RIB 5/2), Doolabh et al [17] showed regeneration across treated nerve allograft recipients that was significantly greater than untreated allograft recipients and near that of nerve isograft (autograft) recipients. Importantly, when successfully regenerated nerve allografts were retransplanted into a second naive recipient, rejection occurred by naive donor strain, but not recipient strain. This finding suggested that

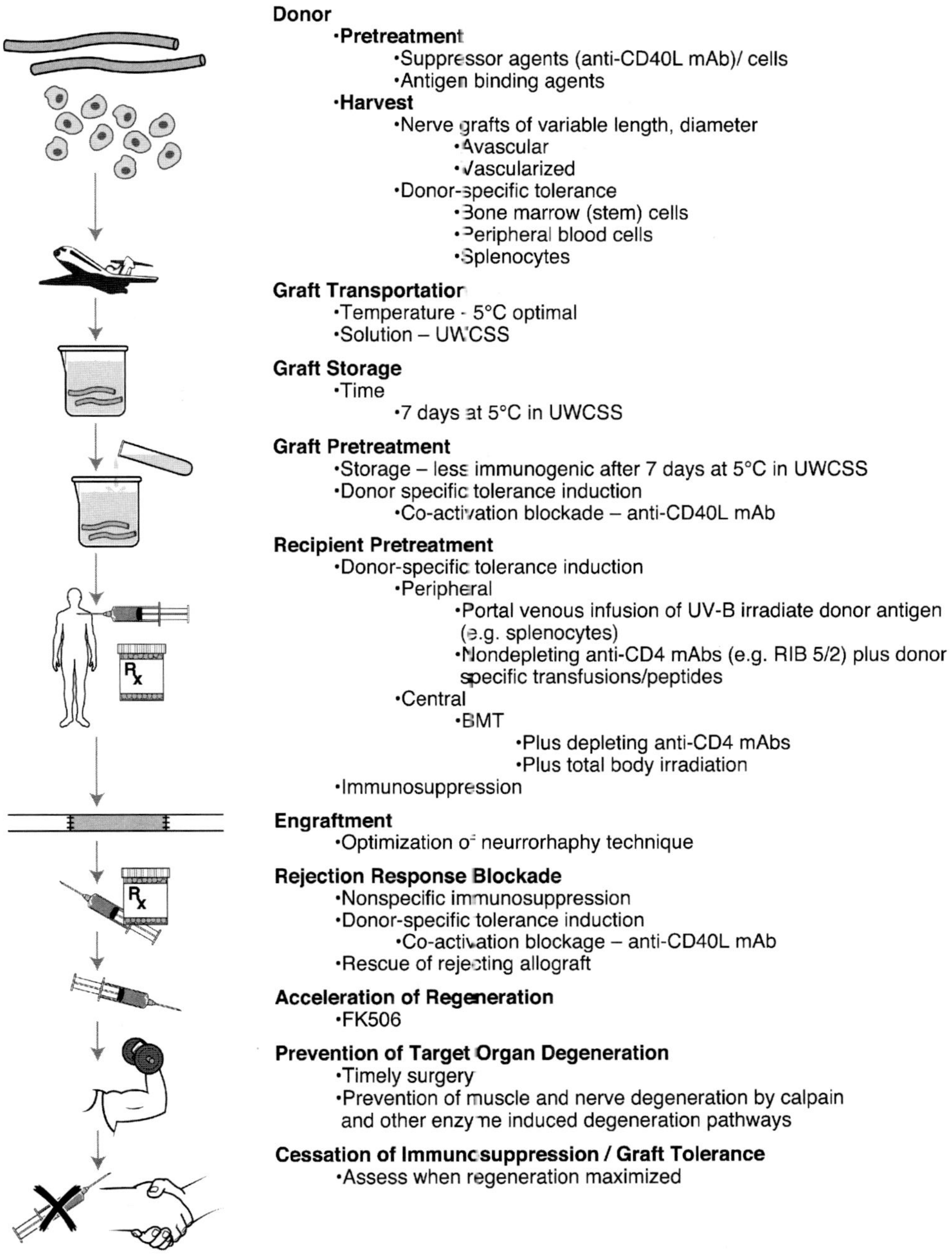

Fig. 4. Nerve Allograft Procedure. Systematic analysis of each step in the procedure helps to optimize regeneration and minimize patient morbidity.

allografts were completely replaced by host tissue. When pretreated recipients of successful nerve allografts were rechallenged 8 and 16 weeks later with a second nerve allograft, the previously unresponsive recipients rejected the new allograft [15]. The loss of the previous intrahepatic-induced unresponsive (tolerance) state is thought to be further evidence of the replacement of the original donor allograft by host tissue and the loss of continued host exposure to donor antigen. This evidence lends support to a DST mechanism of T-cell suppression or anergy that may require persistence of donor antigen versus a mechanism of peripheral or central clonal deletion of donor-specific T cells, which should result in permanent tolerance [18,19]. This finding also underscores the uniqueness of nerve allografts and indicates that this method of DST, although only temporary, is sufficient for successful regeneration, but limiting in the duration and subsequent degree of morbidity of immunosuppression.

Graft transportation, storage, and pretreatment

A necessary adjunct to clinical nerve allografting is the ability to store harvested nerves during transport. Prolonged storage would increase access and allow time to test donor tissue, initiate DST protocols, and facilitate elective planning providing less costly reconstructive procedures. Methods of nerve allograft storage [20] and pretreatment [21] date back to the turn of the twentieth century and are not mutually exclusive. Numerous strategies have been employed, including graft storage in various solutions, freezing, irradiation, freeze-thawing, predegeneration, lyophilization, and combinations thereof [1]. Although strategies that render grafts acellular provide a nonimmunogenic scaffold for regenerating host axons, they have failed to show regeneration equivalent to nerve autografts or allografts with cyclosporine host immunosuppression [1,22].

A practical storage solution was sought, and the University of Wisconsin (UW) cold storage solution was found to be optimal at 5°C (versus 22°C and 37°C), maintaining graft basal lamina and resulting in regeneration across nerve autografts stored at 5°C for 3 weeks that was comparable to that across fresh nerve autografts [23,24]. Cold storage in UW solution maintained cellular viability at near-normal levels for 7 days with progressive reduction thereafter, but viable and functional Schwann cells remained after 3 weeks [25]; this correlated with reduced allograft expression of class II MHC and ICAM-1 antigens [26], reduced immunogenicity [25,27–29], but inferior regeneration compared with autografts [30]. Further results showed that with cold preservation a decrease in the dose of cyclosporine was required for successful regeneration across nerve allografts [31]. Cold preservation was shown to work synergistically with tacrolimus, resulting in superior regeneration than either treatment alone [32].

At present, storage for 7 days at 5°C in the UW solution seems to be the optimal tradeoff between a mild reduction in immunogenicity and preservation of viable allogeneic Schwann cells required for optimal regeneration. There may be a role in the future for immersion of the nerve allograft in anti-CD40L mAB, which theoretically could block the *costimulatory pathway* of Th cell activation (see Fig. 3), but results are pending [4].

Recipient pretreatment

As noted, immunosuppressive strategies to pretreat the potential recipient can be undertaken during the time of graft storage. DST induction with portal venous host pretreatment with donor-specific antigen (splenocytes) typically is initiated at 7 days before transplantation [15–17]. Addition of anti-ICAM-1 and anti-LFA-1 mABs to this regimen [14] involves 10 daily injections, starting 2 days before transplantation.

Alternatively, nondepleting anti-CD4 mABs (eg, RIB 5/2) can be used to block one of the costimulatory pathways by interfering in an as yet to be defined way with the interaction between class II MHC complex on the APC and the CD4 molecule on Th cells rendering them unresponsive. In a murine model, a single dose of RIB 5/2 and donor antigen was given 7 days before nerve allograft transplantation and resulted in donor-specific down-regulation of Th cells. Nerve regeneration was markedly improved compared with allograft controls, but not as robust as nerve autografts [17].

Caution has been raised concerning human recipients who have received multiple recent transfusions of blood products because they may possess anti–human lymphocyte antigen antibodies [33]. Time may decrease antibody titers, and retesting is recommended.

Engraftment

The basic principles of a tension-free microsurgical repair used for nerve autografts apply to allografts.

Rejection response blockade

Contrary to vascularized allograft tissue, nonvascularized nerve allografts remain inert immediately after engraftment. Revascularization of nerve grafts is prompt and occurs via inosculation, not neovascularization, resulting in patent epineurial vessels within 48 hours and endoneurial vessels within 72 hours [34,35]. Host immunocompetent Th cells enter the nerve graft and interact with donor APCs (Schwann, endothelial, and other cells) with peak alloreactivity occurring at day 4, as assessed by mixed lymphocyte culture assays, and peak cytotoxicity occurring at day 11, as determined by cell-mediated lymphocytolysis reaction [36].

In the 1990s, new hope for nerve allograft procedures came with the introduction cyclosporine, a calcineurin inhibitor (see Fig. 3). The minimum dose required to suppress the immune response to nerve allografts and the optimal preparation and route of delivery of cyclosporine were determined [37–39]. Regeneration across nerve allografts in hosts immunosuppressed with cyclosporine was found to be equivalent to nerve autografts in rat [8] and primate [40,41] models. This work led to the world's first nerve allograft in the modern era [42] followed by four other cases [33,43]. Motor and sensory recovery was found in all but one patient, who rejected the radial nerve allograft. Long-term use of cyclosporine in rats and sheep has resulted in side effects causing weight loss and death in many animals [39,44]. This discovery stimulated the quest for adjuvant therapies and alternative immunosuppressants and raised the question of the possibility of discontinuing therapy (see later) after regeneration was accomplished.

As mentioned, cold preservation originally was employed as a means of graft storage [24], but results found that graft antigenicity also was reduced [25–28], which led to further experiments showing a synergistic effect with cyclosporine, decreasing the dose required for successful regeneration across nerve allografts and potentially less toxicity [31]. Another means of decreasing the required cyclosporine dose was to block *secondary signaling* by the use of mABs to ICAM-1 and LFA-1α found on APCs and Th cells (see Fig. 3). Initial success [45–47] was refuted later [48] by differing animal models in the same laboratory, and subsequently these investigators confirmed that these mABs alone were insufficient to block the rejection process, but they were synergistic with cyclosporine, allowing for a reduction of the dose required [49].

As an alternative to cyclosporine, tacrolimus showed promise in other organ transplant models, and it was tested for its efficacy and safety for use with nerve allografts. Initial experimental success [50,51] was confirmed in subsequent studies [52–54] when tacrolimus was given continuously in small animal models, then across an 8-cm nerve graft in swine [4]. To improve safety and efficacy, the minimum dose of tacrolimus required to permit regeneration equivalent to control autografts was determined [55,56]. Cold preservation was shown again to work synergistically, resulting in superior regeneration than tacrolimus alone and allowing for equivalent regeneration to isografts with even subtherapeutic doses [32].

Contrary to the global, pan T-cell immunosuppressive effects of cyclosporine or tacrolimus, DST attempts to produce selective inhibition of the APC–Th cell interaction. Another *costimulatory pathway* target for DST are the CD40 receptor and CD40 ligand (CD40L), which reside on the APC and Th cell (see Fig. 3). In a murine model, anti-CD40L mAB was administered topically to the harvested nerve grafts and intraperitoneally immediately preoperatively and on postoperative days 1, 3, 10, and 18. Anti-CD40L mAB induction successfully blocked the rejection response and allowed for significantly improved parameters of regeneration similar to isografts, but it did not induce a state of long-lasting and specific tolerance as evidenced by rejection of secondary allografts.

Based on solid-organ transplantation research and one clinical case of clinical nerve allograft rejection, Mackinnon's group investigated the ability of cyclosporine and tacrolimus to rescue nerve allografts after rejection had begun. Tacrolimus was able to prevent rejection of nerve allografts after 7 or 10 days but not 14 days of rejection and resulted in regeneration similar to autografts [57]. After 3 weeks without treatment following nerve allograft, cyclosporine was unable to halt rejection and resulted in significantly poorer regeneration than in controls [58].

Acceleration of regeneration

If a method of permanent immune tolerance cannot be found, nerve allografts will continue to function as a scaffold consisting of donor Schwann and other cells that aid in regeneration only temporarily, being replaced by host cells on discontinuation of immunotherapy. It would be desirable to develop a means of accelerating nerve regeneration to decrease the duration of immunotherapy, minimizing its side effects. Although a thorough discussion of neuroenhancing therapies is beyond the scope of this article, one of the most promising agents is tacrolimus, which has been shown to accelerate nerve regeneration after a nerve crush injury [59,60] neurorrhaphy [61], and nerve grafting [62]. Its mechanism later was shown not to occur via calcineurin inhibition based on findings that two tacrolimus analogues, FKBP-12 and FKBP-52, enhanced regeneration without causing immunosuppression.

An alternative means of enhancing nerve regeneration used a previous notion [63] of autologous nerve segments interposed in the center of an allograft with the presumption of providing more viable Schwann cells of host origin to repopulate the allograft segments over time [64]. Despite having to cross more sites of neurorrhaphy, this technique resulted in better regeneration compared with allograft segments alone.

Prevention of target organ degeneration

Paramount to any nerve injury is the assurance that neuromuscular junctions and muscle and sensory nerve endings are viable when axons finally reach them. Schwann cell basal lamina tubes contract after nerve transaction and wallerian degeneration and never regain their full diameter even after successful regeneration, limiting ultimate function. Neuromuscular junctions and muscle atrophy, and although results vary, function is superior if reinnervation occurs within the 18 months postinjury. Sensory nerve endings are more resilient, and sensory recovery can occur even years after injury. Advances in basic science research have translated into clinical trials with agents used to maintain the integrity of muscle during the lag time required for reinnervation. Potentially, embryonic stem cells may play a role in the future in replenishing myocytes and neuromuscular junctions.

Cessation of immunosuppression and graft tolerance

It was postulated that perhaps only short-term immunosuppression may be required, until host axons traversed the graft and successfully innervated motor and sensory targets. This idea was borne out by a series of experiments that showed transient loss of function on cessation of cyclosporine and rapid return in function to that seen previously. It was shown that only a portion of the axons traversing the graft are rejected, with axons from pure cutaneous sensory nerve grafts and smaller diameter motor fibers from pure motor nerve grafts more resistant to rejection compared with mixed motor/sensory grafts and larger diameter motor fibers from pure motor grafts [11]. Axon death was in part due to graft cell (Schwann cells, others) rejection, and the rapid return in function was due to host cell repopulation/remyelination of the graft [9,10,65]. Graft repopulation by host cells was confirmed when regenerated allograft nerve grafts from hosts receiving temporary cyclosporine immunosuppression were rejected on regrafting back into the original donor strain, but not into untreated recipient strain rats, showing a change to recipient graft antigenicity (cellular makeup). Regenerated grafts from continuously immunosuppressed hosts were accepted on regrafting into donor and host strains, indicating migration of host cells into the graft and persistence of donor and host allodeterminants during immunosuppression [65]. Fewer studies using adequate and comparable animal models have been performed studying tacrolimus, and they have shown conflicting results of either equivalent [54] or inferior [50,51,53] regeneration after short-course therapy versus continuous therapy or autografts.

Clinical results

Mackinnon et al [33] reviewed their clinical results of seven patients (mean age 15) who received peripheral nerve allografts ranging from 72 to 350 cm in total graft length per patient. Immunosuppression consisted initially of either cyclosporine (in five patients) or tacrolimus combined with azathioprine and prednisone (see Fig. 3), which was stopped at 6 months after there was evidence of regeneration distal to the nerve allograft. Six patients had return of motor function and sensation, and one had rejection as a result of subtherapeutic immunosuppression.

No patients showed loss of neural function after cessation of immunosuppression, differing from animal experiments and indicating a gradual turnover of donor graft cells with cells of host origin.

Nerve allografting has direct application to CTAs because nerve regeneration is paramount to motor and sensory function of transplanted limbs. The first human hand transplant was performed without success in 1964 [66]. The first in the modern era of immunotherapy was performed in France in 1998 [67,68]; this transplant also failed, owing to patient noncompliance with immunosuppressive therapy. This failure was followed by successes in other countries with varying degrees of functional recovery [69–71]. The first human double-hand transplant was performed in a 33-year-old man using hands from an 18-year-old man 6 years after bilateral amputations. Immunosuppression included induction with antithymocyte globulins and anti-CD25 mAB, followed by tacrolimus, prednisone, and mycophenolate mofetil. Sensory recovery was remarkable with 12 to 14 cm of regeneration after 3 months and pain and temperature sensation and palmar paresthesias by 6 months. By 15 months, Semmes-Weinstein 4.56 monofilaments were detected in all fingers, active wrist motion was 45° to 50°, pinch was 300g, and grip was 150g with single finger motions discernable. If permanent tolerance to nonneural tissue can be achieved in the future, results from nerve allograft studies would predict maintenance of these functional gains.

Summary and future directions

The past decade has seen a greater expansion in the strategies to solve the nerve allograft question than during the previous century by the incorporation of advances in transplantation immunology. A systematic approach to the transplantation process (see Fig. 1) will lead to further successes. Investigation into a different facet of immunology and inflammation may offer clues. Chemokines are chemotactic cytokines that recruit leukocytes to tissues, which is crucial in the initiation and maintenance of inflammatory events, such as rejection. Induction of chemokine genes (*MIP-1α, MIP-1,* and *RANTES*) responsible for recruitment of macrophages, granulocytes, and lymphocytes was shown to occur before nerve allograft infiltration by immunocompetent cells [72]. Potential blocking agents exist and require testing in future studies.

Other more recent alternatives to nerve allografts include synthetic nerve conduits alone, conduits prefilled with autologous or allogeneic Schwann cells, and allografts made acellular and repopulated with autologous Schwann cells [73–75]. This work has shown promise but has not consistently shown regeneration equivalent to autografts even over relatively short (<5 cm) distances. Based on the advances in the 1990s, with continued research into nerve and other organ transplantation immunology and inflammation, the next decade undoubtedly will offer more progress toward making nerve allografting a mainstream procedure.

References

[1] Evans PJ, Midha R, Mackinnon SE. The peripheral nerve allograft: a comprehensive review of regeneration and neuroimmunology. Prog Neurobiol 1994;43:187–233.

[2] Ide C, Osawa T, Tohkyama K. Nerve regeneration through allogeneic nerve grafts, with special reference to Schwann cell basal lamina. Prog Neurobiol 1990;34:1–38.

[3] Siemionow M, Ozer K. Advances in composite tissue allograft transplantation as related to the hand and upper extremity. J Hand Surg 2002;27A:565–80.

[4] Myckatyn TM, Mackinnon SE. A review of research endeavors to optimize peripheral nerve reconstruction. Neurol Res 2004;26:124–38.

[5] Bain JR. Peripheral nerve and neuromuscular allotransplantation: current status. Microsurgery 2000;20:384–8.

[6] Trumble TE, Shon FG. The physiology of nerve transplantation. Hand Clin 2000;16:105–22.

[7] Zalewski AA, Gulati AK. Survival of nerve and Schwann cells in allografts after Cyclosporin A treatment. Exp Neurol 1980;70:219–25.

[8] Bain JR, Mackinnon SE, Hudson AR, Falk RE, Falk JA, Hunter DA. The peripheral nerve allograft: an assessment of regeneration across nerve allografts in rats immunosuppressed with Cyclosporin A. Plast Reconstr Surg 1988;82:1052–66.

[9] Midha R, Mackinnon SE, Evans PJ, et al. Comparison of regeneration across nerve allografts with temporary or continuous cyclosporin A immunosuppression. J Neurosurg 1993;78:90–100.

[10] Midha R, Evans PJ, Mackinnon SE, Wade JA. Temporary immunosuppression for peripheral nerve allografts. Transplant Proc 1993;25:532–6.
[11] Midha R, Nag S, Munro CA, Ang LC. Differential response of sensory and motor axons in nerve allografts after withdrawal of immunosuppressive therapy. J Neurosurg 2001;94:102–10.
[12] Liu Z, Sun Y-K, Zi Y-P, Maffei A, Reed E, Harris P. Contribution of direct and indirect recognition pathways to T-cell alloreactivity. J Exp Med 1993;177:1643–50.
[13] Billingham RE, Brent L, Medawar PB. Actively acquired tolerance. Nature 1953;172:603–6.
[14] Genden EM, Mackinnon SE, Yu S, Flye MW. Induction of donor-specific tolerance to rat nerve allografts with portal venous donor alloantigen and anti-ICAM-1/LFA-1 monoclonal antibodies. Surgery 1998;124:448–56.
[15] Tung TH, Doolabh VB, Mackinnon SE, Hunter DA, Flye MW. Immune unresponsiveness by intraportal UV-B-irradiated donor antigen administration requires persistence of donor antigen in a nerve allograft model. J Reconstr Microsurg 2004;20:43–51.
[16] Genden EM, Mackinnon SE, Yu S, Hunter DA, Flye MW. Pretreatment with portal venous ultraviolet B irradiated donor alloantigen promotes donor-specific tolerance to rat nerve allografts. Laryngoscope 2001;111:439–47.
[17] Doolabh VB, Tung TH, Flye MW, Mackinnon SE. Effect of nondepleting anti-CD4 monoclonal antibody (RIB 5/2) plus donor antigen pretreatment in peripheral nerve allotransplantation. Microsurgery 2002;22:329–34.
[18] Wekerle T, Blaha P, Koporc Z, Bigenzahn S, Pusch M, Muehlbacher F. Mechanisms of tolerance induction through the transplantation of donor hematopoietic stem cells: central versus peripheral tolerance. Transplantation 2003;75: 21S–5S.
[19] Wekerle T, Sykes M. Induction of tolerance. Surgery 2004;135:359–64.
[20] Bethe A. Zwei neue Methoden der Uberbruckung gro Berer Nervenlucken. Dtsch Med Wschr 1916;42:1277–80.
[21] Huber GC. Transplantation of peripheral nerves. Arch Neurol Psychiatry 1919;2:466–80.
[22] Fansa H, Lassner F, Kook PH, Keilhoff G, Schneider W. Cryopreservation of peripheral nerve grafts. Muscle Nerve 2000;23:1227–33.
[23] Carvalho A, Evans PJ, McKee NH, Mackinnon SE. Differences between contractions of fast and slow muscles after nerve grafting. J Reconstr Microsurg 1997;13:351–9.
[24] Evans PJ, Mackinnon SE, Best TJ, et al. Regeneration across preserved peripheral nerve grafts. Muscle Nerve 1995; 18:1128–38.
[25] Evans PJ, Mackinnon SE, Levi AD, et al. Cold preserved nerve allografts: changes in basement membrane, viability, immunogenicity, and regeneration. Muscle Nerve 1998;21:1507–22.
[26] Atchabahian A, Mackinnon SE, Hunter DA. Cold preservation of nerve grafts decreases expression of ICAM-1 and class II MHC antigens. J Reconstr Microsurg 1999;15:307–11.
[27] Hare GMT, Evans PJ, Mackinnon SE, Wade JA, Young AJ, Hay JB. Phenotypic analysis of migrant, efferent lymphocytes after implantation of cold preserved, peripheral nerve allografts. J Neuroimmunol 1995;56:9–16.
[28] Hare GMT, Evans PJ, Mackinnon SE, et al. Effect of cold preservation on lymphocyte migration into peripheral nerve allografts in sheep. Transplantation 1993;56:154–62.
[29] Strasberg SR, Mackinnon SE, Hare GMT, Narini PP, Hertl MC, Hay JB. Reduction in peripheral nerve allograft antigenicity with warm and cold temperature preservation. Plast Reconstr Surg 1996;97:152–60.
[30] Evans PJ, Mackinnon SE, Midha R, et al. Regeneration across cold preserved peripheral nerve allografts. Microsurgery 1999;19:115–27.
[31] Strasberg SR, Hertl MC, Mackinnon SE, et al. Peripheral nerve allograft preservation improves regeneration and decreases systemic Cyclosporin A requirements. Exp Neurol 1996;139:306–16.
[32] Grand AG, Myckatyn TM, Mackinnon SE, Hunter DA. Axonal regeneration after cold preservation of nerve allografts and immunosuppression with tacrolimus in mice. J Neurosurg 2002;96:924–32.
[33] Mackinnon SE, Doolabh VB, Novak CB, Trulock EP. Clinical outcome following nerve allograft transplantation. Plast Reconstr Surg 2001;107:1419–29.
[34] Best TJ, Mackinnon SE, Evans PJ, Hunter DA, Midha R. Peripheral nerve revascularization: histomorphometric study of small- and large-caliber grafts. J Reconstr Microsurg 1999;15:183–90.
[35] Best TJ, Mackinnon SE, Maeda T, Midha R, Evans PJ. Revascularization of perhipheral nerve autografts and allografts. Plast Reconstr Surg 1999;104:152–60.
[36] Ishida O, Ochi M, Ikuta Y, Akiyiama M. Peripheral nerve allograft: cellular and humoral immune responses of mice. J Surg Res 1990;49:233–8.
[37] Bain JR, Mackinnon SE, Hudson AR, Falk RE, Falk JA, Hunter DA. The peripheral nerve allograft: a dose-response curve in the rat immunosuppressed with Cyclosporin A. Plast Reconstr Surg 1988;82:447–57.
[38] Midha R, Mackinnon SE, Evans PJ, Best TJ, Wong P-Y. Subcutaneous injection of oral Cyclosporin A solution. Microsurgery 1992;13:92–4.
[39] Midha R, Mackinnon SE, Wade JA, Evans PJ, Best TJ, Wong P-Y. Chonic Cyclosporin A therapy in rats. Microsurgery 1992;13:273–6.
[40] Bain JR, Mackinnon SE, Hudson AR, et al. The peripheral nerve allograft in the primate immunosuppressed with Cyclosporin A: Part I. histological and electrophysiological assessment. Plast Reconstr Surg 1992;90:1036–46.
[41] Fish JS, Bain JR, McKee NH, Mackinnon SE. The peripheral nerve allograft in the primate immunosuppressed with Cyclosporin A: Part II. functional evaluation of reinnervated muscle. Plast Reconstr Surg 1992;90:1047–52.
[42] Mackinnon SE, Hudson AR. Clinical application of peripheral nerve transplantation. Plast Reconstr Surg 1992;90: 695–9.
[43] Mackinnon SE. Nerve allotransplantation following severe tibial nerve injury. J Neursurg 1996;84:671–6.
[44] Matsuyama T, Midha R, Mackinnon SE, Munro CA, Wong P-Y, Ang LC. Long nerve allografts in sheep with Cyclosporin A immunosuppression. J Reconstr Microsurg 2000;16:219–25.

[45] Nakao Y, Mackinnon SE, Hertl MC, Miyasaka M, Hunter DA, Mohanakumar T. Monoclonal antibodies against ICAM-1 and LFA-1 prolong nerve allograft survival. Muscle Nerve 1995;18:93–102.
[46] Nakao Y, Mackinnon SE, Mohanakumar T. Monoclonal antibodies against ICAM-1 and LFA-1 (CD11A) induce specific tolerance to peripheral nerve allograft in rats. Transplant Proc 1995;18:373–7.
[47] Nakao Y, Mackinnon SE, Strasberg SR, et al. Immunosuppressive effect of monoclonal antibodies to ICAM-1 and LFA-1 on peripheral nerve allograft in mice. Microsurgery 1995;16:612–20.
[48] Hertl MC, Strasberg SR, Mackinnon SE. The dose-related effect of monoclonal antibodies against adhesion molecules ICAM-1 and LFA-1 on peripheral nerve allograft rejection in a rat model. Restor Neurol Neurosci 1996; 10:147–59.
[49] Fox DJ, Doolabh VB, Mackinnon SE, Genden EM, Hunter DA. Decreased Cyclosporin A requirement with anti-ICAM and anti-LFA-1alpha in a peripheral nerve allotransplantation model. Restor Neurol Neurosci 1999;15: 319–26.
[50] Buttemeyer R, Jones NF, Rao UN. Peripheral nerve allotransplant immunosuppressed with FK506: preliminary results. Transplant Proc 1995;27:1877–8.
[51] Buttemeyer R, Rao UN, Jones NF. Peripheral nerve allograft transplantation with FK506: functional, histological, and imunological results before and after discontinuation of immunosuppression. Ann Plast Surg 1995;35:396–401.
[52] Myckatyn TM, Ellis RA, Grand AG, et al. The effects of rapamycin in murine peripheral nerve isografts and allografts. Plast Reconstr Surg 2002;109:2405–17.
[53] Udina E, Gold BG, Navarro X. Comparison of continuous and discontinuous FK506 administration on autograft or allograft repair of sciatic nerve resection. Muscle Nerve 2004;29:812–22.
[54] Weinzweig N, Grindel S, Gonzalez M, Kuy D, Fang J, Shahani B. Peripheral-nerve allotransplantation in rats immunosuppressed with transient or long-term FK506. J Reconstr Microsurg 1996;12:451–9.
[55] Udina E, Voda J, Gold BG, Navarro X. Comparative dose-dependence study of FK506 on transected mouse sciatic nerve repaired by allograft or xenograft. J Periph Nerv Syst 2003;8:145–54.
[56] Yang RK, Lowe JB, Sobol JB, Sen SK, Hunter DA, Mackinnon SE. Dose-dependent effects of FK506 on neuroregeneration in a rat model. Plast Reconstr Surg 2003;112:1832–40.
[57] Feng FY, Ogden MA, Myckatyn TM, et al. FK506 rescues peripheral nerve allografts in acute rejection. J Neurotrauma 2001;18:217–29.
[58] Chen DL, Mackinnon SE, Jensen JN, Hunter DA, Grand AG. Failure of cyclosporin A to rescue peripheral nerve allografts in acute rejection. Ann Plast Surg 2002;49:660–7.
[59] Gold BG, Storm-Dickenson T, Austin DR, Katoh K. FK-506, an immunosuppressant, increases functional recovery and axonal regeneration in the rat following axotomy of the sciatic nerve. Soc Neurosci Abstr 1993;19: 1316.
[60] Gold BG, Villafranca JE. Neuroimmunopilin ligands the development of novel neuroregenerative/neuroprotective compounds. Curr Top Med Chem 2003;3:1368–75.
[61] Jost SC, Doolabh VB, Mackinnon SE, Lee M, Hunter DA. Acceleration of peripheral nerve regeneration following FK506 administration. Restor Neurol Neurosci 2000;17:39–44.
[62] Doolabh VB, Mackinnon SE. FK506 accelerates functional recovery following nerve grafting in a rat model. Plast Reconstr Surg 1999;103:1928–36.
[63] Maeda T, Mackinnon SE, Best TJ, Evans PJ, Hunter DA, Midha R. Regeneration across stepping-stone nerve grafts. Brain Res 1993;618:196–202.
[64] Sugita N, Ishida O, Ikuta Y, et al. Interposed autologous nerve segment stimulates nerve regeneration in peripheral nerve allografts in a rat model. J Reconstr Microsurg 2004;20:167–74.
[65] Atchabahian A, Doolabh VB, Mackinnon SE, Yu S, Hunter DA, Flye MW. Indefinite survival of peripheral nerve allografts after temporary Cyclcosporin A immunosuppression. Restor Neurol Neurosci 1998;13:129–39.
[66] Gilbert R. Transplant is successful with a cadaver forearm. Med Tribune Med News 1964;5:20.
[67] Dubernard JM, Owen E, Herzberg G. Human hand allograft: report on first 6 months. Lancet 1999;353:1315–20.
[68] Dubernard JM, Owen E, Lefrancois N. First human hand transplantation. Transpl Int 2000;13:521–4.
[69] Francois CG, Bredeneinbach WC, Maldonado C. Hand transplantation: comparison and observations of the first four clinical cases. Microsurgery 2000;20:360–71.
[70] Jones JW, Gruber SA, Barker JH, et al. Successful hand transplantation: one year follow-up. N Engl J Med 2000; 342:468–73.
[71] Piza H. Transplantation of hands in Innsbruck. [German] Wien Klin Wochenschr 2000;7:563–5.
[72] Midha R, Munro CA, Ramakrishna V, Matsuyama T, Gorczynski RM. Chemokine expression in nerve allografts. Neurosurgery 2004;54:1472–9.
[73] Accioli-de-Vaconcellos ZA, Kassar-Duchossoy L, Mira J-C. Long term evaluation of experimental median nerve repair by frozen and fresh nerve autografts, allografts and allografts repopulated by autologous Schwann cells. Restor Neurol Neurosci 1999;15:17–24.
[74] Mosahebi A, Fuller P, Wiberg M, Terenghi G. Effect of allogeneic Schwann cell transplantation on peripheral nerve regeneration. Exp Neurol 2002;173:213–23.
[75] Rodriguez FJ, Verdu E, Ceballos D, Navarro X. Nerve guides seeded with autologous Schwann cells improve nerve regeneration. Exp Neurol 2000;161:571–84.

Changing Your Address?

Make sure your subscription changes too! When you notify us of your new address, you can help make our job easier by including an exact copy of your Clinics label number with your old address (see illustration below.) This number identifies you to our computer system and will speed the processing of your address change. Please be sure this label number accompanies your old address and your corrected address—you can send an old Clinics label with your number on it or just copy it exactly and send it to the address listed below.

We appreciate your help in our attempt to give you continuous coverage. Thank you.

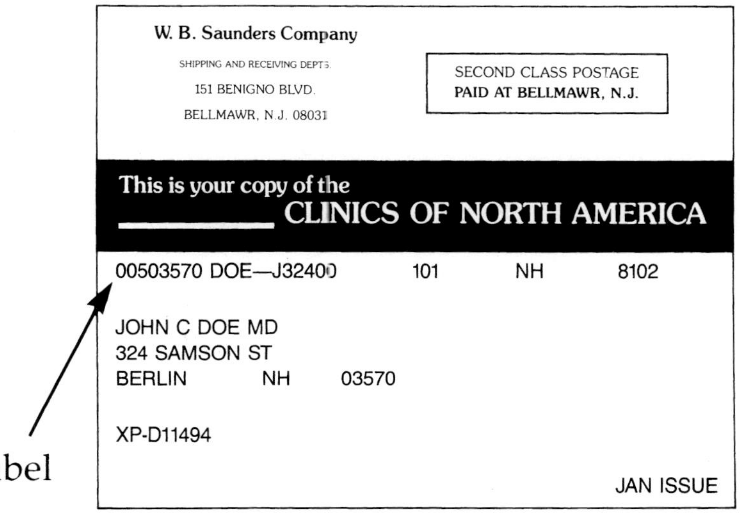

Your Clinics Label Number

Copy it exactly or send your label along with your address to:
W.B. Saunders Company, Customer Service
Orlando, FL 32887-4800
Call Toll Free 1-800-654-2452

Please allow four to six weeks for delivery of new subscriptions and for processing address changes.